Handbook of HIV Prevention

AIDS Prevention and Mental Health

Series Editors:

David G. Ostrow, M.D., Ph.D.
Loyola Health System, Maywood, Illinois

Jeffrey A. Kelly, Ph.D.
Center for AIDS Intervention Research (CAIR), Milwaukee, Wisconsin

---

Coping with HIV Infection:
Psychological and Existential Responses in Gay Men
Lena Nilsson Schönnesson, Ph.D., and Michael W. Ross, Ph.D.

Evaluating HIV Prevention Interventions
Joanne E. Mantell, Ph.D., M.S.P.H., Anthony T. DiVittis, M.A.,
and Marilyn I. Auerbach, A.M.L.S., Dr. P.H.

Handbook of Economic Evaluation of HIV Prevention Programs
Edited by David R. Holtgrave, Ph.D.

Handbook of HIV Prevention
Edited by John L. Peterson, Ph.D., and Ralph J. DiClemente, Ph.D.

Methodological Issues in AIDS Behavioral Research
Edited by David G. Ostrow, M.D., Ph.D., and Ronald C. Kessler. Ph.D.

Preventing AIDS: Theories and Methods of Behavioral Interventions
Edited by Ralph J. DiClemente, Ph.D., and John L. Peterson, Ph.D.

Preventing HIV in Developing Countries:
Biomedical and Behavioral Approaches
Edited by Laura Gibney, Ph.D., Ralph J. DiClemente, Ph.D.,
and Sten H. Vermund, Ph.D., M.D.

Psychosocial and Public Health Impacts of New HIV Therapies
Edited by David G. Ostrow, M.D., Ph.D., and Seth C. Kalichman, Ph.D.

Social Networks, Drug Injectors' Lives and HIV/AIDS
Samuel R. Friedman, Ph.D., Richard Curtis, Ph.D., Alan Neaigus, Ph.D., Benny Jose, Ph.D., and Don D. Des Jarlais, Ph.D.

Women and AIDS: Coping and Care
Edited by Ann O'Leary, Ph.D., and Loretta Sweet Jemmott, R.N., Ph.D., F.A.A.N.

Women at Risk: Issues in the Primary Prevention of AIDS
Edited by Ann O'Leary, Ph.D., and Loretta Sweet Jemmott, R.N., Ph.D., F.A.A.N.

A Continuation Order Plan is available for this series. A continuation order will bring delivery of each new volume immediately upon publication. Volumes are billed only upon actual shipment. For further information please contact the publisher.

Handbook of HIV Prevention

Edited by

John L. Peterson, Ph.D.

Georgia State University
Atlanta, Georgia

and

Ralph J. DiClemente, Ph.D.

Emory University
Atlanta, Georgia

Kluwer Academic/Plenum Publishers
New York, Boston, Dordrecht, London, Moscow

Library of Congress Cataloging-in-Publication Data

Handbook of HIV prevention/edited by John L. Peterson and Ralph J. DiClemente.
     p. cm. — (AIDS prevention and mental health)
    Includes bibliographical references and index.
    ISBN 0-306-46223-0
    1. AIDS (Disease)—Prevention—Handbooks, manuals, etc. I. Peterson, John L. II.
DiClemente, Ralph J. III. Series.

RA644.A25 H365 2000
616.97′9205—dc21

                                          99-053994

ISBN 0-306-46223-0

© 2000 Kluwer Academic / Plenum Publishers
233 Spring Street, New York, N.Y. 10013

http://www.wkap.nl

10 9 8 7 6 5 4 3 2 1

A C.I.P. record for this book is available from the Library of Congress.

Printed in the United States of America

Contributors

Peter Aggleton • Thomas Coram Research Unit, Institute of Education, University of London, London, WC1H 0AA England

Alex Carballo-Diéguez • HIV Research Center, New York, New York 10032

Julia Dayton • Department of Epidemiology and Public Health, Yale University School of Medicine, New Haven, Connecticut 06511

Don Des Jarlais • Chemical Dependency Institute, Beth Israel Medical Center, New York, New York 10003

Ralph J. DiClemente • Department of Behavioral Sciences and Health Education, Rollins School of Public Health, Emory University, Atlanta, Georgia 30322

Jeffrey D. Fisher • Center for HIV Intervention and Prevention, Department of Psychology, University of Connecticut, Storrs, Connecticut 06269

William A. Fisher • University of Western Ontario, Social Science Center, London, Ontario, Canada N6A 5C2

Samuel R. Friedman • National Development and Research Institutes, New York, New York 10048

Joseph Guydish • Institute for Health Policy Studies, University of California, San Francisco, California 94109

Holly Hagan • Seattle/King County Department of Health, Seattle, Washington 98104

David R. Holtgrave • Division of HIV/AIDS Prevention, Intervention Research and Support, National Center for HIV, STD, and TB Prevention, Centers for Disease Control and Prevention, Atlanta, Georgia 30333

John B. Jemmott, III • Annenberg School for Communication, University of Pennsylvania, Philadelphia, Pennsylvania 19104

Loretta Sweet Jemmott • School of Nursing, University of Pennsylvania, Philadelphia, Pennsylvania 19104

Seth Kalichman • Center for AIDS Intervention Research, Medical College of Wisconsin, Milwaukee, Wisconsin 53202

Jeffrey A. Kelly • Center for AIDS Intervention Research, Medical College of Wisconsin, Milwaukee, Wisconsin 53202

Douglas Kirby • ETR Associates, Santa Cruz, California 95061

Marguerita Lightfoot • Department of Social and Community Psychiatry, University of California, Los Angeles, California 90024

Sana Loue • Department of Epidemiology and Biostatistics, Case Western Reserve University, MetroHealth Medical Center, Cleveland, Ohio 44109

Michael H. Merson • Department of Epidemiology and Public Health, Yale University School of Medicine, New Haven, Connecticut 06511

David S. Metzger • Center for Studies of Addiction, Opiate/AIDS Research Division, University of Pennsylvania/VA Medical Center, Philadelphia, Pennsylvania 19104

Helen Navaline • Center for Studies of Addiction, Opiate/AIDS Research Division, University of Pennsylvania/VA Medical Center, Philadelphia, Pennsylvania 19104

Ann O'Leary • Department of Psychology, Rutgers University, New Brunswick, New Jersey 08903

David G. Ostrow • Loyola University Medical School, Maywood, Illinois 60153

John L. Peterson • Department of Psychology, Georgia State University, Atlanta, Georgia 30303

Steven D. Pinkerton • Center for AIDS Intervention Research, Medical College of Wisconsin, Milwaukee, Wisconsin 53202

Kim Rivers • Thomas Coram Research Unit, Institute of Education, University of London, London, WC1H 0AA England

Everett M. Rogers • Department of Communication and Journalism, University of New Mexico, Albuquerque, New Mexico 87131

Michael W. Ross • WHO Center for Health Promotion Research and Development, School of Public Health, University of Texas, Houston, Texas 77225

Mary Jane Rotheram-Borus • Department of Social and Community Psychiatry, University of California, Los Angeles, California 90024

Ronald O. Valdiserri • National Center for HIV, STD, and TB Prevention, Centers for Disease Control and Prevention, Atlanta, Georgia 30333

Gina M. Wingood • Department of Behavioral Sciences and Health Education, Rollins School of Public Health, Emory University, Atlanta, Georgia 30322

George E. Woody • Center for Studies of Addiction, Opiate/AIDS Research Division, University of Pennsylvania/VA Medical Center, Philadelphia, Pennsylvania 19104

Preface

In the nearly two decades since the HIV pandemic began, the rapid expansion of behavioral research on HIV prevention has prompted a crucial need for a sourcebook more advanced than an introductory textbook and broader and more readily accessible than a review periodical. The *Handbook of HIV Prevention* is intended as the first attempt to meet this need. The current state of affairs led us to edit a book that would represent the major areas of HIV behavioral research at a level appropriate for graduate students and experienced researchers in public health, medicine, nursing, education, and the social and behavioral sciences. In addition, we expect that the handbook will be useful in advanced undergraduate courses and as a reference book for health care professionals.

Our plans to assemble the Handbook began in the fall of 1996 when we prepared a tentative outline of chapters and invited a large number of distinguished researchers in the field to be the authors of various chapters. We received an overwhelmingly favorable response from potential authors to our letters of invitation. After considerable effort by both the contributors and the editors the volume was completed in 1999, when all chapters went to press.

Every effort was made to select contributors who were scholars that were well-qualified to prepare their chapter because of their knowledge and research experience in the field. We are especially pleased that the contributors represent extensive areas of research in HIV prevention, including those outside the United States, and a diverse range of professional backgrounds including psychologists, sociologists, epidemiologists, nurses, and physicians. Of course, there are emerging areas of research that could not be included in the current edition. However, we feel fortunate that of the chapters included in the handbook, all those that we consider essential chapters are included, except one on the implications of HIV prevention research for social policy.

Our rationale should be offered for the organization of the content in the volume. In particular, it seemed necessary to begin the book with a description and critique of theoretical models which explain HIV risk behaviors and are used to develop interventions at the individual and community level. Taken together, these theories increase understanding of the complex interaction between individual determinants and social contextual factors that may influence risk behaviors. Moreover, it seemed appropriate to discuss the methods and proce-dures typically used to conduct the empirical research in the field. With theories and methods covered, the subsequent chapters could then identify, describe, and critique the findings from prior intervention studies, especially those demonstrated as most effective in HIV prevention. Similarly, it seemed reasonable to conclude the handbook with several chapters that addressed the implications of HIV prevention research for technology transfer, cost-effectiveness, ethics, and directions for future research. Hence, as organized, the content of this volume provides information about the ways to conduct a rigorous intervention, about the scientific results from those interventions, and about the uses of those findings for community organizations and researchers.

The *Handbook of HIV Prevention* was prepared to provide the most comprehensive compilation of HIV prevention research available in one source today. We admit that any limitations of this volume are our own responsibility in spite of the exceptional contributions of the authors. Also, and of great importance, we express our enormous gratitude to Mariclaire Cloutier, at Kluwer Academic/Plenum Publishers, for her indispensable assistance throughout the editorial process and in final preparation of the manuscripts. Also, we express our gratitude to Tina Marie Greene for her indispensable assistance in the final preparation of the manuscripts.

John L. Peterson
Ralph J. DiClemente

Contents

Chapter 2. Diffusion Theory: A Theoretical Approach to Promote Community-Level Change

Everett M. Rogers

Chapter 3. Methodological Issues in HIV Behavioral Interventions

David G. Ostrow and Seth Kalichman

Part II. Applications to Behavioral Interventions

Chapter 4. School-Based Interventions to Prevent Unprotected Sex and HIV among Adolescents

Douglas Kirby

Chapter 5. HIV Behavioral Interventions for Adolescents in Community Settings

John B. Jemmott, III, and Loretta Sweet Jemmott

Chapter 6. Interventions for High-Risk Youth

Marguerita Lightfoot and Mary Jane Rotheram-Borus

Chapter 7. The Role of Drug Abuse Treatment in the Prevention of HIV Infection

David S. Metzger, Helen Navaline, and George E. Woody

Chapter 8. HIV/AIDS Prevention for Drug Users in Natural Settings

Don C. Des Jarlais, Joseph Guydish, Samuel R. Friedman, and Holly Hagan

Chapter 9. Interventions for Sexually Active Heterosexual Women

Ann O'Leary and Gina M. Wingood

Chapter 10. Interventions to Reduce HIV Transmission in Homosexual Men

Michael W. Ross and Jeffrey A. Kelly

Chapter 11. HIV Prevention among African-American and Latino Men Who Have Sex with Men

John L. Peterson and Alex Carballo-Diéguez

Chapter 12. HIV Prevention in Developing Countries

Julia Dayton and Michael H. Merson

Chapter 13. HIV Prevention in Industrialized Countries

Kim Rivers and Peter Aggleton

Part III. Implications of HIV Intervention Research

Chapter 14. Technology Transfer: Achieving the Promise of HIV Prevention
Ronald O. Valdiserri

Chapter 15. The Economics of HIV Primary Prevention
David R. Holtgrave and Steven D. Pinkerton

Chapter 16. Ethical Issues of Behavioral Interventions for HIV Prevention
Sana Loue

Chapter 17. Looking Forward: Future Directions for HIV Prevention Research

Ralph J. DiClemente

Handbook of HIV Prevention

Theoretical and Methodological Issues

Theoretical Approaches to Individual-Level Change in HIV Risk Behavior

JEFFREY D. FISHER and WILLIAM A. FISHER

INTRODUCTION

Over the course of the human immunodeficiency virus (HIV) epidemic, large numbers of HIV prevention interventions have been implemented in a broad array of settings. Unfortunately, there typically has been an enormous gap between what is known about effective HIV prevention interventions and HIV prevention practice as typically implemented.[1] To date, the vast majority of interventions targeting groups that practice high-risk behavior have been enacted by the public health sector and are government-funded projects. Generally, these are either implemented directly by state or provincial health departments, or funded by them and administered by community-based organizations (CBOs). All too often, neither behavioral scientists nor well-tested theories of behavior change are incorporated into the intervention design process,[2,3] and rigorous evaluations of the efficacy of these programs are rare. A large number of additional HIV prevention interventions have been undertaken by the public schools,[4] and in many jurisdictions there are laws mandating that HIV education be provided but without stipulations concerning how this should be done. Primary and secondary educational institutions generally have fielded extremely weak, atheoretical interventions designed not to offend the religious right wing, with content that is highly unlikely to effectively change HIV risk behavior.[4] Until recently, of the entire "portfolio" of HIV prevention interventions that have been implemented, most have focused primarily—and in many cases solely—on providing information about HIV. Such information consistently has been shown to be unrelated to HIV risk behavior change.[5–8]

In the past few years, a somewhat greater level of sophistication than that described above has begun to emerge in public health sector programs (e.g., in the United States), especially since the US Centers for Disease Control (CDC) mandated that behavioral scientists become involved in intervention design, implementation, and evaluation.[3,9] Recently, greater sophistication also can be found in some school-based programs.[4,10] Nevertheless, over the course of the epidemic, the primary domain in which "cutting-edge" research has been done consistently involves interventions designed, implemented, and evaluated by behavioral scientists—generally based at academic institutions—with funding from government agencies. This work has been much more theoretically elegant and much more likely to have been rigorously

JEFFREY D. FISHER • Center for HIV Intervention and Prevention, Department of Psychology, University of Connecticut, Storrs, Connecticut 06269.   *WILLIAM A. FISHER* • University of Western Ontario, Social Science Center, London, Ontario, Canada N6A 5C2.

Handbook of HIV Prevention, edited by Peterson and DiClemente.
Kluwer Academic / Plenum Publishers, New York, 2000.

evaluated and proven to be effective than other interventions that have been conducted. Unfortunately, such interventions comprise only a very small percentage of those that have been undertaken and only a small proportion of the total HIV prevention intervention funds spent. Further, very few of these interventions have been broadly disseminated (or disseminated at all) beyond the research setting.[2]

When one reviews the entire body of HIV prevention intervention work conducted to date, a number of limitations that curtail impact become clear.[1,2,7,11] First, while relevant conceptual frameworks for HIV-risk behavior change have been proposed (e.g., the health belief model,[12] the HIV risk reduction model,[13] the theory of reasoned action,[14] social cognitive theory,[15] the information–motivation–behavioral skills model of HIV risk behavior change,[7] and the transtheoretical model[16]), most interventions have been intuitively and not conceptually based and have failed to benefit from the substantial theoretical literature that is available to provide guidance for them (see Coates,[11] deWit,[17] Fisher and Fisher,[7] Fisher and Fisher,[18] Gluck and Rosenthal,[1] Holtgrave et al.,[3] and Wingwood and DiClemente[19] for discussion of this issue). Second, relatively few interventions have systematically assessed target group members' preintervention information base, their HIV risk reduction motivation, and their behavioral skills with respect to HIV prevention in order to "tailor" interventions to target group needs; consequently, most interventions have involved empirically untargeted "shooting in the dark" (see Fisher and Fisher[7] and Fisher and Fisher[18] for discussion of this issue). Third, interventions often focus on efforts to change general patterns of behavior (e.g., encouraging people to practice "safer sex") as opposed to focusing on increasing individuals' inclination and ability to practice specific risk reduction acts, even though a great deal of social psychological research suggests that it would be more effective to focus on specific acts than on general patterns of behavior (see Ajzen and Fishbein,[20] Fishbein and Ajzen,[21] and Fishbein et al.[14] for discussion of this issue). Fourth, as noted earlier, most existing interventions focus solely on providing information about HIV. Even within this narrow focus, the information that they provide is often completely irrelevant to preventive behavior (e.g., information about T cells is not directly relevant to HIV prevention) or difficult to comprehend, unnecessarily frightening, and/or sexist (see Fisher and Fisher[18] for discussion of this issue). Fifth, interventions often fail to motivate individuals to change their risky behavior or to provide training to help them acquire, rehearse, and refine the behavioral skills necessary for HIV risk behavior change.[7,15,18,22] Sixth, existing interventions often have not been evaluated with sufficient rigor to determine whether intended changes in mediating factors (e.g., knowledge, behavioral skills) and in HIV preventive behavior actually have occurred in the short or long term and in relation to both direct and indirect and nonreactive indicators of intervention outcome (see Exner et al.,[6] Gluck and Rosenthal,[1] Johnson et al.,[23] Kelly et al.,[2] Leviton and Valdiserri,[24] Oakley et al.,[25] and Wingwood and DiClemente[19] for discussion of this issue).

Many of the limitations described above are addressed, to a greater or lesser extent, by one or more of the theoretical approaches to individual-level behavior change that are described in this chapter. We will review several conceptualizations, some of which were formulated in other domains and later applied to HIV preventive behavior, and some of which were formulated to focus specifically on behavior change in the HIV arena. The models to be reviewed in this chapter include: the health belief model, the AIDS risk reduction model, the transtheoretical model, social cognitive theory, the theory of reasoned action, the theory of planned behavior, and the information–motivation–behavioral skills model. For each conceptual framework, we first discuss the fundamentals of the model and its application to HIV risk and preventive behavior. Next, we discuss relevant research that is based on the model (e.g., testing its assumptions, using it to predict risky and safer behavior, and using it as a framework for intervention design and evaluation) to the extent that such research is available, and finally, we offer a critique and conclusions with respect to the model. We will conclude the chapter with an overall critique and conclusions concerning the models that have been discussed.

THE HEALTH BELIEF MODEL

The health belief model (HBM), the grandparent of all health behavior change models, has been accepted uncritically by many health researchers[26] and probably has been used more than any other health behavior change model over the past decades. It is an expectancy value model developed in the 1950s by psychologists in the US Public Health Service who were attempting to understand why people failed to participate in programs designed to prevent or detect disease.[27–29] The HBM was later extended to account for why people may not respond to symptoms by obtaining necessary medical care[30] and to help explain why people do not follow medical regimens.[31] In effect, the HBM is a model of conscious decision making that has been applied to a variety of health threats in both healthy and ill populations.

Fundamental Assumptions

As originally formulated, the HBM asserted that people will engage in preventive behavior if they feel susceptible to a health condition, if they believe the condition is characterized by a high level of severity (e.g., negative health outcomes), and if they feel that the costs of engaging in the preventive behavior are outweighed by the benefits. Since its inception, the HBM has been subject to a number of conceptual modifications, to be described later.

The original HBM constructs can be elaborated on as follows. *Perceived susceptibility* involves one's subjective perception of the risk of contracting the health threat in question. *Perceived severity* refers to perceptions of both the physical (e.g., death, pain) and social consequences (e.g., effects on social relations, family life) of contracting a condition or of leaving it untreated. *Perceived vulnerability*, which determines "readiness to act," is thought to be some type of (unspecified) joint function of perceived susceptibility and perceived severity. According to Rosenstock et al.,[12] beyond some threshold, perceived vulnerability provides the energy or force to act. Given perceived vulnerability, health behavior options are evaluated in terms of their perceived benefits and costs. *Benefits* involve beliefs about the effectiveness of available options for reducing the threat of disease. Unless a behavioral option is viewed as likely to be effective, it is unlikely to be enacted. *Costs* involve any potentially negative aspect of a particular health action (e.g., pain, expense, danger, stigma, side effects, inconvenience). Even if individuals feel vulnerable to a potentially serious condition, they will not change their behavior (e.g., adopt preventive measures) unless the perceived cost–benefit ratio for doing so is favorable. Further, among available behavior change options, the HBM asserts that individuals generally choose the one with the most favorable perceived cost–benefit ratio.

Following the initial presentation of the HBM, amended versions of the model have included the notion of a *cue stimulus*, which is assumed to be helpful in promoting action. Such a stimulus might be internal (e.g., experiencing symptoms) or external (e.g., knowing a close other who has the disease, being exposed to mass media communications). In HBM research to date, the effects of cue stimuli have not frequently been studied.[12] While individuals' levels of susceptibility, severity, costs, and benefits are viewed as the primary determinants of health behavior, HBM formulators also assume that diverse demographic, sociological, psychological, and structural variables can affect these critical variables and in this way affect preventive behavior indirectly.

Since about 1988, the notion of *self-efficacy* has been added to the HBM to help increase its explanatory power.[32] Self-efficacy involves the perceived likelihood that one can personally perform the preventive behavior successfully and experience expected positive outcomes.[15] Rosenstock et al.[12] explain that self-efficacy was not included in early versions of the HBM because they focused on simple preventive behaviors (e.g., getting an injection) rather than more complex ones (e.g., negotiating safer sex). Even today, most health conditions the HBM has been applied to are less threatening and require less complex responses than those involved in changing HIV risk behavior. It has been suggested that the model may be more useful with the former types of problems than with threatening problems requiring complex responses, such as HIV prevention.[33,34] The elements in the present version of the HBM are represented in Fig. 1.

Empirical Support

Several HBM studies in the HIV prevention area[35] have focused on elicitation research (i.e., assessing existing levels of HBM constructs such as perceived susceptibility to HIV infection in particular populations). However, most research has used the HBM in attempts to predict levels of risky and safer sex and injection drug use behavior. In this domain, the relationship between individual HBM constructs and levels of HIV prevention is generally the focus of study, despite the fact that the HBM assumes (but does not adequately specify) interrelations among its several constructs.[12] Overall, there has been mixed support for the association between individual HBM constructs and levels of HIV preventive behavior. For example, higher levels of perceived susceptibility to HIV infection have been related to increased HIV preventive behavior in several studies.[36–41] Nevertheless, the positive relation between perceived susceptibility and HIV prevention (e.g., condom use) has not been con-

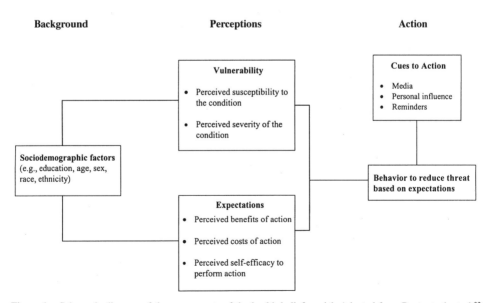

Figure 1. Schematic diagram of the components of the health belief model. Adapted from Rosenstock et al.[32]

firmed in other studies.[42–52] (For a complete review of this literature, see Gerrard et al.[53]) One reason for these inconsistent findings is that while perceptions of susceptibility to HIV may cause preventive behavior, these perceptions also may be a result of risky behavior[5,53] (for other explanations, see Gerrard et al.[53] and Flowers et al.[54]). Prospective research could help to clarify these conflicting findings on the relation between perceived susceptibility to HIV and HIV preventive behavior, but to date, little has been done.

In research on HIV prevention, perceived severity has rarely been operationalized in a manner consistent with the HBM's definition of the construct, in part because perceptions of the severity of HIV are generally very high. For this reason, researchers have sometimes turned to inappropriate operationalizations of the construct.[12] When perceived severity has been measured relatively appropriately, support for the HBM prediction that greater perceived severity will be associated with increased HIV prevention has been inconsistent at best (see Yep[55] for research supporting the proposed relationship; see Brunswick and Banaszak-Holl,[5] Rimberg and Lewis,[56] Wilson et al.,[51] and Yep[41] for findings inconsistent with the proposed relationship). These inconsistent findings may be due in part to a ceiling effect with respect to the perceived severity of HIV.

Perceived benefits of HIV preventive behaviors also have been positively linked with prevention in some studies[37,38,46,51,57–61] but not in others.[5,41,62] Consistent with the HBM, perceived costs of HIV prevention generally have been negatively associated with HIV preventive behavior[38,41,46,51,56,57,59] (for an exception, see Steers et al.[40]). Overall, perceived costs seem to be a particularly strong predictor of HIV preventive behavior. This strong inverse relation between perceived costs and prevention has been found with other health behaviors as well.[34,63]

Concerning constructs that have been added to the HBM since its initial formulation, little work in the HBM tradition has explicitly examined the proposed facilitating effect of cue stimuli on HIV preventive behavior. Nevertheless, three studies[37,64,65] show support for the notion of a link between exposure to a cue stimulus (e.g., another individual who has HIV) and HIV prevention, while another study[57] does not. On the other hand, there is a great deal of consistent evidence, mostly from outside the domain of HBM research, that the self-efficacy construct is related to HIV prevention.[15,40,66–70]

Overall, support for HBM predictions with respect to the practice of HIV preventive behavior has been inconsistent. Outside of the domain of HIV prevention (e.g., cardiovascular risk screening and compliance with public health immunization requests), there also has been equivocal support for HBM constructs as predictors of behavior (see, e.g., Arnold and Quine,[71] Cummings et al.,[72] and Haefner and Kirscht,[73] for findings that are supportive of HBM assumptions; see Becker,[31] Janz and Becker,[63] Montano,[74] Pirie et al.,[75] and Seydel et al.[76] for inconsistent findings).

To date, most HBM research on HIV prevention has involved using individual HBM constructs to predict levels of safer behavior. The model has rarely been used to design HIV risk behavior change interventions, though its formulators and other researchers[12,77,78] have suggested that more HBM research be focused in this area. They assert that collecting initial, preintervention elicitation data on health beliefs with respect to perceived susceptibility, costs, benefits, and the like and then creating targeted interventions to modify antiprevention perceptions in a more favorable direction would constitute a fruitful route to intervention-induced behavior change. For example, if elicitation research showed high levels of vulnerability to HIV but a high perception of the costs of prevention relative to the benefits, an intervention could focus on increasing the perceived benefits of prevention and decreasing the perceived costs. HBM theorists believe that interventions based on the model also should include a strong self-efficacy component. To date, however, the few attempts to use the HBM to intervene to change HIV risk behavior either do not incorporate all of the HBM constructs,[79] mix HBM constructs with constructs from other models,[80] or do not measure behavioral outcomes.[79] Thus, the HBM has not been used faithfully or often, nor has it received empirical support in the behavioral intervention arena. Further, some investigators[81] believe that without more scientifically sound studies demonstrating the HBM's predictive validity, using the HBM to design interventions might be premature.

Conclusions/Critique

While HBM constructs have been shown to be useful in predicting behavior in some health domains, they have proved to be less helpful in others.[31,34,63] Within the area of HIV prevention, the relations between most HBM constructs (e.g., the perceived susceptibility, perceived severity, and perceived benefits constructs) and prevention have generally been inconsistent, while the relations between the perceived costs and self-efficacy constructs and HIV prevention have been much more consistent. Nevertheless, when HBM variables have been shown to be related to health outcomes, the percentage of variance accounted for has generally been quite low.[81,82]

Even the equivocal findings described above are to some extent suspect. Reviews of HBM research find it to be consistently weak from a methodological and a measurement perspective.[26,81] For example, of 147 HBM citations obtained in searches, only 16 studies met minimal criteria for valid representation of the HBM constructs (i.e., they measured all the HBM constructs, the authors assessed reliability for each of the four original HBM constructs, and there was a criterion measure associated with a health behavior). In these studies, effect sizes were small, and in many cases homogeneity was rejected and mean effect sizes may not reflect a single underlying construct.[81] In addition, inconsistent (and often inappropriate) operationalizations of HBM constructs are a common problem[57] and studies are often retrospective rather than prospective,[83] though some support has been found for HBM constructs in both types of research design.

In addition to equivocal findings with the HBM and serious methodological weaknesses, it is important to note that the relationships between the variables in the model remain unconceptualized and unspecified. In our view and that of others,[26] the HBM is essentially a listing of constructs rather than a model per se. Even the HBM authors, Rosenstock et al.,[12] admit that the relationships among the key variables in the model have "never been adequately addressed" (p. 9). For that reason, the HBM has not been tested as a fully integrated multivariate model (studies typically simply correlate individual HBM constructs with criterion behaviors). This approach is problematic, in part since it fails to yield information on whether the individual variables that are found to be related to HIV preventive behavior (e.g., perceived costs of prevention; self-efficacy) make an orthogonal or an overlapping contribution to the prediction of HIV preventive behavior. There has been a recent attempt at specification of the relations between the HBM constructs.[12] From our perspective, this attempt at specification remains inadequate and could not be used as a basis for a test of the HBM as an integrated model. In effect, more than 40 years after its formulation, the HBM as a model has not received empirical support, and due to its lack of specification it really cannot be tested.[81]

Complementing the difficulties with attempting to test the HBM (due to lack of specification) and to use it to predict behavior (due to equivocal results), there would be difficulties in attempting to use the model in behavior change interventions. According to the HBM, anything that leads to the attainment of any of the HBM constructs (e.g., perceived susceptibility, a favorable cost–benefit ratio) will lead to HIV risk behavior change. This makes intervention design difficult, since HBM theorists give us little sense of what will impact most heavily on a given construct, and thus on behavior change. Similarly, the HBM does not specify what constructs will be most important in a particular HIV prevention intervention context (e.g., in a particular population, or for a given high-risk behavior).

Rather than a model that specifies (or even suggests) what would comprise an effective behavior change intervention, we view the HBM as more of a model that suggests conditions that prompt one to seek health-relevant services (e.g., to sign up to attend an HIV risk behavior change intervention). In effect, the HBM may imply more about how to compel an individual to attend an intervention than about what the intervention should involve. For health behaviors that merely involve "getting to" a health care site (e.g., having an immunization), the HBM is clearly more useful than for contexts that require going through some type of behavior change process (e.g., learning how to change risky sexual behavior).

Several additional criticisms have been leveled against the HBM (see Rosenstock[77]). These include the fact that in social psychological work in general, the empirical relationship between beliefs and behavior is generally somewhat inconsistent, and that it has rarely if ever been shown that beliefs per se are sufficient to promote action. A related criticism is that attempts to change beliefs are not uniformly successful. In general, HBM authors concede that more constructs than those in the original HBM are necessary for behavior change and challenge others to supply such variables (see also Abraham et al.[57]). Their addition of self-efficacy to more recent versions of the HBM is an attempt to increase its explanatory power. Other variables that may be critical for HIV prevention, at least in some cases, such as knowledge of HIV transmission and prevention, social normative support for prevention, and the possession of an adequate behavioral skills repertoire[7] currently have no direct expression even in more recent HBM iterations. For all the above reasons, while the HBM was used for some of the early studies exploring predictors of HIV risk and prevention, recent HIV-relevant work with the model is quite limited.

THE AIDS RISK REDUCTION MODEL

The AIDS risk reduction model (ARRM),[84] and the next model we will discuss, the transtheoretical model (TM),[85] are both stage models of behavior change. Both assume that change is a process that individuals must go through and that different factors affect movement through different stages of the process. Both the ARRM and TM distinguish between conceptualizing change as a process characterized by several stages, the achievement of each of which may be seen as a meaningful outcome, and viewing actual behavioral change per se as the *only* critical outcome of a behavior change attempt (as do most of the other models we will discuss). In effect, the ARRM and TM view progress through the stages of change as an important intervention outcome that can be more realistically achieved in the short term than changes in actual overt behavior. According to stage theorists, viewing actual behavioral change as the only critical intervention outcome may miss important variables (e.g., perceptions of susceptibility to HIV; perceptions of HIV risk behavior as being problematic) that may affect the process of change, but which may not directly affect behavioral outcomes. ARRM formulators believe the predominant focus on behavioral outcomes in HIV prevention research to date also may explain why some variables (e.g., knowledge, response efficacy, perceived susceptibility to HIV) have had an inconsistent effect on behavioral outcomes, and assert that they may still be important elements in the change process by affecting movement through the stages of change. In the ARRM, intervention-induced movement through the stages of change is presumed to facilitate eventual behavior change even if a given intervention does not result in changes in behavior per se at a particular point in time. The ARRM proposes that the further in the stage continuum an intervention helps one to progress, the more likely he or she is to exhibit behavior change when exposed to a subsequent intervention attempt.

Fundamental Assumptions

The ARRM includes elements from the HBM, self-efficacy theory,[15] and psychological theory and research on interpersonal processes and attitude change.[84] Catania et al.[84] stipulate that the model is applicable to sexually active or injection-drug-using individuals with a nonzero risk for HIV, and that in order to avoid HIV risk behavior, an individual must pass through three stages (see Fig. 2). First, one must label his or her actions as risky for contracting HIV (i.e., as problematic). Second, he or she must make a commitment to reducing HIV risk behavior and to increasing safer behavior. As in the HBM, the commitment process involves deciding whether the behavior in question can be changed and whether the benefits of doing so outweigh the costs. In the third stage of the ARRM, the individual must seek and enact strategies to attain HIV risk behavioral change. These may be many and varied, may involve multiple steps, and may require overcoming different types of barriers (e.g., financial, interpersonal).

In terms of the ARRM (and other stage theories), change processes are not necessarily

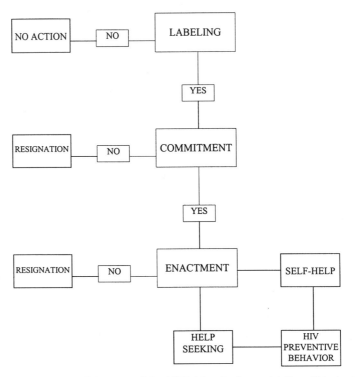

Figure 2. Flow chart of the stages of the AIDS risk reduction model. From Catania et al.[84]

unidirectional or irreversible. For example, one could initially label his or her HIV risk behavior as problematic, experience tremendous costs attempting to be safer, and subsequently decide that his or her behavior was not really problematic in the first place. Further, an individual may not label his or her HIV risk behavior problematic, yet commit to change it to please a significant other (e.g., a relationship partner). In either case, Catania et al.[84] view the ARRM stages as useful for suggesting important "markers" in the change process. They construe the model as providing insights into the process of HIV risk reduction behavior change and how to move people through the process of change, as well as concerning why people fail in the change process.

We will discuss each of the stages of the ARRM in turn, as well as factors posited to be critical to attain each stage and to be prepared to move on to the next. With respect to an individual's labeling his or her risky behavior as problematic, three elements are necessary: knowledge about how HIV is transmitted and prevented, perceiving oneself as susceptible to HIV, and believing that HIV is undesirable. Appropriate information (e.g., that HIV is transmitted by blood and bodily fluids and can be prevented by procedures such as condom or clean needle use; that HIV is generally a fatal disease) is critical to realizing each of these elements. Sexual or needle-sharing partners and social networks also can affect the amount and the accuracy of information (e.g., about HIV transmission and prevention) that one might have,[86] and thus may affect labeling. In addition to the importance of certain types of information, the ARRM asserts that labeling can be affected by the pro- or antiprevention attitudes and norms of one's sexual partner, of one's social network, and by pro- or antiprevention social norms in general. Finally, factors such as a need for denial and avoidance, fear, anxiety, and other aversive emotions can have effects on labeling.[84]

Once an individual has labeled his or her behavior as problematic, he or she may proceed to make a commitment to change. In the ARRM, commitment is essentially a decision-making stage that may result in one of several outcomes: making a firm commitment to deal with the problem, remaining undecided, waiting for the problem to resolve itself, or simply resigning oneself to the problem. Because HIV risk behavior change is a complex process involving the termination of one or more pleasant (but high-risk) activities and the substitution of one or more less pleasant (but safer) activities, the decision to commit to it can be very difficult. According to Catania et al.,[84] commitment decisions are based on a consideration of the perceived psychological and social costs and benefits of the high- and low-risk behaviors in question. The major factors that affect perceived costs and benefits, and thus commitment to change, are: (1) response efficacy (or perceived effectiveness of the behavior change in averting risk), (2) perceived enjoyment of the acts being added to or eliminated from one's repertoire, (3) self-efficacy or the perception that one can successfully enact the change at issue, and (4) relevant informational and social normative factors.

With respect to response efficacy, to the extent that safer behaviors are perceived to be effective in preventing HIV, their perceived benefits are higher and individuals' commitment to behavior change should become greater. Another critical factor affecting perceived costs and benefits of prevention and thus commitment to change is the perceived enjoyment of the behaviors one is being asked to discontinue and of the behaviors one must substitute. To the extent that the behaviors to be discontinued and/or substituted represent a loss of enjoyment, perceived costs will rise and commitment will become less likely. Self-efficacy also affects perceived costs and benefits, and thus commitment to safer practices.[87–89] To the extent one believes he or she can perform safer behaviors and derive the desired outcomes (e.g., protection from infection without damaging one's relationship with their partner), the perceived benefits of safer behaviors increase, as does the likelihood of a commitment to change.

Catania et al.[84] assume that perceived costs and benefits of behavior change (and thus commitment to change) also can be affected by informational and social normative factors. They propose that knowledge of possible health benefits and other favorable outcomes of safer behaviors (e.g., preventing HIV; worrying less about having sex or "shooting up") can affect the perceived cost–benefit ratio of prevention and the likelihood of commitment to change. In addition, since people generally expect costs (e.g., social rejection) for performing nonnormative behaviors, social factors (e.g., antiprevention reference group norms) can affect the perceived costs and benefits of prevention, and thus commitment. Reference groups also can affect costs and benefits in other ways. For example, to the extent that safer behaviors are perceived to be normative, friends may inform others that they have enjoyed condom use and that condoms are not so difficult to use after all.[86]

The final ARRM stage is taking action and the enactment of solutions. According to Catania et al.,[84] this stage involves three phases: seeking information, obtaining remedies, and enacting solutions. Though practiced most often in sequence, these phases may occur in order or simultaneously and some may even be skipped. With respect to seeking information, people intending to take action search for ideas and opinions about how to modify their behavior. At this stage, health education messages that indicate sources of effective help and how to obtain it can be critical.[84] Concerning obtaining remedies, as we have noted, there are several helping styles that one may adopt (e.g., engaging in self-help, getting help from others, resignation to the problem). Based on the help-seeking literature,[90,91] people often attempt self-help initially, followed by seeking help from friends, and finally engaging in formal help-seeking from professionals, although this sequence is by no means invariant. After obtaining remedies, people enact solutions. Catania et al.[84] say relatively little about this phase, and there has been little research on variables associated with the enactment stage (see Flowers et al.[54]). Nevertheless, Catania et al.[84] suggest that behavior change will be enacted more successfully if one has social support for it, if the change attempt involves one's partner, and if one has good communication skills. They also point out that enacting solutions is often difficult because it may involve a dyad and require complex negotiations between partners who have different feelings about behavior change. (For an expanded discussion of relationship issues and risky sexual and drug use behavior, see Misovich et al.[92]) Overall, Catania et al.[84] specify few conditions affecting enactment of behavior change (and thus suggest little in the way of content for effective interventions to decrease HIV risk behavior).

In addition to discussion of how to complete the requirements for attainment of each stage, the ARRM conceptualizes how individuals move from stage to stage. Catania et al.[84] point to both internal (e.g., negative emotions) and external motivators (e.g., external cues) as stimuli for movement between stages. An example of an internal motivator is one's level of distress with a problem such as HIV risk behavior. Distress that is too high may negatively affect self-efficacy and inhibit movement between stages, while a moderate level of distress may facilitate movement. Moderate levels of other negative emotional states (e.g., fear, anxiety) may facilitate movement between stages as well. Examples of external motivators that may facilitate movement are public health education campaigns that make it clear that individuals are susceptible to HIV, and having support for change from one's social network. Another external factor which may affect movement between stages is environmental cues that cause people to think about their risky behavior, and their options for change.

The ARRM suggests that different intervention messages will have greater impact on movement between stages at different stages of change. For individuals at stage one—labeling—messages should focus on factors causing one to identify his or her behavior as problematic (e.g., on how HIV is transmitted to persons like the individual in question; that it is a devastating disease one can get). For individuals at stage two—commitment—interventions should focus on improving the perceived cost–benefit ratio of the desired change. At stage three—enactment—Catania et al.[84] propose that interventions should focus on where to get help with behavior change and on how to actually achieve it.

Empirical Support

The ARRM has been used in elicitation research in several populations to determine the extant levels of factors that are hypothesized to be associated with attaining each of the ARRM stages and to identify the distribution of ARRM stages in populations of interest. Concerning the latter, Yep[62] reported that Asian Pacific Islanders were primarily at the "labeling" phase of the ARRM and suggested intervention components that might be necessary to bring them to the enactment stage. Similar work was done by Bertrand et al.[93] and Ireland et al.[94] The former study reported that most women in Bas-Zaire had not yet labeled HIV risk as a problem, and the latter reported the same finding among indigent US cocaine-abusing women. Knowing what stage a population is at can be useful in effectively targeting future intervention resources and strategies for that population.

A major series of studies has involved partially testing the assumptions of the ARRM. However, because the ARRM is not specified so as to permit it to be tested as an integrated model, as with the HBM, tests have generally consisted of examinations of univariate correlations between levels of individual ARRM components (or subcomponents) and attainment of ARRM stages, or of correlations between levels of ARRM components (or subcomponents) and levels of safer behaviors. In the first line of research, Catania et al.[95] found that perceived susceptibility to HIV predicted individuals' likelihood of labeling their behavior as a problem. In a similar vein, Kowalewski et al.[96] found that for both condom-using and non-condom-using injection drug users (IDUs), labeling behavior as problematic was predicted by greater perceived susceptibility to HIV; for condom-using IDUs, it was also predicted by greater HIV knowledge. Inconsistent with additional ARRM assumptions about factors affecting labeling, normative support and aversive emotional states did not predict labeling one's behavior as problematic. Similar mixed findings for ARRM assumptions about factors affecting labeling were reported by Longshore and Anglin[97] with HIV-negative IDUs who reported recently sharing needles. In another study, Ireland et al.[94] reported that ARRM variables were less predictive of labeling one's behavior as problematic than were psychosocial functioning and contextual variables (e.g., having a primary sexual partner, addiction).

As they did for the stage of labeling, Catania et al.[95] have studied whether elements posited by the ARRM to affect the commitment stage actually affect attaining this stage. Most factors affecting commitment are proposed to exert influence because they affect perceived costs and benefits of prevention. Consistent with this assumption, Catania et al.[95] found that both enjoyment of condoms and supportive norms predicted individual's commitment to change. On the other hand, neither response efficacy nor perceived barriers to prevention (e.g., embarrassment) were related to commitment. Kowalewski et al.[96] assessed the relations between self-efficacy, response efficacy, enjoyment of condoms, normative support for change, and individuals' commitment to change. Findings indicated that for both condom users and nonusers, greater self-efficacy and more normative support for safer practices were associated with greater commitment to safer sex behaviors. Response efficacy was not associated with commitment, nor was the perceived enjoyment associated with using condoms. In a similar study by Longshore and Anglin,[97] neither self-efficacy nor response efficacy were associated with IDUs making a commitment to change.

Catania et al.[84] assert that completing the enactment stage involves seeking information, obtaining remedies, and enacting solutions. While these predictions are generally consistent with the help-seeking literature,[91] they have not been tested in the HIV risk reduction domain. Other ARRM assumptions about enactment have been tested with respect to HIV prevention. Catania et al.[84] suggest that enacting solutions may be affected by relationship characteristics (e.g., ability to engage one's partner in the change process) and by communication skills of the dyad (for supportive research, see Adib et al.,[98] Catania et al.,[95] Hays et al.,[99] Malow et al.,[100] and Misovich et al.[92]). Also, Kline and Van Landingham[101] have reported that in HIV-infected women, number of arguments between partners directly predicted level of risky sexual practices, such that partners who had more arguments were less likely to practice safer sex.

Aside from the line of research just discussed, studies have typically not tested the Catania et al.[84] proposition that the ARRM elements associated with attaining a stage are actually associated with stage attainment. Rather, most studies have correlated the levels of variables associated with attaining a stage to preventive behavior per se.* Note that this approach is inconsistent with Catania and co-workers'[84] assertion that factors that will help individuals attain a particular ARRM stage may *not* directly affect behavioral outcomes. Nevertheless, with respect to labeling, studies have assessed the relation between factors proposed by the ARRM to be associated with attaining this stage and actual behavior change. In this work, findings have typically shown that knowledge about HIV is necessary but not sufficient for prevention (see Fisher and Fisher,[7] Flowers et al.,[54] and Helweg-Larson and Collins[8] for reviews of this literature). Studies also have found that perceiving oneself as susceptible to HIV is inconsistently associated with safer behavior (for reviews of this literature, see Flowers et al.[54] and Gerrard et al.[53] and the review of the perceived susceptibility variable presented for the earlier HBM). Further, it also has been observed that perceived severity of HIV is inconsistently related to safer behavior (again, see the review of the relation between this variable and safer behavior presented earlier for the HBM). Finally, the ARRM proposes that motivational factors such as denial can affect the attainment of labeling. While this assertion has not yet been verified, denial has been related to actual levels of HIV preventive behavior.[102,103]

Other studies have related factors associated with attainment of the commitment stage to behavior change. In the ARRM, costs and benefits are proposed to be important determinants of commitment. Major factors proposed by the model to affect costs and benefits and thus commitment are response efficacy, perceived enjoyment of the acts being added to or eliminated from one's repertoire, self-efficacy, and relevant informational and social network factors. In research with the ARRM, Flowers et al.[54] reported that only about 25% of the studies relating response efficacy to safer behavior reported a positive association. Additional work[104] has similarly failed to find a relation between response efficacy and prevention. Other safer and risky sex costs and benefits have been shown to more strongly predict safer sex practice.[54] For example, Catania et al.[105] report that enjoyment of anal intercourse is positively correlated with the frequency of its practice, and Connell et al.[106] found that for those for

---

*It has been suggested[54] that there will be more significant associations between variables associated with the attainment of a particular ARRM stage and behavioral outcomes as one moves from labeling to enactment, since the variables become more proximate precursors of actual behavior change. Flowers et al.[54] find support for the notion. Further, Flowers et al.[54] assert that the ARRM would predict different findings for the relation between variables associated with a particular stage and behavior changes as a function of what stage of change the individual is at. For example, a negative correlation might be expected between perceived vulnerability and prevention for those at the labeling stage, whereas a positive correlation between perceived vulnerability and preventive behavior might occur for those at the enactment stage.[54]

whom anal sex was less important, protected anal sex was more likely. Others report that feeling that condoms decrease sexual pleasure is negatively related to condom use.[101,104] With respect to self-efficacy, it has been consistently found that this variable is highly predictive of preventive behavior.[101,104] Finally, Catania et al.[84] propose and find support for the notion that knowledge about favorable outcomes of safer behavior and unfavorable outcomes of risky behavior can affect levels of such behavior. A degree of support has also been found for the notion that reference group norms can affect perceived costs and benefits of prevention.[54] Again, inconsistent with the ARRM, these factors have been studied in relation to behavioral outcomes, rather than attainment of the commitment stage.

There have been only a few studies that have attempted to relate elements associated with attaining the enactment stage with the ultimate practice of safer behavior. The ARRM assumption that enacting solutions involves seeking information and obtaining remedies has not been explicitly tested in the HIV prevention literature, but receives support in the help-seeking literature.[91] The ARRM assertions that actually enacting solutions (e.g., practicing safer sex) may be affected by characteristics of one's relationship and by one's communication skills have also been corroborated.[95,98,101]

In their discussion of the ARRM, Catania et al.[84] posit that movement between ARRM stages may be affected by levels of distress, by social support for change, and by alcohol and/ or drug use. Again, the studies relevant to this prediction focus on the relation between variables assumed to affect movement between the stages and ultimate behavioral outcomes, rather than the relation between these variables and actual stage movement. Nevertheless, it has been found that greater distress is related to greater use of condoms among IDUs and to lower overall numbers of sexual partners among college students.[42,107] Further, several studies have related normative support for change to levels of safer behavior.[37,108] Finally, a number of studies report that safer behaviors are negatively associated with drug and/or alcohol use.[101]

In addition to testing the assumptions of the ARRM, there have been limited attempts to conduct behavior change interventions based on this model. Basically, the ARRM assumes that the presence of elements in an intervention posited by the model to be associated with the realization of the labeling, commitment, and enactment stages should be associated with ultimate behavior change. Malow et al.[100] constructed an intervention for recovering drug abusers that addressed a number of critical ARRM valuables (e.g., perceived susceptibility, self-efficacy, training communication and other skills, and discussion of perceived costs and benefits associated with behavior change). This was compared to a standard "information only" intervention. It was found that the intervention containing some ARRM variables led to greater changes in self-efficacy, communication skills, and condom use skills at the posttest compared with the information-only condition. Inconsistent with the ARRM, the two groups did not vary on HIV-related susceptibility, anxiety, or response efficacy, or on overall post-intervention HIV risk behavior, since both groups improved. Nevertheless, additional analyses found that individuals' postintervention increase in the ARRM variables described above predicted their levels of subsequent safer behavior. A second intervention described as based on the ARRM (but reflective of other behavior change models described in this chapter as well) was conducted with African-American homosexual and bisexual men.[109] In this study an intensive, three-session intervention including some ARRM elements (e.g., knowledge, skills training, self-efficacy, attitude change, normative support) yielded stronger safer sex outcomes than a briefer single-session intervention using the same ARRM elements.

While several additional ARRM-based interventions are currently in the field (J. Catania, personal communication, January 1998), the interventions discussed herein represent the only published ARRM-based intervention research work to date. It should be noted that neither of the intervention studies reviewed above contained the full range of ARRM variables, neither was targeted to individuals' stage of change, and neither yielded unequivocal results. In addition to being used to design interventions, Catania et al.[84] also state that the ARRM offers insights that can be useful for conserving intervention resources and for keeping intervention dropout rates low. They believe that when interventions are targeted to the appropriate stage of change, they can be more effective, cost-effective, and apt to retain participants. While we agree with these claims in principle, they have not yet been subject to empirical tests.

Conclusions/Critique

In contrast to several of the models described in this chapter, the ARRM was developed specifically in context of HIV prevention, and it appears to provide a number of insights concerning HIV preventive behavior. The model has been used in one way or another with a broad array of populations.[110] It conceptualizes HIV prevention as a process of change involving multiple intermediate stages, specifies numerous factors that may affect the various stages of change, and reminds us that factors that do not have a direct impact on behavior change per se may have important implications earlier in the change process. At the same time, the ARRM provides somewhat more clarity concerning the milestones of change (labeling, commitment, and enactment) than it does concerning the process involved in reaching each of these milestones. In one sense, the ARRM posits very few ideas about how to actually change behavior, since its description of factors associated with realizing the enactment stage is sparse (see also Flowers et al.[54]). In another sense, the critical variables associated with attaining the three ARRM stages incorporate many of those found in the literature to be critical for behavior change to occur, though the model generally associates them with attainment of a single stage rather than with behavior change per se. With respect to the ARRM, there are areas where additional work is needed. Research on the interrelations between the variables specified as necessary for the attainment of the various stages is necessary.[54] Also, the model says little about how individuals move between stages, and little work has explored this issue. Finally, little work has been done on the issue of the extent to which the ARRM stages are or are not sequential and all necessary for behavior change to occur.

Overall, the ARRM posits a multitude of relevant factors, some of which are assumed to affect attainment of a particular stage of the change process and some of which are assumed to affect more than one stage. Moreover, research has empirically supported the notion that factors associated with the attainment of one stage may be associated with the attainment of other stages.[95] This characteristic makes the ARRM potentially nonparsimonious and relatively complex to test or to use to design specific HIV risk reduction interventions. Even more importantly, the relations among the elements in the ARRM have not been specified sufficiently to permit the ARRM to be empirically tested as an integrated, multivariate model (for attempts at this, which posit relations *beyond* those implied in the ARRM as originally formulated by Catania et al.,[84] see Breakwell et al.[111] and Kowalewski et al.[96]).

In the absence of adequate tests of the complete ARRM, attempts to relate even the elements posited to be associated with the attainment of a given ARRM stage with stage attainment have been equivocal.[95,96] In defense of the model, Catania et al.[95] suggest that such elements may be more predictive of stage attainment for some populations and in some contexts than others (e.g., for condom use with secondary rather than with primary sexual partners). In research that has tested the relations between individual ARRM components and subcomponents and actual behavior, results also are inconsistent.[54] While such research has identified a number of individual ARRM elements that are associated with safer behavior, such a univariate approach does not provide data concerning which ARRM elements make an orthogonal contribution to safer sexual or injection drug use behavior. If there is overlap between ARRM constructs, it is possible that fewer ARRM elements may contribute to HIV prevention than it appears. Overall, while the ARRM has some distinct conceptual strengths, it has conceptual weaknesses as well, and empirical support for it has been somewhat equivocal.

THE TRANSTHEORETICAL MODEL

The second stage model we will consider is the transtheoretical model (TM).[85] Both the ARRM and the TM assume that change is best viewed as a *process* (e.g., that healthy behavior such as increased condom use is ultimately achieved through a series of incremental, smaller changes), and for this reason change should not be viewed solely as a discrete overt behavioral outcome (Fig. 3). The ARRM and TM each assert that change is not linear. During the change process, relapse and "recycling" through the stages of change is the rule, rather than the exception.

Fundamental Assumptions

According to the TM, there are six stages of change that can be observed in individuals who change on their own (self-changers), as well as in those who participate in change-oriented interventions. The first stage of change is termed *precontemplation*. Precontemplators are people who do not intend to change their behavior in a given domain in the foreseeable future. For safer sex and injection drug use, precontemplators are those who are not practicing safer behavior now and who have no intention to do so. Typically, about 35 to 55% of individuals ranging from college students to high-risk women are in the precontemplation stage for condom use with their primary partner at a given point in time. This may be because they are uninformed or misinformed about HIV, because they know about the negative health effects of HIV but minimize them (e.g., believe contracting HIV "could never happen to them"), because they have previously attempted to change unsuccessfully and have become demoralized, or for some other reason. Generally, precontemplators avoid reading, talking, or thinking about their unhealthy behaviors and resist outside pressures to get them to change.[16]

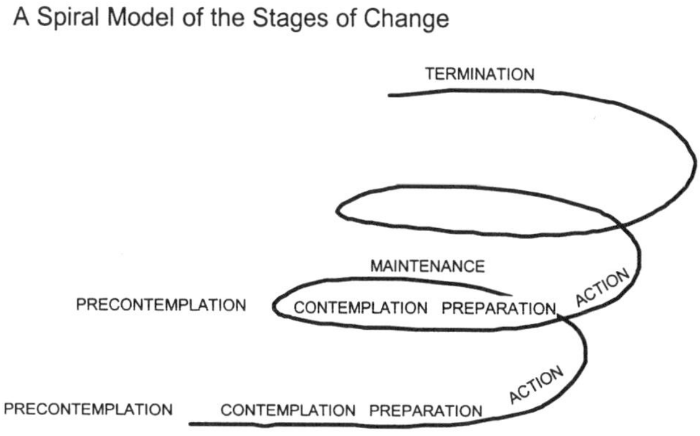

A Spiral Model of the Stages of Change

Figure 3. Transtheoretical model. From Prochaska et al.[113]

Prochaska and Velicer[85] argue that traditional action-oriented intervention programs (e.g., HIV prevention interventions that assume some degree of readiness to change) cannot deal successfully with precontemplators and are not likely to engage them.

People in the *contemplation* stage intend to modify their behavior in the next 6 months and have thought about the pros and cons of changing. For them, the pros and cons of changing are somewhat balanced, which can produce ambivalence that can keep individuals in the contemplation stage for some time. For HIV prevention, contemplators are people who know what constitutes risky behavior and are considering practicing safer behaviors in the future, but are not doing so at present. At any point in time, about 5 to 30% of individuals ranging from college students to high-risk women are in the contemplation stage with respect to condom use with their primary partners. Because they are not sufficiently ready to change, contemplators will not be well served by traditional action-oriented interventions.[85] Neverthe-less, contemplators are much more open to information about their problem behavior and how to change it than precontemplators.[16]

In the *preparation* stage, people seriously intend to take effective action to change, usually in the next month. At any point in time, about 5 to 30% of people ranging from college students to high-risk women are in the preparation stage with respect to condom use with a primary partner. Generally, individuals in the preparation stage have previously attempted change, and this often has occurred in the past year. They may even be currently attempting to reduce their frequency of unsafe sex. Even though they may have reduced their problem behavior, they have not met a criterion for effective change (e.g., condom use during every sexual encounter), but they intend to in the next month. People in preparation frequently have an "action plan" (i.e., a plan of what they will do to implement effective change) and, in contrast to those in precontemplation or contemplation, are appropriate recruits for traditional "action-oriented" interventions.

In the *action* stage, individuals have made modifications in their health behavior that have been effective in significantly reducing their risk during the previous 6 months. People are classified in this stage if they have met some behavioral criterion for efficacy (e.g., using condoms during every sexual encounter, or consistently abstaining from sex or from sharing unclean needles) for up to 6 months. The behavioral changes made during the action stage are often highly visible to others and necessitate a great deal of commitment and energy. Changes that are inefficacious (e.g., practicing unsafe sex only with partners whom one "knows well") would not qualify a person for the action stage. At any point in time, about 5 to 30% of populations ranging from college students to high-risk women are in the action stage for condom use with primary partners.

Maintenance begins six months after the initiation of consistent behavior change that is effective at reducing risk. In this stage people work to prevent relapse. For HIV prevention, those in maintenance have consistently practiced safer sexual and/or injection drug use behavior for more than 6 months. According to Prochaska and Velicer,[85] individuals in the maintenance stage are less tempted than those in the action stage to relapse and are more confident they can continue to practice their changed behaviors. Fortunately, across health behavior change domains, only about 15% of relapsers become totally disenchanted and forego any subsequent change attempt; most return to thinking about or attempting another cycle of change.[112] Typically, about 20% of people ranging from college students to high-risk women are in the maintenance stage for condom use with primary partners. Maintenance is followed by the termination stage, in which individuals are presumed to have no temptation to relapse and a complete sense of self-efficacy concerning their ability to maintain healthy behavior.

While at any point in time a person is viewed as being in one of the six stages of change for a particular problem behavior (e.g., risky sexual behavior or injection drug use), according to Prochaska et al.,[113] there are ten processes of change that assist individuals in progressing through the stages of change. These processes can be used by individuals engaged in self-change activities, as well as by outside intervenors, to promote change for a diverse set of problem behaviors. According to the TM, these processes reflect the critical common elements in the hundreds of extant models of change. They also have been validated in the context of safer sex and condom use[114,115] and can provide a context for the development of HIV prevention interventions.[16] The processes of change that are envisioned by the TM are presented and defined in Table 1; each includes an example of its use in HIV risk behavior change.

The specific processes of change that are used in a given attempt to move forward in the change continuum may vary as a function of one's preexisting stage of change and as a function of the type of unhealthy behavior being addressed. In the earlier stages of change, people typically apply the more experiential processes (e.g., consciousness-raising, dramatic relief, and self-reevaluation) to move forward; in the latter stages, they rely on the more behavioral processes (e.g., reinforcement management, counterconditioning, and helping relationships).[16] A challenge for interventionists is to ascertain the best ways to assist pre-contemplators to process information more effectively (consciousness-raising), to increase their emotional awareness of the problem (dramatic relief), and to realize that their self-image can be affected by reducing risk (self-reevaluation). For people in later stages of change, interventionists must find ways to reinforce individuals for small steps in the appropriate direction (reinforcement management), for replacing unhealthy behaviors with healthy ones

Table 1. Titles, Definitions, and Representative Interventions of the Processes of Change[a]

Process	Definitions: Interventions	Sample item
1. Consciousness raising	Increasing level of awareness and more accurate information processing	I seek information related to AIDS risk reduction
2. Dramatic relief	Experiencing and releasing feelings	Articles about the risks of unsafe sex upset me
3. Environmental reevaluation	Affective and cognitive reexperiencing of one's environment and problems	I think the world would be a better place if more people practiced safer sex
4. Self-reevaluation	Affective and cognitive reexperiencing of one's self and problems	I feel that being a responsible person includes my practicing safer sex
5. Self-liberation	Belief in one's ability to change and commitment to act on that belief	I make a commitmment to avoid risky sexual situations
6. Helping relationships	A relationship involving openness, caring, trust, genuineness, and empathy	I have someone who listens when I need to talk about my sexual behavior and AIDS
7. Social liberation	Noticing social changes that support personal changes	I notice society changing in ways that make is easier to practice safer sex
8. Counterconditioning	Substituting more positive behaviors and experiences for problem ones	Instead of risky sex, I engage in other safer sexual activities
9. Reinforcement management	Reinforcing more positive behaviors and punishing negative ones	I can expect to be praised by others if I practice safer sex
10. Stimulus control	Restructuring one's environment or experience so that problem stimuli are less likely to occur	I keep condoms with me to remind me to practice safer sex

[a]Prochaska et al.[16]

(counterconditioning), and for increasing their social support for a safer lifestyle (helping relationships). Applying the wrong processes of change to people at a particular stage of change can inhibit further progress from occurring.

Just as different processes of change are more appropriate for use at some stages than others, according to the TM, decisional balance varies by stage. This refers to the pattern of pro (positive) and con (negative) beliefs held by individuals at different stages of change about the consequences of changing an unhealthy behavior. For condom use, pros may include beliefs that condoms provide one with protection from pregnancy and sexually transmitted diseases (STDs), provide protection for ones' partner, and so forth. Cons could include beliefs about decreased sensation and perceived problems (e.g., rejection from partners) if condoms are introduced. In general, pros can be viewed as facilitators of change and cons as barriers. Changes in pros and cons are associated with progress (or lack thereof) through the stages of change, and individuals at different stages of change exhibit different profiles of pros and cons. Prochaska et al.[116] reported that across 12 different problem behaviors, the perceived cons of changing a behavior outweighed the pros for people in precontemplation. The reverse was the case for those in action. Generally, the pros began to outweigh the cons around the stage of contemplation. These findings have been replicated in studies of contraceptive behavior and condom use.[117]

Overall, people must decide that the pros of changing a behavior outweigh the cons before they act to change it. This suggests that to facilitate people's movement from pre-contemplation to action with respect to safer sexual or injection drug use behaviors, interventions should target the pros and cons of changing. Prochaska[118] found that across multiple problem behaviors (including safer sex) progressing from precontemplation to action generally involves about a one standard deviation increase in the pros of changing and about a half standard deviation decrease in the cons of changing. The implication is that for change to become likely, the pros of changing must increase about twice as much as the cons must decrease, so more emphasis should be placed on increasing the perceived benefits of change. Once an individual has begun to change behavior, interventions can focus more on decreasing the cons, which can facilitate further progress in the stages of change continuum and help to prevent relapse.

In addition to decisional balance, self-efficacy may affect movement across the stages, and different levels of self-efficacy characterize different stages of change. In the TM, self-efficacy is operationalized in two ways: situational confidence in one's ability to change a problem behavior and situational temptation to engage in the behavior. The former generally increases from precontemplation to maintenance and the latter generally decreases. Confidence and temptation to engage in the problem behavior generally interact across the stages of change. There is a large gap between the two in precontemplation, which reduces in the contemplation and preparation stages. As people move to action, confidence ratings increase sharply and temptation decreases more slowly. In maintenance, confidence peaks and tempta-tion continues to decline. In termination, temptation tends toward zero and confidence remains high. In addition to reflecting one's stage of change, increasing levels of confidence and decreasing levels of temptation can help facilitate movement across the stages.

The TM has a number of important intervention implications.[85] First, to meet the intervention needs of a particular population for a given problem behavior, we need to know the stage distribution of persons who engage in the problem behavior (e.g., risky sex or injection drug use) in that population. Second, people at risk will be best served by interven-tion strategies that are matched to their stage of change with respect to adopting safer sexual or injection drug use practices. Using the TM, one can create different interventions, highlighting different change processes, for people at each stage of change. Being able to articulate interventions for all stages of change permits intervenors to reach a much larger number of people than can be reached by traditional "action-oriented" programs, which work only for the relatively small percentage of people in the action stage at a given point in time.[113] Stage-matched interventions also have higher rates of retention than typical nonstaged interventions and are more effective.[85] "Mismatching" stages of change and processes of change results in low treatment efficacy, low treatment utilization, and low treatment retention.[119] This is not surprising, since people use different change processes at different stages of change.

According to the TM, an appropriate goal for a single HIV prevention intervention session would be to move people one stage along the change continuum. Moreover, interventionists are less frustrated with an approach that targets a one-stage change per change attempt than with the unrealistic (but common) notion that one should change conceivably from precontemplation to action, or even maintenance, as the result of a single interaction. In TM-based research, treatment programs "tailored" to move people just one stage actually double the chances that in the near future they will take action to change on their own.[120] It also has been found that the further along in the stages of change one is at a given point in time, the more likely he or she is to succeed in a given change attempt.[119,120]

Empirical Support

The TM has been applied in a variety of ways within the HIV prevention context. First, a series of studies has successfully used processes specified by the model to stage individuals or populations with respect to their position on the six stages of change.[114,121–125] Interestingly, and consistent with actual patterns of condom use, individuals were generally much more advanced in stages of change with respect to condom use with nonprimary than primary partners (see also Grimley et al.,[126] Harlow et al.,[123] and Misovich et al.[92]). It also has been found that men and women generally have a similar distribution of stages of change, but that younger people are generally more advanced in their stages of change for safer sex than older people.[127] Importantly, studies have demonstrated that individuals' stage of change for condom use predicts their actual levels of condom use,[126] and that stage of change for clean needle practices predicts safer injection drug use practices.[125] Finally, research has indicated that, as with other problem behaviors, relapse with respect to condom use is very common.[128]

Less work has been done with respect to the process of change used in the context of safer sexual and injection drug use behaviors. Nevertheless, it appears that in addition to the ten processes described earlier, another—assertiveness with regard to condom use—emerges with respect to safer sex.[121,127] According to Prochaska and associates,[121,127] assertiveness is necessary for progressing across the stages of change for condom use and for condom acquisition and condom use maintenance. In addition, for condom use, the way the basic processes of change act across the various stages of change is consistent with that found for other problem behaviors. Specifically, the finding that particular change processes are used at particular stages of change parallels that described for other behaviors.[126] However, while for most behaviors fewer change processes are used in maintenance than in action, for safer behaviors the use of the change processes continues to increase into maintenance. This suggests that for safer behaviors, even in maintenance, people must continue to use change processes actively to prevent relapse, while this is less necessary for other behaviors. Consistent with our earlier observation that people are in different stages of change for condom use in primary and secondary relationships, recent findings suggest that the former type of relationships may require a somewhat different use of the change processes than for the latter type.[126]

In addition to the process of change, the concept of decisional balance has been studied in the context of HIV preventive behaviors. As with other behaviors, it has been reported that people in precontemplation have fewer condom pros and higher condom cons than those at other stages of change.[126,129] While in general, decisional balance findings for safer sex are similar to those of other problem behaviors and the traditional "crossover" between pros and cons occurs before the action stage, the cons of condom use do not appear to decrease as individuals move through subsequent stages of change.[126] Movement across the stages is more a function of increases in the perceived pros of safer sex. Thus, media campaigns or interventions focusing on the negative aspects of HIV might be more effective if they stressed the benefits of prevention (e.g., that it shows your partners you care and keeps you safe[126]). Nevertheless, unless the perceived cons of condom use can somehow be addressed, even when people begin to use condoms, there is significant potential for relapse, which poses a challenge to interventionists. Interestingly, Bowen and Trotter[127] suggest that while an increase in the perceived pros of condom use may be all that is needed to increase this behavior with casual partners, for main partners both an increase in the perceived pros and a decrease in the perceived cons may be necessary.

The TM self-efficacy construct also has been studied in the context of safer sex. It has been found that for women, self-confidence in ability to use condoms is low in contexts where they believe the man may become angry[130] and that it is higher with casual than with main partners[131] (for possible reasons for this, see Misovich et al.[92]). Also, as would be expected based on other TM research,[120] confidence ratings for using condoms increase as individuals progress through the stages of change.[117] Similar findings (although in the opposite direction) occurred for the temptation construct.[132]

The TM has been used to guide HIV prevention interventions as well. Extensive application of the model to developing and evaluating community-based interventions has occurred in the context of the CDC-funded HIV community demonstration projects.[133,134] These used elicitation research to develop printed intervention materials that portrayed the stage-to-stage progression of community role models with respect to safer sexual and injection drug use practices. The print materials were stage-matched to the predominant stages of change at a particular point in time in the community. Other aspects of the TM (e.g., processes of change, decisional balance) were also addressed in the printed intervention materials, which were distributed by peers who reinforced their message and also distributed condom and bleach kits. The primary intervention outcome indicator was progression through the stages of change. It was found that those who recalled recently being exposed to the intervention materials progressed through the stages of change for condom use with main and nonprimary partners and for bleaching of injection drug equipment more than those who did not recall recent exposure to the materials. (While this could be a "real" treatment effect, it also could be due to an experimental artifact, such as self-selection). In addition, over the course of the intervention, stages of change for condom use with nonprimary partners increased among participants overall.[133] In a study currently in progress by the CDC, Cabral et al.[135] are providing "stage of change counseling" to women at high risk. In this program (Project CARES), women are assessed on their stage of change by peer advocates, who help them engage in stage-based processes of change to move them toward the action stage for condom use. A similar stage-based intervention has been developed to increase condom use in men.[126]

Conclusions/Critique

Cross-sectional analyses suggest that the TM and its components—stages of change, processes of change, decisional balance, self-efficacy, and temptation—work in the same way in the area of HIV prevention as in the other domains in which the theory has been applied.

Both the TM and the ARRM, as stage models, offer some very useful theoretical insights on the value of viewing change as a process rather than merely as an outcome. From the perspective of the TM, using condoms or clean needles can be viewed as the endpoint of a five-phase process. Consistent with the TM, it is likely that interventions that are stage-congruent for an individual or target population will be more effective than those that are not. Also, a staged approach probably permits interventions to reach a much broader segment of the population than relying solely on an approach that assumes that all persons are ready to change. In addition, consistent with the TM, a measure of an individual's stage of change is a useful "marker" for where one is in the change process and can be a more sensitive indicator of whether intervention-induced change has occurred than overt behavior change measures.

On the negative side of the ledger, the TM is unspecified as an integrated theoretical model and cannot be tested as such. For the most part, it is unclear how its various components and subcomponents interact. While decisional balance, processes of change, self-efficacy, and temptation have been found to act in accord with the predictions of the model as individual constructs, how all these elements work together is unclear. The lack of multivariate work with TM constructs leaves the extent to which its constructs are orthogonal or overlap and do not contribute uniquely to behavioral prediction an open question. It is also unclear whether each of these constructs are as parsimonious as they might be. The 11 processes of change, for example, all involve processes that can increase information, motivation, or behavioral skills and might be more parsimoniously viewed as such. Even Prochaska and associates[126] suggest that their linking of particular change processes (e.g., consciousness-raising, dramatic relief) with movement from a given stage of change is equivalent to saying that depending on the stage of change in question, movement requires a change process emphasizing information, motivation, and/or behavioral skills.[88,126] Similarly, the pros and cons of change are quite akin to positive and negative beliefs in Fishbein's theory of reasoned action (and Prochaska would not disagree), and the self-efficacy construct is the same as Bandura's (again, Prochaska would not disagree).

To date, the TM has been tested mostly in cross-sectional studies and relatively little longitudinal or experimental work has been done. More importantly, much of the TM, and thus the evidence to support its assumptions, seems rather circular. Given the way the stages of change (e.g., for condom use) are measured (e.g., with questions like, "Do you use condoms every time with all your sex partners?"), it is not at all surprising to find differences in condom use at different stages of change. Given the way the stages of change are defined and assessed, it also is not surprising to find differences in pros and cons, in self-efficacy and in temptation across the various stages. Finally, and very important as well, from an applied perspective sometimes it may be difficult to design interventions based on the TM. While the TM posits certain types of change processes to be most appropriate for particular stages of change, how elements from the array of processes depicted in Table 1 would be chosen and operationalized into the context of an HIV prevention intervention is unclear. It also is somewhat unclear how to use the TM in group-based interventions (e.g., in schools) where there is great diversity of stages of change, although the recent community demonstration projects do suggest a model for doing this.

THE SOCIAL COGNITIVE THEORY

Social cognitive theory (SCT) has been successfully applied in a variety of health domains (for a review, see Bandura[136]), and Bandura[15,137,138] has articulated it to the area of

HIV prevention. According to Bandura, the biggest problem with respect to behavior change is not instructing people in what they need to do (e.g., to use condoms or to clean needles), it is imparting to them the social and self-regulatory skills and the self-beliefs necessary to practice safer behaviors. Even when one possesses the requisite social and self-regulatory skills, in order to use them consistently across contexts, ranging from simple to difficult, one needs a belief in his or her self-efficacy to do so. Self-efficacy is the sense that one can control his or her motivation and environment, and especially his or her behavior. It affects whether people will attempt to change at all, how much effort they will exert, and how much they will persist in a change attempt without giving up. Without a sense of self-efficacy, people will not behave safely even if they know what constitutes safer behavior (e.g., that using condoms can help prevent HIV) and have the requisite skills (e.g., know how to put condoms on properly).

Fundamental Assumptions

According to Bandura,[15,138] an effective behavior change intervention must involve four components, one of which is self-efficacy. The four components are: (1) an informational component to increase awareness and knowledge of health risks and to convince people that they have the ability to change behavior; (2) a component to develop the self-regulatory and risk reduction skills needed to translate risk knowledge into preventive behavior; (3) a component to increase the level of these skills and individuals' level self-efficacy with respect to them; and (4) a component that develops or engages social supports for the individual who is making the change, in order to facilitate the change process and promote maintenance (see Fig. 4). We will review each of these critical elements below.

With respect to HIV risk behavior change, the information component of an intervention should highlight the types of behavior that can cause one to contract HIV, stress what constitutes effective preventive behavior, and include information that disposes individuals to believe that they could effectively engage in prevention.[15,138] In effect, an intervention must inform people that their current behavior may pose a danger, instruct them in how to be safer, and foster a sense of self-efficacy regarding HIV prevention. Bandura believes that the degree of self-efficacy instilled by the informational component of an intervention is a good predictor of whether or not people will even attempt to change unhealthy behavior. He also contends that the information component should stress that successful change requires perseverance, so that one's feelings of self-efficacy are not eroded by a setback. According to SCT, it is *not* necessary for an HIV prevention intervention to include behaviorally irrelevant information (e.g., about T cells and opportunistic infections). Finally, the content of the information component must be well crafted (e.g., it must be understandable, believable, and culturally competent) and it must be targeted to reach the group at focus (i.e., different groups respond better to different media, messages, and messengers).

In terms of SCT, information is necessary but not sufficient for preventive behavior to occur. In addition to an information component, an effective HIV prevention intervention must have an element that develops in individuals the necessary self-regulatory skills to engage in prevention. Self-regulatory skills include knowing one's risk triggers, being able to remind oneself how important safer behavior is, and reinforcing oneself for practicing it. In effect, self-regulation involves recognizing the behavioral sequences that lead to risk, developing internal standards, invoking affective reactions to their being met (or not met), using self-incentives to motivate oneself, and employing other types of cognitive self-guidance. Having these skills creates the ability for an individual to motivate and guide his or her actions. Self-regulation skills determine the types of risky situations in which people find themselves, how

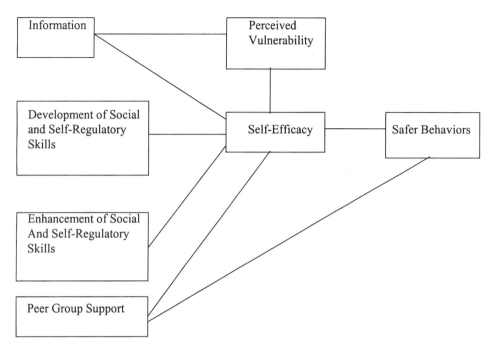

Figure 4.   Social cognitive theory. Adapted from Wulfert and Wan[143] and Bandura[15]. Note that because the TPB is unspecified, Fig. 4 represents a construction by the authors of what is implied by various SCT authors (e.g., Bandura[15]; Wulfert and Wan[143]).

well they deal with them, and how well they can resist social factors (e.g., recalcitrant partners) that coerce them into risky behavior. Once a person's risk triggers have been identified, self-regulatory skills can be trained through cognitive rehearsal (e.g., practicing how to tell oneself that risk triggers should be avoided, practicing reinforcing oneself for successful risk avoidance, and punishing oneself for failure). Showing people role models effectively displaying self-regulatory skills can assist in their development. When individuals have effective self-regulatory skills, they can realize that they are in a risky situation and disentangle themselves before engaging in dangerous behavior. According to Bandura,[15] the earlier that one removes him- or herself from a sequence that can ultimately culminate in risky behavior (e.g., for a gay man, drinking heavily at a gay bar), the more likely it is that he or she will succeed in avoiding risk.

   In addition to self-regulation skills, it is also critical for individuals to develop risk reduction skills. Risk reduction skills can be technical (e.g., knowing how to use a condom), social (e.g., knowing how to negotiate condom use, or how to exit unsafe situations), or both (e.g., knowing how to eroticize safer sex). Until one has developed risk reduction skills and a sense of self-efficacy regarding their use, it is best for the individual to stay out of risky situations entirely.[15,138] HIV risk reduction skills can be acquired by exposing individuals to videos of actors enacting the skills at focus, showing them live role models displaying these skills, or having individuals role-play the skilled behaviors themselves. People generally learn best and develop a greater sense of self-efficacy from exposure to role models similar to themselves in terms of gender, racial or ethnic status, age, or type of HIV risk behavior.

   Once one has developed the necessary skills, according to Bandura, the third essential component of an effective HIV prevention intervention is an element to increase the level of critical HIV prevention skills and to build on individuals' sense of self-efficacy. To increase skills and self-efficacy, individuals need to practice the behavior at focus (e.g., negotiating safer sex) in progressively more difficult contexts ranging from those in which they do not fear making mistakes or appearing inadequate, to more difficult situations that they may encounter in their environment, to the most difficult situations they can imagine. In each practice situation, they should receive constructive feedback on how they could improve their enactment of the necessary skills. According to Bandura,[15] such procedures lead both to greatly enhanced skills and to a greater sense of self-efficacy. The stronger the sense of self-efficacy that results, the more apt people are to use their new skills and to maintain their use in the face of adverse conditions. Beyond the practice that can occur in interventions, using one's skills successfully over time in challenging, "real-life" situations can result in an even greater sense of self-efficacy.

The fourth component of an effective HIV prevention intervention involves developing a context of social support for the behavior change at focus. According to Bandura,[15] since change often must occur in a social context, social influence, especially normative social influence, can assist or detract from its initiation and maintenance. Behavior that violates social norms is generally punished by others, while actions that are consistent with social norms are rewarded.[86] For example, in some segments of the gay community, proprevention social norms exist that result in rewards for those who practice safer sex and sanctions for those who do not. Generally, those more proximate to an individual (e.g., people in one's immediate social network) have greater social influence (i.e., ability to reward or punish) than those who are more distant. Over time, individuals' sensitivity to social norms results in their developing internal self-standards of conduct and an internal self-regulation system. When they conform to these standards, they feel good; when they fail to conform, they feel bad. Because having proprevention sources of support affects the development of proprevention self-standards and directly reinforces one's enactment of preventive behavior, they can play a major role in the initiation and maintenance of safer behavior.

Empirical Support

Since the interrelations between the elements in the SCT have not been specified, it cannot be considered to be an integrated multivariate model and cannot be tested as such. Nevertheless, the relations between some of the individual elements posited to be necessary for HIV prevention in the SCT and HIV preventive behavior have received empirical support. As Bandura[15,138] has suggested, many studies have shown that information is a necessary but not sufficient condition for HIV prevention (for reviews, see Fisher and Fisher,[7] Helweg-Larsen and Collins,[8] and St. Lawrence et al.[139]). While it has not been tested empirically, consistent with Bandura,[15,138] others have similarly contended that only "behaviorally relevant" information (e.g., focusing on HIV transmission and prevention, instead of information about T cells) is likely to be critical for HIV prevention to occur.[7] Further, Bandura's[15,138] assertion that behavior change is more likely to be attempted when the information component of an intervention fosters a sense of self-efficacy has not been tested in the context of HIV prevention, nor has his assertion that information components that stress that perseverance is necessary for successful change will be associated with greater maintenance. The assumptions that for change to occur the contents of the information component must be disseminated effectively (e.g., that they must be understandable, believable, and culturally competent) and that population-specific techniques must be used to reach the target group at focus (e.g., that different populations respond best to particular messages and messengers) have received empirical support at a general level.[140]

According to SCT, to engage in HIV prevention, one needs both self-regulation and risk reduction skills in addition to information. The former involve knowing one's risk triggers, having internal standards that result in affective reactions to their being met (or unmet), and using self-incentives for motivation. The latter refers to possessing both the technical and social skills necessary to practice HIV preventive behavior. The literature to date has not related possessing self-regulation or risk reduction skills per se to individuals' levels of HIV preventive behavior. Nevertheless, lack of support for the direct effect of these variables on HIV prevention is not problematic, since the SCT views them as necessary but not sufficient conditions for prevention. They only become necessary and sufficient when one possesses these skills and has a sense of self-efficacy regarding their use. Not surprisingly, individuals' level of self-efficacy with respect to critical HIV prevention skills has been strongly and consistently related to HIV prevention.

The relationship between feelings of self-efficacy associated with the skills necessary for safer sex and the actual performance of safer sexual behavior has been shown repeatedly. Perceived self-efficacy with respect to practicing safer sex predicts risk-taking behavior in minority and nonminority heterosexual adolescents,[88,89,141,142] university students,[87,88,143] minority and nonminority heterosexual adults,[144,145] IDUs,[104,146] HIV-infected IDUs,[102] men who have sex with men (MSM),[146,147] HIV-infected MSM,[148] and HIV-infected women.[101] Nevertheless, self-efficacy does not always lead to safer sexual behavior.[149] Further, O'Leary et al.[89] reported that the more self-efficacy individuals felt regarding their ability to assess their partner's HIV status through discussions with them, the more apt they were to practice unprotected sex. Similar to the general pattern of findings for safer sex, among IDUs higher self-efficacy generally has been observed to lead to safer injection drug use practices. Specifically, it has been shown to predict cleaning one's needles and works, using new needles, and not sharing needles,[150–153] though this pattern has not been entirely consistent.[154] Finally, HIV prevention interventions that increase individuals' levels of critical prevention skills and their sense of self-efficacy regarding their use (see discussion below) have been consistently shown to increase HIV preventive behavior.[66,68]

SCT asserts that social normative support for HIV prevention behavior change is associated with its initiation and maintenance. The prediction that normative support facilitates HIV prevention has been supported with respect to sexual behavior in heterosexual adults,[108] heterosexual adolescents,[146] MSM in general,[37] and HIV-positive MSM.[102] It also has been corroborated for safer sexual and injection drug use behavior for IDUs in general[134,155–157] and with HIV-infected IDUs.[158]

Changing HIV Preventive Behavior

Many HIV risk behavior change interventions performed to date can be classified as social cognitive in nature. Of these, some have explicitly used SCT as a conceptual framework,[139] while others have simply included some, most, or all of the elements of the theory without the authors explicitly viewing their work as a SCT-based intervention.[66] Kalichman et al.[68] present a meta-analysis of 12 relatively rigorously evaluated HIV prevention interventions that they classify as being formulated on SCT-based principles. While some were explicitly derived from SCT, others were based on alternate theories that included similar elements. Although relatively few of the interventions reviewed by Kalichman et al.[68] included all four SCT components, the authors characterized them as "sharing a core of central components that included such features as risk education, risk sensitization, self-efficacy building, and skills training" (p. 10). The Kalichman et al.[68] meta-analysis concluded that the effect sizes in all 12 interventions that they reviewed were positive, and that six performed with populations ranging from gay and bisexual men, to women, to adolescents demonstrated a significant change in risky sexual behaviors.

A review of two interventions based on SCT principles, one that was included in the Kalichman et al.[68] meta analysis and one that was not, help illustrate the use of SCT in intervention contexts. St. Lawrence et al.[139] conducted a highly effective HIV prevention intervention targeting minority adolescents and employing all four SCT model elements. This intervention involved an HIV education component; separate components for developing the social, technical, and cognitive competencies specified by SCT; extensive role playing; and a social support and empowerment component. The results of a rigorous evaluation indicated that it was highly effective in reducing unprotected sex. As with many of the interventions reviewed by Kalichman et al.,[68] the St. Lawrence et al.[139] intervention can be viewed as containing elements consistent with more than one theory (in fact, the authors view it as based on both the SCT and the information–motivation–behavioral skills models). A second intervention including SCT model-based elements was conducted with MSM by Peterson et al.[109] This intervention involved a knowledge component, a skills training component, a component to increase self-efficacy, and elements to induce more favorable attitudes toward HIV preventive behavior and to create normative support for prevention. The results indicated that risky behavior was reduced only slightly in a brief, single-session version of the intervention, but that a three-session version greatly reduced unprotected anal intercourse. Again, these researchers viewed their intervention as reflecting more than one behavior change model (in this case, SCT and the ARRM).

While several SCT-based interventions have been successful in changing HIV risk behavior across multiple populations (see also Kelly[22]), some interventions using the model have been unsuccessful.[68,159] One such study was performed with inner-city African-American men and followed SCT intervention principles quite closely. Participants were given training in identifying "triggers" for risk, in how to manage these triggers (e.g., by keeping condoms handy), in avoiding sex after drinking, and in remembering information about risk behaviors. They also were instructed in identifying barriers to risk reduction and in how to cope with them, and in how to use condoms. Overall, the SCT-based intervention was not more effective in changing risky behavior than a control condition, and the authors cautioned against assuming that SCT-based interventions will be effective for all at risk populations and argued that they may "miss the mark" with many urban, heterosexual men.[159]

Conclusions/Critique

SCT has received corroboration as a behavior change model for a number of unhealthy behaviors, and it has received support in the area of HIV prevention as well. Because the interrelations between the SCT constructs remain unspecified, it cannot be tested as an integrated multivariate model, which is a distinct weakness. Nevertheless, predicted relations between individual SCT constructs and HIV preventive behavior have been supported. This is particularly true of the relations between self-efficacy and social normative support for change and HIV risk behavior change. It is important to note that without multivariate tests it is not possible to determine the extent to which these constructs make orthogonal or overlapping contributions to prediction. Some of the SCT's other propositions remain untested (e.g., its assertions that information components that focus primarily on HIV transmission and prevention and self-efficacy and highlight the importance of perseverance are more likely to promote the initiation and maintenance of change).

Overall, the most significant work involving the SCT in the HIV risk reduction domain has involved SCT-inspired interventions, not model tests. In this regard, it is clear that the SCT contains most or all the elements typically associated with effective interventions, with the possible exception of an explicit attitude change component. Further, meta-analytic studies suggest that interventions containing SCT elements have been quite successful at changing HIV risk behavior. Nevertheless, it must be remembered that the credit for this must be shared with other models that share elements in common with SCT (e.g., the theory of reasoned action, the theory of planned behavior, and the information–motivation–behavior skills model), and which are more adequately specified. Finally, it should be noted that the SCT does not include an explicit elicitation research component, which can be very useful in targeting the particular intervention needs of the population at focus.

THE THEORY OF REASONED ACTION

The theory of reasoned action (TRA)[20,21] is a well-specified and well-tested model of the psychological determinants of volitional social behavior. As such, it has considerable relevance for understanding and promoting HIV risk reduction behavior change and has been extensively applied in this area.[14,160,161]

Fundamental Assumptions

According to the TRA, an individual's HIV preventive behavior is a function of his or her intention to perform a given preventive act. Behavioral intentions to perform an HIV preventive act in turn are a function of two factors: the individual's attitude toward performance of the preventive act and/or the individual's subjective norm or perception of referent support for performance of the preventive act. Algebraically, the TRA can be expressed by the following formula in which B = behavior, BI = behavioral intention, $Aact$ = attitude toward a preventive act, and SN = subjective norm regarding the preventive act. In this equation, $w1$ and $w2$ are empirically determined regression weights that reflect the degree to which attitudes and norms influence performance of the HIV preventive behavior in question: $B \sim BI = [Aact]_{w1} + [SN]_{w2}$.

The TRA also specifies the basic psychological underpinnings of the attitudinal and normative determinants of intention and behavior. According to the theory, attitudes toward an HIV preventive act are a function of beliefs about the consequences of performing the act (B_i), multiplied by evaluations of these consequences (e_i). Algebraically, $Aact = \Sigma B_i e_i$. Subjective norms concerning HIV preventive acts are viewed as a function of perceptions of whether specific categories of referent other want the individual to perform the act (NB_j), multiplied by the individual's motivation to comply with these referent's wishes (MC_j). Algebraically, $SN = \Sigma NB_j MC_j$.

The TRA asserts that it is critical to elicit salient beliefs about the consequences of preventive acts and salient categories of referents for preventive acts that are important for specific target populations and preventive behaviors, as opposed to attempting to identify such beliefs and referents intuitively.[20,21] Elicitation research is conducted to empirically identify salient perceived consequences of, say, condom use among low-income women and salient sources of referent influence for this behavior in this population, as opposed to researchers attempting to identify such consequences and referents on the basis of their intuition. In addition, it should be noted that the TRA asserts that personality, demographic, and other variables external to the model may only influence behavior indirectly, by way of their influence on *BI*, *Aact*, *SN*, or their basic underpinnings.[20,21] Thus, for example, perceived vulnerability to HIV, degree of hedonic enjoyment of unsafe sex, and other factors that are conceptually relevant to HIV prevention are expected to work through the TRA's components to affect HIV preventive behavior indirectly (see, however, Fisher[162] and Basen-Enquist[163] for evidence of a direct relation of variables external to the model and condom use behavior).

The TRA's hypothesized relationships appear in Fig. 5. The theory has significant implications for predicting, understanding, and changing HIV preventive behavior, and these are discussed in the sections that follow.

With respect to the prediction of HIV preventive behavior, the TRA asserts that preventive behavior will be likely to occur among individuals who have formed intentions to practice such behavior. Intentions to practice HIV preventive behavior in turn will be formed by individuals who have positive attitudes toward the personal performance of preventive acts and/or perceptions of social support for performance of these acts.[20,21,160]

With respect to understanding HIV preventive behavior, the TRA directs our attention to the basic psychological underpinnings of the attitudinal and normative determinants of behavior—specific B_is, e_is, NB_js, and MC_js—and to the relative weights of the attitudinal and normative determinants of behavior. Comparing the particular beliefs, evaluations, perceptions of referent support, and motivation to comply that characterize those who perform HIV preventive acts and those who do not should be informative about specific psychological factors that determine specific preventive behaviors. In such comparisons, for example, we have learned that gay men who use condoms in anal intercourse believe strongly that this practice will reduce their risk and fear of HIV, that they evaluate these consequences very positively, and that specific referent others are perceived as supporting this behavior.[164] Similarly, comparison of the relative weights of the attitudinal and normative determinants of preventive behavior can provide insight into the personal and/or social motivation of specific HIV preventive behaviors within specific populations. Thus, for example, it has been found that gay men's condom use in anal intercourse is influenced by their personal attitudes and by their subjective norms concerning social support for this critical preventive behavior.[164]

With respect to promoting HIV preventive behavior, the TRA holds that it is necessary to

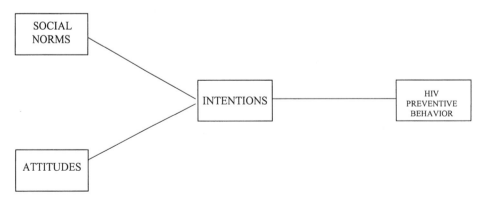

Figure 5.   Theory of reasoned action. From Fishbein et al.[14]

strengthen prevention intentions in order to increase preventive behavior. To strengthen intentions, it is necessary to enhance the individual's attitudes toward preventive acts and/or the individual's subjective norms concerning these acts. Following the TRA's approach, effective means for changing intentions, attitudes, and norms would involve efforts to change the specific B_is, e_is, NB_js, and MC_js that underlie attitudes and norms concerning a particular preventive act and that differentiate between those who perform the act and those who do not. In terms of the example considered earlier, to change gay men's condom use in anal intercourse, it would be necessary to change their intentions to engage in this behavior. To change intentions, interventions should focus on strengthening beliefs that condoms reduce HIV risk to the self and to others, strengthening positive evaluations of these consequences, and strengthening perceptions of social support from referent others found to be salient in this regard.[164]

In practice, the TRA is used to predict, understand, and change HIV preventive behavior along the following lines.[20,21,160] First, elicitation research is conducted to identify salient beliefs and referents for specific preventive behaviors within a population of interest. For example, following standard procedures for elicitation research,[20] a subsample of a high school target population would respond to open-ended measures of the advantages and disadvantages of abstinence from intercourse and of consistent condom use and concerning the categories of referent others who might approve or disapprove of these preventive behaviors. Then, research concerning the prediction and understanding of these preventive behaviors within this target population could proceed. Such research would involve assessment of BI, $Aact$, SN, and salient B_is, e_is, NB_js, and MC_js concerning the HIV preventive behaviors under study. An assessment of students' performance of these HIV preventive behaviors would take place at a later point in time.

Analysis of these data would indicate whether the HIV preventive behaviors under study in this population are in fact determined by behavioral intentions. It would also indicate whether intentions to perform these HIV preventive behaviors are under attitudinal or normative influence or under the influence of both factors. In addition, this research would identify specific B_is, e_is, NB_js, and MC_js that differentiate those who perform these HIV preventive behaviors from those who do not. This set of findings can be used to create an empirically targeted, population and preventive behavior-specific intervention that is designed to strengthen attitudes, norms, and intentions that favor prevention. This would be accomplished by targeting for change the most important B_i, e_i, NB_j, and MC_j underpinnings of the attitudinal and/or normative determinants of preventive behavior in order to change HIV prevention intentions and behavior.

Empirical Support

The TRA has been applied widely over the past two decades in efforts to understand and predict a diversity of behaviors, and research has consistently confirmed the theory's hypothesized relationships among behavior, intention, attitudes, norms, and their underpinnings. The TRA also has been applied widely and successfully in efforts to predict and understand HIV preventive behavior, and less widely but also with some success in efforts to change HIV preventive behavior. (See Sheppard and co-workers'[165] meta-analysis of TRA research outside of the HIV domain; Albarracin and co-workers'[166] meta-analysis of TRA research concerning HIV prevention; and Rye's[167] qualitative review and synthesis of TRA research concerning HIV prevention. See also Fishbein and Middlestadt,[160] Fishbein et al.,[14] and Terry et al.,[161] for discussions of the TRA as a model of HIV preventive behavior.)

With respect to the prediction of HIV preventive behavior, reviews by Albarracin et al.[166] and Rye[167] document the fact that the TRA has been utilized in dozens of published studies, involving thousands of participants, that have predicted condom use as a function of behavioral intentions. Across this research literature, it is consistently observed that condom use intentions predict condom use behavior across prospective time intervals, across the sexes, and across sexual orientation and ethnic group categories. These findings are completely consistent with the results of TRA-based research outside of the area of HIV prevention[165] and may qualify as one of the more robust predictions that psychological science can make within or without the HIV prevention area.

To illustrate research on the prediction of condom use behavior from condom use intentions, consider research reported by Fisher et al.[164] These investigators assessed intentions to use condoms and intentions to engage in related safer sexual behaviors in samples of gay men, heterosexual high school students, and heterosexual university students. Self-reports of condom use and of related safer sexual behaviors were collected 1 to 2 months later. Behavioral intentions proved to be significant predictors of a wide variety of safer sex practices across the prospective intervals employed, across the categories of safer sexual behavior studied (e.g., abstinence, condom use), and across the sexes, ethnicities, sexual orientations, and age ranges represented.

TRA-based investigations also have provided critical information about the attitudinal and normative determinants of intentions to practice safer sex. Research has explored the question of whether intentions to practice safer sexual behavior are a function of attitudes or norms concerning such behaviors or are a function of both factors, and has examined the basic underpinnings of attitudes and norms as well. Across a large number of studies of the determinants of safer sex intentions, it is generally found that attitudes toward safer sex behaviors and subjective norms contribute significantly to the determination of safer sex intentions (see, for example, Doll and Orth,[168] Fishbein et al.,[169] Fisher et al.,[164] Jemmott and Jemmott,[170] Kashima et al.,[171] Morrison et al.[172]). Discrepancies from the pattern of joint attitudinal and normative influence over intentions are relatively uncommon, and when they occur, they somewhat more often involve findings for sole attitudinal than for sole normative influence on intentions to practice safer sex.

It should be emphasized that findings for attitudinal, normative, or mutual attitudinal and normative influence on intentions to practice safer sex have important implications for the empirical targeting of HIV risk reduction interventions. For example, Fisher et al.[164] found that among gay men in a community sample both personal attitudes and perceptions of social support were significantly associated with intentions to use condoms during anal intercourse. These intentions, it will be recalled, were consistently predictive of condom use behavior by gay men. It follows that HIV prevention interventions to promote condom use in anal intercourse in this population should focus on changing attitudes toward condom use in anal intercourse and on changing perceptions of referent support for these practices. In contrast, these investigators found that for heterosexual high school males and heterosexual university males, intentions to use condoms during sexual intercourse were solely under the control of personal attitudes toward the performance of this behavior and were not influenced by perceptions of social support for it. It follows that HIV prevention interventions directed toward promoting condom use in these populations should focus mostly on modification of attitudes toward the personal use of condoms during sexual intercourse. Focus on changing perceptions of social support for condom use should probably be a lesser priority in these later populations, because perceptions of social support for this behavior did not influence intentions to engage in this practice. (See Fishbein et al.[169] for further discussion and illustration of the attitudinal and/or normative determination of safer sex intentions.)

In addition to exploring attitudinal and normative determination of safer sex intentions, a number of studies[164,170,172,173] also have examined the basic underpinnings of these attitudinal and normative factors. This research has identified population- and preventive behavior-specific beliefs, evaluations, perceptions of referent support, and motivation to comply that are associated with the practice of HIV preventive behaviors and comprise an empirically derived roster of targets for HIV prevention interventions attempting to promote such behaviors.

With respect to changing HIV risk behavior, a number of published interventions have applied the TRA to one degree or another in efforts to promote prevention. The results of these intervention studies are broadly supportive of the TRA's postulates and of the utility of applying the theory to promote HIV risk reduction behavior change in applied settings.[66,174–180] For example, in a series of studies guided in part by the TRA, Jemmott et al.[177,178] conducted one-session small-group HIV prevention interventions with African-American inner-city adolescents. Each HIV prevention intervention employed a variety of engaging techniques that were designed to modify attitudes and intentions with respect to risky sex and was compared to an intervention employing parallel techniques with a focus on objectives other than HIV prevention (e.g., career opportunities in Jemmott et al.,[177] general health promotion in Jemmott et al.[178]). In an initial investigation, Jemmott et al.[177] found that the TRA-inspired intervention was effective in changing attitudes toward risky sexual behaviors and intentions to engage in them at an immediate postintervention assessment and confirmed that change in intentions to engage in risky sexual behavior persisted at a 3-month follow-up. Moreover, participants in the TRA-inspired HIV prevention intervention reported engaging in significantly less risky sexual behavior 3 months following the intervention, including reports of increased condom use and decreased anal intercourse in comparison with controls. In an additional study in this research line, Jemmott et al.[178] examined effects of a similar intervention on African-American adolescents' condom use beliefs, intentions, and behaviors across a 6-month prospective interval. Results at an assessment 3 months after the TRA-inspired intervention showed that African-American adolescent participants had more positive beliefs about the ability of condoms to prevent STDs, HIV, and pregnancy, more favorable beliefs about the hedonistic consequences of using condoms, and stronger condom use intentions compared to controls. At a 6-month follow-up, results showed a significant impact of the TRA-inspired intervention on safer sex behavior, including reports of fewer occasions of unprotected coitus and fewer occasions of anal intercourse among intervention versus control subjects.

Beyond demonstration that TRA-guided HIV prevention interventions are capable of changing intentions, attitudes, and behaviors, a small number of studies have directly examined the role of TRA-based constructs in mediating changes in HIV risk reduction intentions and behavior. For example, Jemmott and Jemmott[179] conducted a one-session HIV prevention intervention, guided in part by the TRA, with small groups of African-American adolescent women. Intervention activities were designed to improve beliefs about the hedonistic and prevention consequences of condom use and to improve perceptions of referent support for this behavior. Results of an immediate postintervention assessment demonstrated that the intervention was successful in modifying beliefs that condoms do not interfere with sexual pleasure; condoms effectively prevent pregnancy, STDs, and HIV; and sexual partners would be supportive of condom use. In accord with the TRA, African-American women in the HIV intervention also reported significantly stronger intentions to use condoms in the future. Moreover, correlational analyses revealed that increases in women's beliefs about the consequences of condom use relative to hedonistic pleasure and partner support were significantly related to increases in condom use intentions, in accord with expectations of the TRA. In more recent research, Bryan et al.[66] found that a single 45-minute HIV prevention intervention was successful in modifying female university students' beliefs about the health consequences of using condoms, their attitudes toward condom use, and their self-reported condom use behavior. Moreover, changes in beliefs about the health consequences of using condoms were found to be associated with changes in attitudes toward condom use, which in turn were associated with significant increases in condom use reported across 6-month's time, once again confirming expectations based on the TRA.

Conclusions/Critique

The propositions of the TRA concerning the performance of HIV preventive behavior as a function of intentions, attitudes, norms, and their underpinnings have been confirmed consistently across a large number of prospective studies of diverse subject samples and preventive behaviors. The propositions of the TRA concerning changing HIV preventive behavior by way of changing intentions, attitudes, norms, and their underpinnings have been studied much less extensively and generally have involved TRA-guided or TRA-inspired efforts, as opposed to formal testing of TRA-based hypotheses concerning HIV prevention behavior change. Nonetheless, results of HIV risk behavior change research inspired by the TRA or directly testing TRA behavior change assumptions are quite supportive of the propositions of the theory and provide a reasonable basis for further HIV prevention intervention efforts based on this model. They also provide encouragement for pursuing formal TRA-based HIV risk behavior change research. In such research, elicitation and prediction research would be used to identify and target specific B_is, e_is, NB_js, and MC_js that underlie safer sex attitudes, norms, intentions, and behavior. Interventions would be targeted to influence these factors and evaluation research would assesses success or failure in modifying B_is, e_is, NB_js, and MC_js and associated safer sex attitudes, norms, intentions, and behavior.

A number of criticisms of the TRA also should be noted. First, it is by no means clear that all factors external to the TRA influence behavior only by influencing the components of the model. Especially in the HIV prevention context, the unmediated impact on preventive behavior of factors such as feelings about sexuality,[66,162] HIV-related information and HIV prevention behavioral skills,[7,18] perceptions of vulnerability to HIV,[181] and sex and ethnicity[179] remain critical to consider. Second, it appears to be important to conceptualize explicitly the role of past behavior within the TRA's approach to predicting and understanding HIV preventive actions. To what extent are intentions, attitudes, norms, and their underpinnings malleable causes of future HIV preventive behavior? To what extent do they represent an unmalleable history of factors that originally triggered a pattern of risky or preventive behavior? To what extent are they simply the attitudinal and normative results of chronic patterns of risky or preventive behavior?

An additional critique of the TRA rests on the fact that it is fundamentally a motivational model that, all else being equal, predicts substantial variance in many types of HIV preventive behavior. However, the TRA does not explicitly take into account the degree to which HIV prevention is not entirely under an individual's volitional control, nor does it address the fact that the individual may lack perceived control over HIV preventive acts.[182,183] Moreover, the TRA does not take into account the changing and complex HIV prevention information base that may be necessary to facilitate performance of preventive behaviors, nor does it address the need for specialized behavioral skills that may be required for the initiation and maintenance of preventive behaviors. Against a background of such concerns, the theory of planned behavior[182,183] has been developed to address the possibility that the TRA as originally conceptualized may be too narrow to afford prediction, understanding, and change of less than completely volitional HIV preventive behaviors. Similarly, the information–motivation–behavioral skills model[7,18] has been developed to address the possibility that it may be necessary to conceptualize HIV prevention information and HIV prevention behavioral skills, in addition to HIV prevention motivation, as fundamental to the prediction, understanding, and change of HIV preventive behavior. These two theories are discussed in turn in the sections that follow.

THE THEORY OF PLANNED BEHAVIOR

The theory of planned behavior (TPB)[182,183] is an extension of the TRA that adds the construct of perceived behavioral control to the model's original assertions concerning intentions, attitudes, and norms as determinants of behavior. The TPB was developed on the basis of the TRA to achieve enhanced ability to predict, understand, and change behavior in domains of action that are not entirely under volitional control. The TPB has considerable relevance for HIV preventive behavior since HIV preventive acts are arguably not always under an individual's complete personal control, given the influence of factors such as sexual arousal, gender-based power differentials, and alcohol and drug use.

Fundamental Assumptions

From the perspective of the TPB,[182,183] HIV preventive behaviors are determined by intentions, attitudes, norms, and perceived control over the performance of preventive behaviors, when perceived control over preventive behavior is not complete. Perceived control is conceptualized as an individual's assessment of the ease or difficulty of performing a given preventive behavior and is seen as reflecting an individual's control beliefs or assessments of the degree to which he or she possesses the resources and opportunities necessary for performing the preventive behavior in question.[184]

According to the TPB,[182,183] perceived control may affect the performance of HIV preventive behavior indirectly, as a determinant of HIV prevention intentions, or it may affect HIV preventive behavior directly. With respect to indirect effects on behavior, the TPB theorizes that perceptions of control can add to the influence of attitudes and norms to incline an individual to intend to perform HIV preventive acts. All else being equal, an individual who has positive attitudes toward an HIV preventive act, positive norms concerning performance of the act, and perceptions of control over the performance of the act should intend to practice the HIV preventive behavior in question. In contrast, an individual who has positive attitudes toward an HIV preventive act and positive norms in this regard but who perceives performance of this behavior to be entirely out of his or her control (due, say, to intractable partner resistance) should be less inclined to intend to practice the preventive behavior. Perceptions of control also are thought to be capable of directly affecting performance of HIV preventive behaviors, insofar as persons who believe they have control over a preventive behavior are more likely to be able to enact the behavior. Finally, it seems intuitively obvious that perceptions of control should interact with attitudes, norms, and intentions, such that perceived control should affect behavior when attitudes and norms and intentions are favorable to behavior and should not affect behavior when attitudes and norms and intentions to a behavior are unfavorable. Ajzen,[183] however, suggests that perceptions of control motivate behavioral performance in the presence of positive as well as negative attitudes and norms. The constructs and relationships of the TPB are presented in Fig. 6.

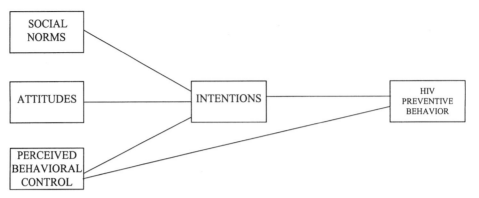

Figure 6. Theory of planned behavior. From Ajzen.[182]

It should be noted that when an HIV preventive behavior is perceived to be under the complete control of the individual, the TPB reverts to the TRA. In addition, the perceived control construct is expected to make a greater contribution to the prediction of behavior when perceived control approximates actual control over behavior. Finally, it is noted that factors which affect perceived control (e.g., resources and opportunities) can be identified in the context of elicitation research.

Empirical Support

The TPB has been applied widely in efforts to understand and predict a number of social and health-related behaviors (see Ajzen[183] and Godin and Kok[185] for reviews of this literature). The TPB also has been used extensively as a basis for understanding and predicting HIV preventive behavior (see Albarracin and co-workers'[166] meta-analysis and Rye's[167] qualitative review of this literature). The TPB's emphasis on perceived behavioral control also has guided efforts to change HIV preventive behavior in diverse populations (see, for example, Basen-Enquist,[186] Bryan et al.,[66] Fisher et al.,[176] and Jemmott and Jemmott[179]). Further, the TPB and the TRA also have been tested competitively against one another within the HIV prevention domain[187,188] and without.[189,190]

The TPB's assertion that perceived control over behavioral performance adds significantly to the influence of attitudes and norms in the formation of behavioral intentions has been confirmed consistently in research conducted outside of the HIV prevention area[183,185] as well as in research focusing specifically on HIV prevention.[166,167] For example, Ajzen[183] reported that perceived control contributed significantly to the prediction of intention in all studies reviewed, and Godin and Kok[185] relate that perceived control contributed to determining intentions to perform an array of health-related behaviors in the vast majority of cases reviewed. Similarly, in TPB-based research on HIV preventive behaviors, Rye[167] reported that perceived control contributed to the prediction of intention in approximately 75% of the cases examined, and Albarracin et al.[166] reported a significant correlation of perceived control with intention over a large number of studies in the HIV prevention area.

The TPB's assertion that perceived control over behavior is directly related to behavior has been confirmed inconsistently in research conducted outside the HIV prevention area[183,185] and has been confirmed erratically[167] or not at all[166] in TPB-based research focusing on HIV preventive behavior. For example, Ajzen[183] reported that perceived behavioral control contributed significantly to the prediction of behavior over and above intention in 64% of the studies reviewed, and Godin and Kok[185] related that perceived behavioral control contributes to the prediction of health-related behaviors over and above intention in about 50% of the cases examined. In reviewing TPB-based research on HIV preventive behaviors, however, Rye[167] reported that perceived behavioral control contributed to the prediction of preventive behavior over intention erratically and Albarracin et al.[166] reported that perceived behavioral control contributed negligibly to the prediction of HIV preventive behavior when intentions, attitudes, and norms were factored into consideration in the context of a path analysis. Also in the context of a path analytic approach to the TPB and the TRA, Albarracin et al.[166] reported that across existing research, the overall fit of the TRA and the TPB in the prediction of condom use behavior is equivalent.

A number of HIV prevention interventions have been guided, at least in part, by the TPB's emphasis on the importance of strengthening perceptions of control in efforts to promote performance of preventive behaviors (see, for example, Basen-Enquist,[186] Bryan et al.,[66] Jemmott and Jemmott[179]). These interventions have been broadly supportive of the TPB's focus on perceived control and of the utility of intervening to change perceptions of control in efforts to promote HIV risk reduction behavior change. For example, Basen-Enquist[186] conducted a 3-hour safer sex self-efficacy workshop with university students in which mastery experiences, role-playing, and persuasive messages were used to bolster students' perceptions of safer sex self-efficacy. Results showed that the safer sex self-efficacy workshop was effective in increasing perceptions of safer sex self-efficacy assessed 1 week postintervention, and significantly increased reported condom use assessed 8 weeks postintervention, compared to controls. To the extent that safer sex self-efficacy and perceived behavioral control in this domain are related constructs, such intervention research is supportive of the TPB's proposed effects of perceived behavioral control on behavior.

In addition to demonstrating that HIV prevention interventions are capable of changing perceptions of self-efficacy or control with respect to safer sexual practices and that such changes may be implicated in HIV risk reduction behavior change, a few interventions have examined directly the role of changes in safer sex self-efficacy as mediators of change in HIV prevention intentions and behavior. For example, in a study that was guided in part by the TPB's emphasis on changing perceptions of control, Jemmott and Jemmott[179] conducted a one-session HIV prevention intervention, focused partly on improving safer sex self-efficacy, with small groups of African-American adolescent women. Results of an immediate postintervention assessment demonstrated that the intervention was successful in modifying self-efficacy to use condoms. Further, correlational analyses showed that intervention-induced increases in women's sense of self-efficacy for condom use were significantly related to increases in women's condom use intentions. Again, to the extent that safer sex self-efficacy and perceived behavioral control are related constructs, these findings are in accord with the assumptions of the TPB. In a related study, Bryan et al.[66] found that a 45-minute HIV prevention intervention was successful in modifying female university students' condom use self-efficacy and perceptions of control over sexual encounters. These changes in turn were associated with increases in condom use intentions and ultimately with increases in condom use behavior across a 6-month time span, again confirming the expectations of the TPB.

Conclusions/Critique

The TPB's assertion that HIV prevention intentions are a function of attitudes and norms and perceived control has been confirmed consistently across a number of studies.[166,167] The TPB's assertion that HIV preventive behavior may be directly influenced by perceived control over such behavior has been subject to serious question,[166,167] however, and the ability of the constructs of the TPB to predict HIV preventive behavior over and above the constructs of the TRA seems negligible.[166,167] Finally, the TPB's emphasis on changing HIV preventive behavior by way of changing perceptions of control over such behavior is consistent with the fairly limited amount of intervention research that is relevant to this proposition.

A number of generalities emerge from this consideration of the TPB. First, it is apparent that perceptions of control play a significant role in influencing intentions to practice HIV preventive behavior. Second, it is apparent that perceptions of control generally exert their influence on HIV prevention by influencing intentions to engage in such behavior as opposed to having direct independent effects on behavioral performance. Further research is needed to confirm the conditions under which perceptions of control may be expected to have greater or lesser effect on HIV prevention intentions. Such research should test directly the TPB's assumptions about the impact of perceptions of control at varying levels of perceived control over preventive behavior. Third, research suggests that promoting perceptions of control is helpful in promoting HIV preventive behavior, a fact that is consistent with the TPB. Fourth, it is evident that more research directly testing the behavior change implications of the TPB (and for that matter the behavior change implications of the TRA) is needed. In such research, a special focus might be on monitoring mediators of change and examining whether changes in perceived control influence preventive behavior directly or by way of changes in intentions to practice prevention.

A number of conceptual issues concerning the TPB should be raised as well. For example, it is possible to critique the TPB, in common with the TRA, as an essentially motivational model that directs insufficient explicit attention to the specific information and specific sets of behavioral skills that are required for the initiation and maintenance of HIV preventive behaviors. The information–motivation–behavioral skills model[7,18] addresses this issue directly in the section to follow. In addition, in an attempt to integrate the TRA and the TPB, Rye[167] has suggested conceptualizing control beliefs as cognitive underpinnings of the TRA's *Aact* and *SN* components. In this fashion, an individual's assessment of the resources and opportunities available for the performance of preventive behavior may be seen as affecting attitudes and norms rather than as comprising an additional theoretical construct. Whether perceptions of control merit consideration as basic underpinnings of attitudes and norms in a TRA approach to HIV prevention or whether they merit consideration as an independent construct in a TPB approach might be explored further from this perspective.

THE INFORMATION–MOTIVATION–BEHAVIORAL SKILLS MODEL

The information–motivation–behavioral skills (IMB) model conceptualizes the psychological determinants of HIV preventive behavior and provides a general framework for understanding and promoting prevention across populations and preventive behaviors of interest.[7,18,88,191] The IMB model is based on an analysis and integration of theory and research in the HIV prevention and social psychological literatures,[7,18,176,191] and focuses comprehensively on the set of informational,[192] motivational,[160] and behavioral skills[193] factors that are conceptually and empirically associated with HIV prevention but often are dealt with in isolation.[7] The model specifies a set of causal relationships among these constructs and a set of operations to be utilized in translating this approach into conceptually based and empirically targeted HIV prevention interventions.[7,18,194]

Fundamental Assumptions

The IMB model asserts that HIV prevention information, HIV prevention motivation, and HIV prevention behavioral skills are the fundamental determinants of HIV preventive behavior.[7,18,176,191] To the extent that individuals are well-informed, motivated to act, and possess the behavioral skills required to act effectively, they will be likely to initiate and maintain patterns of HIV preventive behavior.

According to the IMB model, HIV prevention information that is directly relevant to preventive behavior and can be enacted easily in the social ecology of the individual is a prerequisite of HIV preventive behavior.[7,195] HIV prevention information that is closely related to preventive behavior enactment can include specific facts about HIV transmission (e.g., "Oral sex is a much safer alternative to vaginal intercourse") and HIV prevention (e.g., "Consistent condom use can prevent HIV") that serve as guides for personal preventive actions. In addition to easy-to-translate-into-behavior facts, the IMB model recognizes additional cognitive processes and content categories that significantly influence performance of preventive behavior. Individuals often rely heavily on HIV prevention heuristics (simple decision rules which permit automatic and cognitively effortless decisions about whether or not to engage in HIV preventive behavior) and endorsement of such heuristics appears to be strongly negatively related to HIV preventive practices.[103,196–198] For example, reliance on HIV prevention heuristics that hold that "monogamous sex is safe sex" and "known partners are safe partners" is ubiquitous and substantially interferes with performance of preventive behavior.[196,197] Individuals also operate on the basis of implicit theories of HIV risk that hold that it is possible to detect and avoid HIV risk on the basis of assessment of a partner's externally visible characteristics such as dress, demeanor, personality, or social associations. Based on estimates of HIV risk made by assessing a partner's overtly accessible profile of risk cues, individuals often decide that the partner poses no risk and that preventive behaviors are not warranted.[92,103,196–198]

Motivation to engage in HIV preventive acts is an additional determinant of preventive behavior and influences whether even well-informed individuals will be inclined to act on what they know about prevention. According to the IMB model,[7,18] HIV prevention motivation includes personal motivation to practice preventive behaviors (e.g., attitudes toward practicing specific preventive acts[21]), social motivation to engage in prevention (e.g., perceptions of social support for performing such acts[21]), and perceptions of personal vulnerability to HIV infection.[28]

Behavioral skills for performing HIV preventive acts are an additional prerequisite of HIV preventive behavior and determine whether even well-informed and well-motivated individuals will be capable of practicing prevention effectively. The behavioral skills component of the IMB model is composed of an individual's objective ability and his or her perceived self-efficacy concerning performance of the sequence of HIV preventive behaviors that is involved in the practice of prevention.[7,15,137,193,195] Behavioral skills involved in HIV prevention can include objective and perceived abilities to purchase and to put on condoms effectively; to negotiate consistent condom use before, or during, sexual contact; to negotiate HIV testing and monogamy; and the ability to reinforce the self and the partner for maintaining patterns of preventive behaviors across time, among many other such behaviors.

The IMB model specifies that HIV prevention information and HIV prevention motivation work primarily through HIV prevention behavioral skills to influence HIV preventive behavior. In essence, effects of prevention information and prevention motivation are expressed mainly as a result of the development and deployment of prevention behavioral skills that are directly applied to the initiation and maintenance of preventive behavior. The IMB model also specifies that prevention information and prevention motivation may have direct effects on preventive behavior, in cases in which complicated or novel behavioral skills are not necessary to effect prevention. For example, HIV prevention information may have a direct effect on preventive behavior when a pregnant women learns of the benefits of prenatal HIV antibody testing and agrees with her physician's suggestion that she undergo such testing. Motivation may have a direct effect on behavior as when a motivated adolescent maintains a sexually abstinent pattern of behavior as opposed to consistently using condoms, which might require relatively complicated and/or novel behavioral skills including those involved in condom acquisition, discussion, negotiation, and consistent use. Finally, from the perspective of the IMB model, information and motivation are regarded as generally independent constructs, in that well-informed individuals are not necessarily well-motivated to practice prevention and well-motivated individuals are not always well-informed about prevention.[7,88] The IMB model's basic constructs and the relationships among them are depicted in Fig. 7.

The IMB model's information, motivation, and behavioral skills constructs are regarded as highly generalizable determinants of HIV preventive behavior across populations and preventive behaviors of interest.[7,18,199] At the same time, however, it is asserted that these constructs should have specific content that is most relevant to the prevention needs of particular populations and particular preventive practices. Thus, within the IMB model, it is presumed that specific HIV prevention information, motivation, and behavioral skills will be especially relevant to understanding and promoting prevention among males (as compared to females), among African Americans (as compared to whites), and among members of particular ethnic groups and persons of particular sexual orientation, chemical dependency status, and the like. Similarly, specific HIV prevention information, motivation, and behavioral skills content will be especially relevant to specific HIV preventive practices, such as abstinence, condom use, and HIV antibody testing, within specific populations of interest. Also following this logic, the IMB model proposes that particular constructs of the model, and particular causal pathways among them, will emerge as more or less powerful determinants of HIV preventive practices for specific populations and specific preventive behaviors.[7,18,199]

The IMB approach specifies measurement and statistical procedures for eliciting infor-

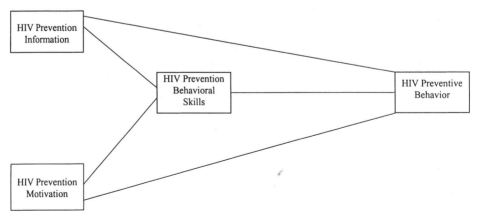

Figure 7. IMB model of HIV preventive behavior. From Fisher and Fisher.[7]

mation, motivation, and behavioral skills content that are relevant to HIV prevention for particular populations and behaviors of interest. These procedures may then be used for the purpose of identifying specific causal elements and paths in the model that are especially influential in determining a given population's practice of a particular preventive behavior.[7,18,88,199] According to the IMB model, specification of the information, motivation, and behavioral skills content most relevant to a population's practice of a particular preventive behavior and identification of IMB model constructs that most powerfully influence the population's practice of the preventive behavior are crucial to the design of conceptually based and empirically targeted prevention interventions that are effective for the population and preventive behavior of interest.[7,18,199]

The IMB approach to understanding and promoting HIV preventive behavior specifies a set of generalizable operations for constructing, implementing, and evaluating HIV prevention interventions for particular target populations and behaviors.[7,18,199] On the basis of the IMB model, the first step in the process of changing HIV preventive behavior involves elicitation research conducted with a subsample of a population of interest, to empirically identify population-specific deficits and assets in HIV prevention information, motivation, behavioral skills, and HIV risk and preventive behavior. The use of open-ended data collection techniques such as focus groups and open-ended questionnaires to avoid providing occasions for prompted responses is advocated, in addition to the use of close-ended techniques that lend themselves to quantitative analyses.[18] The second step in this process of changing HIV risk behavior involves the design and implementation of conceptually based, empirically targeted, population-specific interventions, constructed on the basis of elicitation research findings. These targeted interventions address identified deficits in HIV prevention information, motivation, behavioral skills, and behavior and capitalize on assets in these factors that may be identified within a population. The third step in the process of HIV risk behavior change involves methodologically rigorous evaluation research conducted to determine whether an intervention has had significant and sustained effects on the information, motivation, and behavioral skills determinants of HIV preventive behavior and on HIV preventive behavior per se. The IMB approach advocates evaluation research reliance on multiple convergent sources of data, at least some of which are relatively nonreactive and at least some of which are collected in a context that appears to participants to be unrelated to the intervention per se.[7,18,176]

The IMB model has been used as a basis for understanding HIV risk and HIV prevention across populations and behaviors of interest and for the focused conceptual analyses of heightened HIV risk behavior seen among individuals in close relationships[92] and the severely mentally ill.[200,201] The IMB model also has been used as a basis for understanding and promoting adolescent contraception,[202] STD risk reduction,[194] and reproductive health promotion education.[10,203] Standardized measures of the IMB model's constructs have been developed and validated for use within a number of populations and for a number of behaviors of interest.[18,88,176,197,204,205]

Empirical Support

Considerable empirical support for the fundamental assumptions of the IMB model has been provided in multivariate correlational research concerning informational, motivational, and behavioral skills determinants of HIV preventive behavior across populations and preventive behaviors of interest.[88,206–209] Confirmatory evidence concerning the IMB model's risk reduction behavior change implications also has been accumulated in model-based experimental intervention research that has resulted in significant and sustained increases in HIV risk reduction information, motivation, behavioral skills, and preventive behavior over time and across diverse populations.[176,210,211]

Multivariate correlational evidence consistently supports the IMB model's assumptions concerning the determinants of HIV preventive behavior. In an initial study in this research line, Fisher et al.[88] used a structural equation modeling approach to empirically test the IMB model's assumptions concerning the determinants of HIV preventive behavior within a heterosexual university student sample. In this sample, HIV prevention information and HIV prevention motivation were statistically independent factors; HIV prevention information and HIV prevention motivation were each related to HIV prevention behavioral skills; and HIV prevention behavioral skills were related to HIV preventive behavior per se. Each relationship was precisely as predicted by the IMB model. In an additional study in this series, Fisher et al.[88] examined HIV preventive behavior from the perspective of the IMB model within a community sample of adult homosexual men. Once again, it was found that information and motivation were independent constructs, that they were each associated with behavioral skills, and that behavioral skills were associated with preventive behavior, as predicted by the model. A direct link between HIV prevention motivation and HIV preventive behavior was observed as well, also in accord with the model's assumptions. Subsequent research has substantially confirmed the IMB model's propositions concerning the determinants of HIV preventive behavior in populations of sexually active minority high school students,[209] among African-American and white very-low-income women,[206] and in a cohort of gay men in the Netherlands.[207]

Beyond these confirmatory findings, a recent study by Bryan et al.[208] adopted a fine-grained approach to empirically testing the IMB model's assumptions about the determinants of HIV preventive behavior, using a sample of urban minority high school students. Male and female urban minority high school students completed measures of HIV prevention information, motivation, and behavioral skills, and at a 1-month follow-up indicated whether they had enacted a preparatory HIV preventive behavior (discussing condom use with their partner) and an actual HIV preventive behavior (condom use). Results showed that HIV prevention information and motivation were independent constructs; that prevention information and prevention motivation were each associated with prevention behavioral skills; that prevention behavioral skills were associated with enactment of the preparatory preventive behavior; and that enactment of the preparatory preventive behavior was associated with enactment of actual HIV preventive behavior. These results provide consistent and detailed evidence that information and motivation stimulate the application of preventive behavioral skills that result in the practice of actual preventive behavior.

The relationships observed across multiple empirical tests of the IMB model's relationships are summarized in Table 2. It is clear that the central propositions of the IMB model are consistently supported and that the data are in accord with the assertion that HIV prevention information and HIV prevention motivation stimulate the application of HIV prevention behavioral skills to effect HIV preventive behavior. It also is clear that there often is a direct link between HIV prevention motivation and HIV preventive behavior, in accord with the model's supposition that motivation may directly influence the practice of preventive behaviors that are not complicated or novel. In addition, it is evident that the IMB model's constructs generally account for a very substantial proportion of the variance in HIV preventive behavior. Potential criticisms of the IMB model also are suggested in Table 2. For example, information appears to be a somewhat unstable contributor to the prediction of HIV preventive behavior, and HIV prevention information and HIV prevention motivation seem occasionally to be correlated constructs.

Table 2. Tests of the IMB Model: Summary of Relevant Findings

Sample	Information—motivation	Information—behavioral skills	Motivation—behavioral skills	Behavioral skills—behavior	Information—behavior	Motivation—behavior	Percent variance
Heterosexual university males and females (Fisher et al.[88])		✓	✓	✓			10%
Homosexual adult males (Fisher et al.[88])		✓	✓	✓		✓	35%
Urban minority high school males (Fisher et al.[209])			✓	✓		✓	75%
Urban minority high school females (Fisher et al.[209])		✓	✓	✓			46%
Netherland adult homosexual males (deVroom et al.[207])	✓	✓	✓	✓	✓	✓	26%
Low-income African-American females (Anderson et al.[206])	✓	✓	✓	✓		✓	36%
Low-income white females (Anderson et al.[206])	✓		✓	✓		✓	57%
Urban minority high school males and females (Bryan et al.[208])		✓	✓	✓		✓	75%

With respect to HIV risk reduction behavior change, IMB model-based experimental intervention research has demonstrated the utility of this approach and has produced sustained and significant changes in HIV prevention information, motivation, behavioral skills, and behavior. In research reported by Fisher et al.,[176] samples of heterosexual university students participated in elicitation studies to identify deficits in their HIV prevention information, motivation, and behavioral skills and to determine their most significant HIV risk behaviors. Based on elicitation findings, an IMB model-based, empirically targeted HIV risk reduction intervention was designed to address HIV prevention information gaps, motivational obstacles, and behavioral skills deficits related to this population's primary HIV risk behaviors. The intervention comprised a field experiment in which paired male and female dormitory floors received an IMB model-based intervention consisting of information, motivation, and behavioral skills-focused slide shows, videos, group discussions, and role-plays delivered by a health educator and peer educators, or they were assigned to a control condition. Evaluation research showed that the intervention had significant effects on multiple measures of HIV prevention information, motivation, and behavioral skills at 4 weeks postintervention and significant effects on discussing condom use with sexual partners, keeping condoms accessible, and using condoms during sexual intercourse at this time. Results of a follow-up assessment conducted later indicated that the intervention had significant and sustained effects on condom accessibility and condom use and on HIV antibody testing, 2 to 4 months after the end of the intervention.

In a related experimental intervention, Carey et al.[210] used the IMB model to guide HIV risk reduction elicitation, intervention, and evaluation research in a sample of primarily African-American, economically disadvantaged, urban women. The IMB model-based intervention focused on education concerning HIV transmission and prevention, on increasing motivation to practice HIV preventive behavior, and on the development of HIV prevention behavioral skills and was delivered in the context of four, 90-minute intervention sessions. Evaluation research indicated that the intervention had a significant impact on HIV risk reduction information, motivation, and behavioral skills and on HIV risk behavior, such that participants were significantly less likely than controls to engage in unprotected vaginal intercourse at a 3-week follow-up. The mean effect size for the behavioral outcome measures at this time was reported to be a robust .94, and most effects of the intervention persisted at a 12-week follow-up assessment. In addition, in a study described earlier in the SCT section of this chapter, St. Lawrence et al.[139] found strong experimental support of the intervention efficacy of that model and the IMB model with minority adolescents. In a further HIV risk reduction application of the IMB model, Weinhardt et al.[211] conducted an uncontrolled pilot investigation of an IMB model-based intervention for seriously mentally ill men and women. Results of this pilot study indicated that this approach to HIV risk reduction among chronically mentally ill individuals resulted in pre- to postintervention increases in HIV prevention information and trends toward enhanced prevention behavioral skills and preventive behavior. These findings are consistent with the IMB model and the investigators suggest that IMB model-based risk reduction research with larger, controlled samples has promise for the amelioration of the high levels of HIV risk behavior seen among chronically mentally ill individuals.

Conclusions/Critique

The IMB model provides a comprehensive conceptual approach to understanding the determinants of HIV preventive behavior and a generalizable methodology for intervening to promote such behavior. The IMB model's assumptions concerning the determinants of HIV preventive behavior have been consistently confirmed in multivariate correlational research conducted across a diversity of populations at risk, ranging from university students to gay men to inner-city minority women,[88,206,209] and the model's constructs account for a substantial proportion of the variance in HIV preventive behavior. The IMB model's approach to HIV risk reduction behavior change has been similarly supported in elicitation, experimental intervention, and evaluation research conducted with university students, minority adolescents, and inner-city minority women[139,176,210] and in pilot research with chronically mentally ill individuals.[211] Results of this research are consistent with the IMB model's focus on identifying and addressing deficits in HIV prevention information, motivation, and behavioral skills as an effective means for promoting HIV preventive behavior. Effects of IMB model-based interventions on risk reduction behavior change have been significant and sustained.[176,210]

Empirical tests of the IMB model also have suggested criticisms of the IMB approach to understanding and promoting HIV preventive behavior that need to be addressed in future conceptual and empirical work. First, given the relatively recent provenance of the IMB model, first published in 1992, it is not surprising that some areas of IMB model-based research are somewhat sparse. Prospective studies of the determinants of HIV preventive behavior[208] are far fewer in number than cross-sectional studies,[88] and experimental intervention research, while consistently confirmatory and dealing with very diverse populations,[176,210] remains limited. Moreover, much IMB-based research is still in the process of being submitted for publication and is not yet widely available, although this too should be seen in light of the recency of this model.

Second, on a conceptual level, this review raises questions about the role of the IMB model's information construct, which across studies appears to be a relatively inconsistent contributor to the prediction of preventive behavior. Although the IMB model has specified situations in which information is expected to be a substantial contributor to HIV preventive behavior (e.g., early in epidemics) and when it will not (e.g., later on in epidemics[7,212]), further conceptualization of the role of information in stimulating the development and application of behavioral skills and as a direct determinant of HIV preventive behavior appears necessary. This review also raises questions concerning the relationship of the information and motivation constructs, which are sometimes independent and sometimes not. The model's logic, which holds that well-informed people are not necessarily well-motivated to practice prevention and vice versa,[7] would appear to permit at least the possibility of a relationship between informational and motivational factors. Other questions remaining for future conceptual and empirical consideration involve specification of when, in terms of populations at risk and preventive behaviors of interest, specific model constructs may prove to be most important.

COMPARISON AND CRITIQUE OF THE MODELS DISCUSSED

The conceptual models of HIV preventive behavior that have been discussed vary considerably in terms of comprehensiveness, specification, parsimony, empirical support, ease of translation into risk reduction interventions, and a number of other significant characteristics.

With respect to comprehensiveness, several of the models reviewed—the HBM, the TRA, and to an extent the TPB—focus on a relatively narrow range of primarily motivational factors to conceptualize the determinants of HIV preventive behavior. Other models, such the ARRM, TM, SCT, and IMB, are conceptually broader accounts of a wider range of factors that may ultimately prove necessary for understanding and changing HIV preventive behavior.

With respect to specification, some models, such as the HBM, the ARRM, the TM and SCT, are not specified in terms of clear statements of the relationships that are proposed among the hypothesized determinants of HIV preventive behavior. Other models, such as the TRA, TPB, and IMB, completely specify all relationships among constructs proposed, although these specifications are sometimes subject to question and revision on the basis of the findings examined. Degree of specification of a model, however, places fundamental limits on the precision of model testing research, on the ability to conduct multivariate tests of models, and on the ability to apply models to understanding, predicting, and changing HIV preventive behavior.

With respect to parsimony, some of the models discussed, including the ARRM and TM, posit such a multiplicity of constructs and processes that on rational grounds alone they appear to be less than parsimonious explanations of HIV preventive behavior. Adding to the difficulty of assessing model parsimony, we find that some of the models discussed (TRA, TPB, IMB) have been subjected to multivariate testing and some (HBM, ARRM, TM, SCT) have not and probably cannot be at their current state of specification. The lack of multivariate research is a fundamental conceptual and empirical problem at this point in the development of models of HIV preventive behavior. Lacking multivariate testing, we have no information on the unique contributions of the individual constructs of these models to prediction of HIV risk behavior. In such cases, discussion of model constructs "as if" unique links between such constructs and preventive behavior have been demonstrated is inappropriate. Adding still more to the problem of assessing model parsimony, there is considerable overlap of constructs across models, with multiple models claiming information, attitudes, social norms, self-efficacy, perceived vulnerability, and other constructs. Thus, we often do not know whether a particular factor makes a unique contribution to the determination of HIV preventive behavior (lack of multivariate testing), and we often do not know within which model the particular construct might uniquely fit, conceptually and empirically speaking. Only a very small subset of the models discussed herein begin to identify a discrete and parsimonious set of necessary and sufficient constructs as an account of the determinants of HIV risk reduction behavior change.

With respect to empirical support, the models reviewed are uneven. The HBM cannot be tested as an integrated multivariate model, and individual postulated relationships within the HBM have received mixed support. The ARRM remains mostly untested, although particular univariate relationships posited by the model have received support. While a fair amount of support is available for individual relationships proposed by the TM, important individual relationships asserted by this theory have not been tested, and it cannot be examined as an integrated multivariate whole at its present state of development. The SCT also is untested as an integrated multivariate model, although considerable support for particular univariate relationships has been reported, and again it may not be testable as an integrated multivariate model at its present state of development. In contrast with these models, the TRA, TPB, and IMB models have been thoroughly tested as integrated multivariate models. Each has achieved a considerable degree of support and each explains considerable variance in HIV preventive behaviors across populations of at risk.

With respect to empirical support for the behavior change implications of the models collected in the context of intervention research, it is important to note that such research is much more often inspired by a model than devoted to direct tests of the behavior change implications of the model. Intervention research rarely directly examines changes in a model's hypothesized determinants of HIV risk behavior in relation to HIV risk behavior change to fully test behavior change implications of a given model. Nonetheless, it is clearly the case that interventions inspired by the SCT, TRA, TPB, and IMB models have created sustained changes in critical HIV preventive behaviors, and intervention research evidence has also directly confirmed a number of the behavior change implications of the models. The TM has primarily received support in the context of changing individuals' HIV risk reduction stages of change, rather than behavior change per se. Nevertheless, taken together, there is considerable support for the power of theory to guide successful individual-level HIV risk behavior change interventions, although much more work in this area is still needed.

With respect to translation of the models into HIV risk reduction interventions, no single model readily translates into a comprehensive intervention, although elements of each contain valuable suggestions for constructing components of a comprehensive intervention, and different models generate suggestions for interventions in different ways. For example, the ARRM and TM suggest targeting interventions to stages of change and discuss processes that are thought to be particularly important at each stage of change. The TRA, TPB, and the IMB models specify elicitation research procedures that can readily be applied to create a conceptually based and empirically identified roster of targets for focused intervention attempts. Also in relation to translating the models into behavior change interventions, it is important to note that most of the models are actually better at providing a roster of objectives for change (e.g., change attitudes, norms, perceived behavioral control, behavioral skills) than they are at directly informing intervenors about specific strategies for achieving change in postulated determinants of HIV risk behavior and in HIV risk behavior per se.

Another conceptual point emerging from this review is the fact that some of the models discussed are actually models of the determinants of stages of behavior change (e.g., ARRM, TM) and some of them are simply models of the determinants of behavior in general (e.g., TRA, TPB, and in some respects the IMB model). The latter are applied to the issue of risk reduction behavior change under the assumption that changing the proposed determinants of behavior will be an effective means of changing behavior. Whether the models that focus on stages of behavior change or on behavior in general prove to be superior remains to be seen. At present, there is less intervention outcome research supportive of the intervention efficacy of the "stage models" than of the "determinants of behavior" models as far as overt behavior change is concerned.

Another conceptual issue that must be raised involves the fact that while HIV preventive behavior is a heavily dyadic activity, the models discussed in this chapter are not dyadic. It is clear that each of the models must be articulated to accommodate the fact that HIV preventive behavior is often dyadic activity. Specification of how factors posited by models to be crucial to HIV prevention function within the dyadic context is a critical conceptual and empirical challenge for future research. Considerations of the contribution of sex differences and power differentials to the unilateral or dyadic determination of HIV risk reduction behavior change should be a special focus within this approach. In addition, each of the models discussed assume that individuals behave rationally and that certain theoretically relevant elements affect their behavior. They also assume that individuals are free to choose a rational course of action and that they have the necessary resources (e.g., money to purchase condoms, or to obtain clean needles). Especially with certain populations, these assumptions are open to question.

A final point to be raised is that competitive tests of each of the HIV prevention conceptualizations discussed in this chapter remain fundamentally important objectives for research in this field. Such competitive tests should be based on multiple empirical and conceptual criteria, including competitive tests of predictive power, parsimony, and ease of translation into effective intervention strategy and content.

ACKNOWLEDGMENTS. Work on this chapter was supported in part by NIMH grant MG54378 and by a Health Canada Research Scientist Award.

REFERENCES

1. Gluck M, Rosenthal E. *OTA Report: The Effectiveness of AIDS Prevention Efforts*. Washington, DC: American Psychological Association; 1995.
2. Kelly JA, Murphy DA, Sikkema KL, et al. Psychological interventions to prevent HIV infection are urgently needed: New priorities for behavioral research in the second decade of AIDS. *Am Psychol* 1993; 48:1023–1034.
3. Holtgrave DR, Qualls NL, Curran JW, et al. An overview of the effectiveness and efficiency of HIV prevention programs. *Public Health Rep* 1995; 110:134–146.
4. Kirby D, DiClemente RJ. School-based interventions to prevent unprotected sex and HIV among adolescents. In: DiClemente RJ, Peterson JL, eds. *Preventing AIDS: Theories and Methods of Behavioral Interventions*. New York: Plenum Press; 1994:117–139.
5. Brunswick AF, Banaszak-Holl J. HIV risk behavior and the health belief model: An empirical test in an African American community sample. *J Community Psychol* 1996; 24:44–65.
6. Exner TM, Seal DW, Ehrhardt AA. A review of HIV interventions for at-risk women. *AIDS Behav* 1997; 1:93–124.
7. Fisher JD, Fisher WA. Changing AIDS risk behavior. *Psychol Bull* 1992; 111:455–474.
8. Helweg-Larsen M, Collins BE. A social psychological perspective on the role of knowledge about AIDS in AIDS prevention. *Curr Dir Psychol Sci* 1997; 6:23–53.
9. US Department of Health and Human Services, Public Health Service, Centers for Disease Control Prevention. *Planning and Evaluating HIV/AIDS Prevention Programs in State and Local Health Departments: A Companion to Program Announcement 300*. Atlanta, GA: Centers for Disease Control: 1993.
10. Health Canada. *Canadian Guidelines for Sexual Health Education*. Ottawa: Health Canada; 1994.
11. Coates TJ. Strategies for modifying sexual behavior patterns for primary and secondary prevention of HIV disease. *J Consult Clin Psychol* 1990; 58:57–69.
12. Rosenstock IM, Stretcher VJ, Becker MH. The health belief model and HIV risk behavior change. In: DiClemente RJ, Peterson JL, eds. *Preventing AIDS: Theories and Methods of Behavioral Interventions*. New York: Plenum Press; 1994:5–25.
13. Catania JA, Gibson DR, Chitwood DD, et al. Methodological problems in AIDS behavioral research: Influences on measurement error and participation bias in studies of sexual behavior. *Psychol Bull* 1990; 108:339–362.
14. Fishbein M, Middlestadt SE, Hitchcock PJ. Using information to change sexually transmitted disease-related behaviors. In: DiClemente RJ, Peterson JL, eds. *Preventing AIDS: Theories and Methods of Behavioral Interventions*. New York: Plenum Press; 1994:61–78.
15. Bandura A. Social cognitive theory and exercise control of HIV infection. In: DiClemente RJ, Peterson JL, eds. *Preventing AIDS: Theories and Methods of Behavioral Interventions*. New York: Plenum Press; 1994:25–59.
16. Prochaska JO, Redding CA, Harlow LL, et al. The transtheoretical model of change and HIV prevention: A review. *Health Educ Q* 1994; 21:471–486.
17. deWit JBF. The epidemic of HIV among young homosexual men. *AIDS* 1996; 10:(suppl 3):s21–25.
18. Fisher WA, Fisher JD. A general social psychological model for changing AIDS risk behavior. In: Pryor J, Reeder G, eds. *The Social Psychology of HIV Infection*. Hillsdale, NJ: Erlbaum; 1993:127–153.
19. Wingood GM, DiClemente RJ. HIV sexual risk reduction interventions for women: A review. *Am J Prev Med* 1996; 12:(3):209–217.
20. Ajzen I, Fishbein M. *Understanding Attitudes and Predicting Social Behavior*. Englewood Cliffs, NJ: Prentice Hall; 1980.
21. Fishbein M, Ajzen I. *Belief, Attitude, Intention and Behavior: An Introduction to Theory and Research*. Reading, MA: Addison-Wesley; 1975.
22. Kelly JA. *Changing HIV Risk Behavior: Practical Strategies*. New York: Guilford Press; 1995.
23. Johnson RW, Ostrow DG, Joseph J. Educational strategies for prevention of sexual transmission of HIV. In: Ostrow DG, ed. *Behavioral Aspects of AIDS*. New York: Plenum Press; 1990:43–73.
24. Leviton LC, Valdiserri RO. Evaluating AIDS prevention: Outcome, implementation, and mediating variables. *Eval Prog Plan* 1990; 13:55–66.
25. Oakley A, Fullerton D, Holland J. Behavioral interventions for HIV/AIDS prevention. *AIDS* 1995; 9:479–486.
26. Wallston BS, Wallston KA. Social psychological models of health behavior: An examination and integration. In: Baum RJ, Taylor, Singer, eds. *Handbook of Psychology and Health*. NJ: Lawrence Erlbaum; 1984:24–53.

27. Hochbaum GM. *Public Participation in Medical Screening Programs: A Sociopsychological Study*. Public Health Service, PHS Publication 572. Washington, DC: US Government Printing Office; 1958.
28. Rosenstock IM. Why people use health services. *Milbank Mem Fund Q* 1996; 44:94–124.
29. Rosenstock IM. Historical origins of the health belief model. *Health Educ Monogr* 1974; 2:328–335.
30. Kirscht JP. The health belief model and illness behavior. *Health Educ Monogr* 1974; 2:387–408.
31. Becker MH. The health belief model and personal health behavior. *Health Educ Monogr* 1974; 2:324–473.
32. Rosenstock IM, Stretcher VJ, Becker MH. Social learning theory and the health belief method. *Health Educ Q* 1988; 13:73–92.
33. Kirscht JP. The health belief model and predictions of health actions. In: Crochman D, ed. *Health Behavior: Emerging Research Perspectives*. New York: Plenum Press; 1988:27–41.
34. Montgomery S, Joseph J, Becker M, et al. The health belief model in understanding compliance with preventive recommendations for AIDS: How useful? *AIDS Educ Prevent* 1989; 1:303–323.
35. Petosa R, Wessinger J. Using the health belief model to assess the HIV education needs of junior and senior high school students. *Int Q Community Health Educ* 1990; 10:135–143.
36. Basen-Enquist K, Parecel GS. Attitudes, norms and self-efficacy: A model of adolescents' HIV-related sexual risk behavior. *Health Educ Q* 1992; 19:263–277.
37. Fisher JD, Misovich SJ. Social influence and AIDS-preventive behavior. In: Edwards J, Tindale RS, Health L, Posavac EJ, eds. *Social Influence Processes and Prevention*. New York: Plenum Press; 1990:39–70.
38. Hingson RW, Strunin L, Berlin BM, et al. Beliefs about AIDS, use of alcohol and drugs, and unprotected sex among Massachusetts adolescents. *Am J Public Health* 1990; 80:295–299.
39. Povinelli M, Remafedi G, Tao G. Trends and predictors of human immunodeficiency virus antibody testing by homosexual and bisexual adolescent males, 1989–1994. *Arch Pediatr Adolesc Med* 1996; 150:33–38.
40. Steers WN, Elliott E, Nemiro J, et al. Health beliefs as predictors of HIV-preventive behavior and ethnic differences in prediction. *J Soc Psychol* 1996; 136:99–110.
41. Yep GA. Health beliefs and HIV prevention: Do they predict monogamy and condom use? *J Soc Behav Pers* 1993; 8:507–520.
42. Baldwin JD, Baldwin JI. Factors effecting AIDS-related sexual risk taking behavior among college students. *J Sex Res* 1988; 25:181–196.
43. Brown LK, DiClemente RJ, Park T. Predictors of condom use among sexually active adolescents. *J Adolesc Health* 1992; 13:651–657.
44. Catania JA, Dolcini MM, Coates TJ, et al. Predictors of condom use and multiple partnered sex among sexually active adolescent women: Implications for AIDS related health interventions. *J Sex Res* 1989; 26:514–524.
45. Catania JA, Coates TJ, Kegeles SM, et al. Condom use in multi-ethnic neighborhoods of San Francisco: The population based AMEN (AIDS in multi-ethnic neighborhoods) study. *Am J Public Health* 1992; 182:284–287.
46. DiClemente RJ, Durbin M, Siegel D, et al. Determinants of condom use among junior high school students in a minority, inner city, school district. *Pediatrics* 1992; 89:197–202.
47. Joseph JG, Montgomery SB, Emmons C, et al. Magnitude and determinants of behavioral risk reduction: Longitudinal analysis of a cohort at risk for AIDS. *Psychol Health* 1987; 1:73–96.
48. McKusick L, Coates T, Morin S, et al. Longitudinal predictors of reductions in unprotected anal intercourse among gay men in San Francisco: The AIDS behavioral research project. *Am J Public Health* 1990; 80:978–983.
49. Walter H, Vaughan R, Gladis M, et al. Factors associated with AIDS risk behaviors among high school students in an AIDS epicenter. *Am J Public Health* 1993; 82:528–532.
50. Weisman CS, Nathanson CA, Ensminger M, et al. AIDS knowledge, perceived risk and prevention among adolescent clients of a family planning clinic. *Fam Plann Perspect* 1989; 21:213–217.
51. Wilson DJ, Lavelle S, Hood R. Health knowledge and beliefs as predictors of intended condom use among Zimbabwean adolescents in probation/remand homes. *AIDS Care* 1990; 2:267–274.
52. Zielony RD, Wills TA. *Psychosocial predictors of AIDS risk behavior in methadone patients*. Unpublished manuscript, Ferkauf Graduate School of Psychology and Albert Einstein College of Medicine, New York. Forthcoming.
53. Gerrard M, Gibbons FX, Bushman BJ. Relation between perceived vulnerability to HIV and precautionary sexual behavior. *Psychol Bull* 1996; 119:390–409.
54. Flowers P, Sheeran P, Beail N, et al. The role of psychosocial factors in HIV risk reduction among gay and bisexual men: A quantitative review. *Psychol Health* 1997; 12:(2):197–230.
55. Yep GA. HIV prevention among Asian-American college students: Does the health belief model work? *J Am Coll Health* 1993; 14:199–205.
56. Rimberg HM, Lewis RJ. Older adolescents and AIDS: Correlates of self-reported safer sex practices. *J Res Adolesc* 1994; 4:453–464.

57. Abraham C, Sheeran P, Spears R, et al. Health beliefs and promotion of HIV-preventive intentions among teenagers: A Scottish perspective. *Health Psychol* 1992; 11:(6):363–370.

58. Des Jarlais DC, Abdul-Quader A, Tross S. The next problem: Maintenance of AIDS risk reduction among intravenous users. *Int J Addict* 1991; 26:1279–1292.

59. Edem CU, Harvey SM. Use of health belief model to predict condom use among university students in Nigeria. *Int Q Community Health Educ* 1994; 15:3–14.

60. Kegeles SM, Adler NE, Irwin CE, Jr. Adolescents and condoms. *Am J Dis Child* 1989; 143:911–915.

61. Orr DP, Langefeld CD, Katz PB, et al. Factors associated with condom use among sexually active female adolescents. *J Pediatr* 1992; 120:311–317.

62. Yep GA. HIV/AIDS in Asian and Pacific Islander communities in the US: A review, analysis and integration. *Int Q Community Health Educ* 1993; 13:293–315.

63. Janz N, Becker M. The health belief model: A decade later. *Health Educ Q* 1984; 11:1–47.

64. Fisher WA, Fisher JD. Understanding and promoting AIDS preventive behavior: A conceptual model and educational tool. *Can J Hum Sex* 1992; 1:99–106.

65. McKusick L, Wiley JA, Coates TJ, et al. Reported changes in the sexual behavior of men at risk for AIDS. San Francisco, 1982–1984. *Public Health Rep* 1985; 100:622–628.

66. Bryan AD, Aiken LS, West SG. Increasing condom use: Evaluation of a theory-based intervention to prevent sexually transmitted diseases in young women. *Health Psychol* 1996; 15:371–382.

67. Joffe A, Radius SM. Self-efficacy and intent to use condoms among entering college freshmen. *J Adolesc Health* 1993; 14:262–268.

68. Kalichman S, Carey M, Johnson BT. Prevention of sexually transmitted HIV infection: A meta-analytic review of the behavioral outcome literature. *Ann Behav Med* 1996; 18:6–15.

69. McKusick L, Coates T, Wiley JA, et al. *Prevention of HIV Infection among Gay and Bisexual Men: Two Longitudinal Studies.* Paper presented at the III International Conference on AIDS, Washington, DC; 1987.

70. Weisman CS, Plichta S, Nathanson CA, et al. Consistency of condom use for disease prevention among adolescent users of oral contraceptives. *Fam Plann Perspect* 1991; 23:71–75.

71. Arnold L, Quine L. Predicting helmet use among schoolboy cyclists: An application of the health belief model. In: Rutter DR, Quine L, eds. *Social Psychology and Health: European Perspectives.* Aldershot, England UK: Avebury/Ashgate Publishing; 1994:101–130.

72. Cummings K, Jette A, Brock B, et al. Psychosocial determinants of immunization behavior in a swine influenza campaign. *Med Care* 1979; 17:639–649.

73. Haefner D, Kirscht J. Motivational and behavioral effects on modifying health beliefs. *Public Health Rep* 1970; 85:478–484.

74. Montano DE. Predicting and understanding influenza vaccination behavior. *Med Care* 1986; 24:438–453.

75. Pirie P, Elias W, Wackman D, et al. Characteristics of participants and nonparticipants in a community cardiovascular risk factor screening: The Minnesota Heart Health Program. *Am J Prev Med* 1986; 2:20–25.

76. Seydel E, Taal E, Wiegman O. Risk-appraisal, outcome and self-efficacy expectancies: Cognitive factors in preventive behaviour related to cancer. *Psychol Health* 1990; 4:99–109.

77. Rosenstock IM. The health belief model: Explaining health behavior through expectancies. In: Glanz K, Lewis FM, Rimer BK, eds. *Health Behavior and Health Education.* San Francisco: Jossey-Bass; 1990:39–62.

78. Sorensen JL. Preventing HIV transmission in drug treatment programs: What works? In: Stimmel B, Friedman JR, Lipton DS, eds. *Cocaine, AIDS, and Intravenous Drug Use.* Binghamton, NY: Harrington Park Press; 1991:67–79.

79. Rose MA. Effect of an AIDS education program for older adults. *J Commun Health Nurs* 1996; 13:141–148.

80. Ford K, Wirawan DN, Fajans P, et al. Behavioral interventions for reduction of sexually transmitted disease/HIV transmission among female commercial sex workers and clients in Bali, Indonesia. *AIDS* 1996; 10:213–222.

81. Harrison JA, Mullen PD, Green LW. A meta-analysis of studies of the health belief model with adults. *Health Educ Res* 1992; 7:107–116.

82. Montano DE. *Compliance with health care recommendations: A reassessment of the health belief model.* Unpublished doctoral dissertation. University of Washington, Seattle; 1983.

83. Kirscht JP, Joseph JG. The health belief model: Some implications for behavior change, with reference to homosexual males. In: Mays VM, Albee GW, Schneider SF, eds. *Primary Prevention of AIDS.* Newbury Park, CA: Sage; 1989:111–127.

84. Catania JA, Kegeles SM, Coates TJ. Towards an understanding of risk behavior: An AIDS risk reduction model (ARRM). *Health Educ Q* 1990; 17:53–72.

85. Prochaska JO, Velicer WF. The transtheoretical model of health behavior change. *Am J Health Prom* 1997; 12:38–48.

86. Fisher JD. Possible effects of reference group-based social influence on AIDS-risk behavior and AIDS-intervention. [Special issue on *AIDS*] *Am Psychol* 1988; 43:914–920.
87. Bryan AD, Aiken LS, West SG. Young women's condom use: The influence of responsibility for sexuality, control over the sexual encounter and perceived susceptibility to common STDs. *Health Psychol* 1997; 16:468–479.
88. Fisher JD, Fisher WA, Williams SS, et al. Empirical tests of an information–motivation–behavioral skills model of AIDS-preventive behavior with gay men and heterosexual university students. *Health Psychol* 1994; 13: 238–250.
89. O'Leary A, Goodhart F, Jemmott LS, et al. Predictors of safer sex on the college campus: A social cognitive theory analysis. *J Am Coll Health* 1992; 40:254–263.
90. Fisher JD, Nadler A, Whitcher-Alagna S. Recipient reactions to aid. *Psychol Bull* 1982; 91:27–54.
91. Nadler A. Personal characteristics of help seeking. In: DePaulo B, Nadler A, Fisher J, eds. *New Directions in Helping: Help Seeking*. New York: Academic Press; 1983:303–336.
92. Misovich SJ, Fisher JD, Fisher WA. Close relationships and HIV risk behavior: Evidence and possible underlying psychological processes. *Gen Psychol Rev* 1997; 1:72–107.
93. Bertrand JT, Brown LF, Kinzoni M, et al. AIDS knowledge in three sites in Bas-Zaire. *AIDS Educ Prevent* 1992; 4:251–266.
94. Ireland SJ, Malow RM, Alberga L, et al. *A Test of the AIDS Risk Reduction Model with Indigent, Cocaine Abusing Women*. Paper presented at the 56th Annual Scientific Meeting of the College on Problems of Drug Dependence, Palm Beach, FL, June 18–23, 1994.
95. Catania J, Coates TJ, Kegeles S. A test of the AIDS risk reduction model: Psychosocial correlates of condom use in the AMEN cohort survey. *Health Psychol* 1994; 13:548–555.
96. Kowalewski MR, Longshore D, Anglin MD. The AIDS risk reduction model: Examining intentions to use condoms among injection drug users. *J Appl Soc Psychol* 1994; 24:2002–2027.
97. Longshore D, Anglin MD. Intentions to share injection paraphernalia: An empirical test of the AIDS risk reduction model among injection drug users. *Int J Addict* 1995; 30:305–321.
98. Adib SM, Joseph JG, Ostrow DG, et al. Predictors of relapse in sexual practices among homosexual men. *AIDS Educ Prevent* 1991; 3:293–304.
99. Hays R, Kegeles S, Coates T. High HIV risk-taking among young gay men. *AIDS* 190; 4:901–907.
100. Malow RM, West JA, Corrigan SA, et al. Outcome of psychoeducation for HIV risk reduction. *AIDS Educ Prevent* 1994; 6:113–125.
101. Kline A, Vanlandingham M. HIV-infected women and sexual risk reduction: The relevance of existing models of behavior change. *AIDS Educ Prevent* 1994; 6:390–402.
102. Fisher JD, Kimble DL, Misovich SJ, et al. Dynamic of sexual risk behavior in HIV-infected men who have sex with men. *AIDS Behav* 1998; 2:101–113.
103. Offir JT, Fisher JD, Williams SS, et al. Reasons for inconsistent AIDS preventive behaviors among gay men. *J Sex Res* 1993; 30:62–69.
104. Malow RM, Corrigan SA, Cunningham SC, et al. Psychosocial factors associated with condom use among African-American drug abusers in treatment. *AIDS Educ Prevent* 1993; 5:244–253.
105. Catania JA, Coates TJ, Kegeles SM, et al. Implications of the AIDS risk reduction model for the gay community: The importance of perceived sexual enjoyment and help-seeking behaviors. In: Mays VM, Albee GW, Schneider SF, eds. *Primary Prevention of AIDS*. Newbury Park, CA: Sage; 1989:242–261.
106. Connell RW, Crawford J, Kippax S, et al. Facing the epidemic: Changes in the sexual lives of gay and bisexual men in Australia and their implications for AIDS prevention strategies. *Soc Prob* 1989; 36:384–402.
107. Gibson DR, Sorensen JL, Lovelle-Drache J, et al. *Psychosocial Predictors of AIDS: High Risk Behaviors among Intravenous Drug Users*. Paper presented at the Fourth International Conference on AIDS, Stockholm; 1988.
108. Fishbein M, Trafimow D, Middlestadt SE, et al. Using an AIDS KAPB survey to identify determinants of condom use among sexually active adults from St. Vincent and the Grenadines. *J Appl Soc Psychol* 1995; 25:1–20.
109. Peterson JL, Coates TJ, Catania J, et al. Evaluation of an HIV risk reduction intervention among African-American homosexual and bisexual men. *AIDS* 1996; 10:319–325.
110. Boyer CB, Kegeles SM. AIDS risk and prevention among adolescents. *Soc Sci Med* 1991; 33:11–23.
111. Breakwell GM, Millward LJ, Fife-Schaw C. Commitment to "safer" sex as a predictor of condom use among 16–20 year olds. *J Appl Soc Psychol* 1994; 24:189–217.
112. Prochaska JO, DiClemente CC. Toward a comprehensive model of change. In: Miller WR, Heather N, eds. *Treating Addictive Behaviors: Processes of Change*. New York: Plenum Press; 1986:3–27.
113. Prochaska JO, DiClemente CC, Norcross JC. In search of how people change: Application to addictive behaviors. *Am Psychol* 1992; 47:1102–1114.
114. Grimley DM, Riley GE, Prochaska JO, et al. *The Application of the Transtheoretical Model to Contraceptive*

and Condom Use in High Risk Women. Technical Report to the Centers for Disease Control and Prevention (contract grant CSA-92-109). Kingston, RI: Cancer Prevention Research Center; 1992.

115. Redding CA, Rossi JS. The processes of safer sex adoption. *Ann Behav Med* 1993; 15:S106. Abstract.

116. Prochaska JO, Velicer WF, Rossi JS, et al. Stages of change and decisional balance for 12 problem behaviors. *Health Psychol* 1994; 13:39–46.

117. Galavotti C, Cabral RJ, Lansky A, et al. Validation of measures of condom and other contraceptive use among women at high risk for HIV or unintended pregnancy. *Health Psychol* 1995; 14:570–578.

118. Prochaska JO. Strong and weak principles for progressing from precontemplation to action on the basis of twelve problem behaviors. *Health Psychol* 1994; 13:47–51.

119. Ockene J, Ockene I, Kristellar J. *The Coronary Artery Smoking Intervention Study.* Worcester, MA: National Heart Lung Blood Institute; 1988.

120. Prochaska JO, DiClemente CC. Stages of change in the modification of problem behaviors. In: Herson M, Eisler R, Miller PM, eds. *Progress in Behavior Modification.* Sycamore, IL: Sycamore Publishing; 1992:183–218.

121. Grimley DM, Prochaska GE, Prochaska JO. Condom use assertiveness and the stages of change with main and other partners. *J Appl Biobehav Res* 1993; 1:152–173.

122. Grimley DM, Riley GE, Bellis JM, et al. Assessing the stages of change and decision making for contraceptive use for the prevention for pregnancies, STDs and AIDS. *Health Educ Q* 1993; 20:455–470.

123. Harlow LL, Prochaska JO, Redding CA, et al. Stages of condom use in a high HIV-risk sample. *Psychol Health* 1997;1–15.

124. Prochaska JO, Harlow LL, Redding CA, et al. *Stages of Change, Self-Efficacy, and Decisional Balance for Condom Use with a High Risk Sample.* Contract Grant 0-415-486. Atlanta, GA: Centers for Disease Control and Prevention; 1990.

125. Rhodes F, Malotte CK. Using stages of change to assess intervention readiness and outcome in modifying drug-related and sexual HIV risk behaviors of IDUs and crack users. *Drugs Soc* 1996; 9:(1–2):109–136.

126. Grimley DM, Prochaska GE, Prochaska JO. Condom use adoption and continuation: A transtheoretical approach. *Health Educ Res* 1997; 12:61–75.

127. Bowen AM, Trotter R. HIV risk in intravenous drug users and crack cocaine smokers: Predicting stages of change for condom use. *J Consult Clin Psychol* 1995; 63:238–248.

128. Evers KE, Harlow LL, Redding CA, et al. Longitudinal changes in stages of change for condom use in women. *Am J Health Prom* 1998; 13:(1):19–25.

129. Evers KE, Harlow LL. *Predictors of Stage of Condom Use in Women Over a One Year Period.* Washington, DC: Fourth International Congress of Behavioral Medicine (Poster); 1996.

130. Galavotti C, Grimley DM, Cabral RJ. *Condom Acceptability among Women at High Risk for HIV Infection.* Society of Behavioral Medicine, Boston, MA: CDC Perinatal HIV Prevention and Education Demonstration Activities and the CDC Prevention of HIV in Women and Infants Demonstration Projects; 1994.

131. Grimley DM, Prochaska JO, Velicer WF, et al. Contraceptive and condom use adoption and maintenance: A stage paradigm approach. *Health Educ Q* 1995; 22:20–35.

132. Redding CA, Rossi JS. Testing a model of situational self efficacy for safer sex among college students: Stage of change and gender-based differences. *Psychol Health* 1998; 00:1–20.

133. Anonymous. Community-level prevention of human immunodeficiency virus infection among high-risk populations: The AIDS Community Demonstration Projects. *Morb Mortal Wkly Rep* 1996; 45:(RR-6):1–16.

134. Jamner MS, Wolitski RJ, Corby NH. Impact of a longitudinal community HIV intervention targeting injecting drug users' stage of change for condom and bleach use. *Am J Health Prom* 1997; 12:15–24.

135. Cabral RJ, Galavotti C, Gargiullo PM, et al. Paraprofessional delivery of a theory-based HIV prevention counseling intervention for women. *Public Health Rep* 1996; 3:75–82.

136. Bandura A. *Self-Efficacy: The Exercise of Control.* New York: W. H. Freeman and Company; 1997.

137. Bandura A. Perceived self-efficacy in the exercise of control over AIDS infection. In: Mays VM, Albee GW, Schneider SM, eds. *Primary Prevention of AIDS.* Newbury Park, CA: Sage; 1989:128–141.

138. Bandura A. A social cognitive approach to the exercise of control of AIDS infection. In: DiClemente RJ, ed. *Adolescents and AIDS: A Generation in Jeopardy.* Newbury Park, CA: Sage; 1992:89–116.

139. St. Lawrence JS, Brasfield TL, Jefferson KW, et al. Cognitive–behavioral intervention to reduce African American adolescents' risk for HIV infection. *J Consult Clin Psychol* 1995; 63:221–237.

140. Jemmot JBI. Social psychological influences on HIV risk behavior among African-American youth. In: *Understanding and Preventing HIV Risk Behavior: Safer Sex and Drug Use.* Thousand Oaks, CA: Sage; 1996:131–156.

141. DiClemente RJ, Lodico M, Grinstead OA, et al. African-American adolescents residing in high-risk urban environments do use condoms: Correlates and predictors of condom use among adolescents in public housing developments. *Pediatrics* 1996; 98:269–278.

142. Sieving R, Resnick MD, Bearinger L, et al. Cognitive and behavioral predictors of sexually transmitted disease risk behavior among sexually active adolescents. *Arch Pediatr Adolesc Med* 1997; 151:243–251.

143. Wulfert E, Wan CK. Condom use: A self-efficacy model. *Health Psychol* 1993; 12:346–353.

144. Fernandez-Esquer ME, Krepcho MA, Freeman AC, et al. Predictors of condom use among African-American males at high risk for HIV. *J Appl Soc Psychol* 1998; 27:58–74.

145. Kalichman SC, Stevenson LY. Psychological and social factors associated with histories of risk for human immunodeficiency virus infection among African-American inner-city women. *J Women Health* 1997; 6:(2):209–217.

146. Kalichman S, Kelly JA, St. Lawrence JS. Factors influencing reduction of sexual risk behaviors for human immunodeficiency virus: A review. *Ann Sex Res* 1996; 3:129–148.

147. Wulfert E, Wan CK, Backus CA. Gay men's safer sex behavior: An integration of three models. *J Behav Med* 1996; 19:345–366.

148. Wulfert E, Safren SA, Brown I, et al. Cognitive, behavioral, and personality correlates of HIV-positive persons' unsafe sexual behavior. *J Appl Soc Psychol* 1999; 29:(2):223–244.

149. Seal A, Minichiello V, Omodei M. Young women's sexual risk taking behavior: Revisiting the influences of sexual self-efficacy and sexual self esteem. *Int J STD AIDS* 1997; 8:159–165.

150. Falck RS, Siegal HA, Wang J, et al. Usefulness of health belief model in predicting HIV needle risk practices among injection drug users. *AIDS Educ Prevent* 1995; 7:523–533.

151. Gibson DR, Choi KH, Ctania JA, et al. Psychological predictors of needle sharing among intravenous drug users. *Int J Addict* 1993; 28:973–981.

152. Kok G, deVries H, Muddle AN, et al. Planned health education and the role of self-efficacy: Dutch research. *Health Educ Res* 1991; 6:231–402.

153. Krepcho MA, Fernandez-Esquer ME, Freeman AC, et al. Predictors of bleach use among current African-American injecting drug users; A community study. *J Psychoactive Drugs* 1993; 26:135–141.

154. Longshore D, Stein JA, Anglin MD. Ethnic differences in the psychosocial antecedents of needle/syringe disinfection. *Drug Alcohol Depend* 1996; 42:183–196.

155. Des Jarlais DC, Friedman SR. The psychology of preventing AIDS among intravenous drug users: A social learning conceptualization. *Am Psychol* 1988; 43:865–870.

156. Latkin C, Mandell W, Vlahov D, et al. Personal network characteristics as antecedents to needle-sharing and shooting gallery attendance. *Soc Net* 1995; 17:219–228.

157. Neaigus A, Friedman SR, Curtis R, et al. The relevance of drug injectors' social and risk network for understanding and preventing HIV infection. *Soc Sci Med* 1994; 38:67–78.

158. Poku KA, Linn JG. Behavioral and psychosocial factors related to HIV-infected individual's knowingly engaging in high risk-behavior. *J Tenn Med Assoc* 1994; 87:97–100.

159. Kalichman S, Rompa D, Coley B. Lack of positive outcomes from a cognitive–behavioral HIV and AIDS prevention intervention for inner-city men: Lessons from a controlled pilot study. *AIDS Educ Prevent* 1997; 9: 299–313.

160. Fishbein M, Middlestadt SE. Using the theory of reasoned action as a framework for understanding and changing AIDS-related behaviors. In: Mays VM, Albee GW, Schneider SF, eds. *Primary Prevention of Psychopathology.* Newbury Park, CA: Sage; 1989:93–110.

161. Terry D, Gallois C, McCamish M. *The Theory of Reasoned Action: Its Application to AIDS-Preventive Behavior.* Oxford, England: Pergamon Press; 1993.

162. Fisher WA. Predicting contraceptive behavior among university men: The roles of emotions and behavioral intentions. *J Appl Soc Psychol* 1984; 14:104–123.

163. Basen-Enquist K. Psychosocial predictors of "safer sex" behaviors in young adults. *AIDS Educ Prevent* 1992; 4:120–134.

164. Fisher WA, Fisher JD, Rye BJ. Understanding and promoting AIDS preventive behavior: Insights from the theory of reasoned action. *Health Psychol* 1995; 14:255–264.

165. Sheppard BH, Hartwick J, Warshaw PR. The theory of reasoned action: A meta-analysis of past research with recommendations for modifications and future research. *Journal of Consumer Research* 1988; 15:325–342.

166. Albarracin D, Johnson BT, Fishbein M, et al. Theories of reasoned action and planned behavior as models of condom use: A meta-analysis. *Psychol Bull* (in press).

167. Rye BJ. *The theory of reasoned action and the theory of planned behavior in relation to university women's safer sex behaviors: A prospective investigation.* Unpublished manuscript. Department of Psychology, University of Western Ontario, London, Ontario. Forthcoming.

168. Doll J, Orth B. The Fishbein and Ajzen theory of reasoned action applied to contraceptive behavior: Model variants and meaningfulness. *J Appl Soc Psychol* 1993; 23:395–415.

169. Fishbein M, Chan DKS, O'Reilly K, et al. Attitudinal and normative factors as determinants of gay men's

intentions to perform AIDS-related sexual behaviors: A multisite analysis. *J Appl Soc Psychol* 1992; 22:999–1011.

170. Jemmott LS, Jemmott JB. Applying the theory of reasoned action to AIDS risk behavior: Condom use among black women. *Nurs Res* 1991; 40:228–234.

171. Kashima Y, Gallois C, McCamish M. The theory of reasoned action and cooperative behavior: It takes two to use a condom. *J Soc Psychol* 1993; 32:227–239.

172. Morrison DM, Gillmore MR, Baker SA. Determinants of condom use among high-risk heterosexual adults: A test of the theory of reasoned action. *J Appl Soc Psychol* 1995; 25:651–676.

173. Boyd B, Wandersman A. Predicting undergraduate condom use with the Fishbein and Ajzen and the Triandis attitude–behavior models: Implications for public health interventions. *J Appl Soc Med* 1991; 21:1810–1830.

174. Centers for Disease Control. *Project Respect Observation and Feedback Guide.* Atlanta, GA: Project Respect Group; 1993.

175. Centers for Disease Control. *Community Demonstration Projects* (CSI data). Atlanta, GA: Community Demonstration Projects; 1996.

176. Fisher JD, Fisher WA, Misovich SJ, et al. Changing AIDS risk behavior: Effects of an intervention emphasizing AIDS risk reduction information, motivation, and behavioral skills in a college student population. *Health Psychol* 1996; 15:114–123.

177. Jemmott JBI, Jemmott LS, Fong GT. Reductions in HIV risk-associated sexual behaviors among Black male adolescents: Effects of an AIDS prevention intervention. *Am J Public Health* 1992; 82:372–377.

178. Jemmott JBI, Jemmott LS, Fong GT, et al. Reducing HIV risk-associated sexual behavior among African American adolescents: Testing the generality of intervention effects. *Am J Community Psychol* 1999; 27:(2): 161–187.

179. Jemmott LS, Jemmott JBI. Increasing condom use intentions among sexually active inner-city black adolescent women: Effects of an AIDS prevention program. *Nurs Res* 1992; 41:273–279.

180. Kazprzyk D, Montano DE, Fishbein M. Application of an integrated behavioral model to change condom use behaviors: A prospective study among high HIV risk groups. *J Appl Soc Psychol* 1998; 28:(17):1557–1583.

181. Gerrard M, Gibbons FX, Warner TD, et al. Perceived vulnerability to HIV infection and AIDS preventive behavior: A critical review of the evidence. In: Pryor JB, Reeder GD, eds. *The Social Psychology of HIV Infection.* Hillsdale, NJ: Lawrence Erlbaum Associates; 1993:59–84.

182. Ajzen I. From intentions to actions: A theory of planned behaviour. In: Kuhl J, Beckman J, eds. *Action Control from Cognition to Behaviour.* New York: Springer-Verlag; 1985:11–39.

183. Ajzen I. The theory of planned behaviour. *Org Behav Hum Dec Proc* 1991; 50:179–211.

184. Ajzen I, Madden TJ. Prediction of goal directed behavior: Attitudes, intentions, and perceived behavioral control. *J Exp Soc Psychol* 1986; 22:453–474.

185. Godin G, Kok G. The theory of planned behavior: A review of its applications to health-related behaviors. *Am J Health Prom* 1996; 11:87–98.

186. Basen-Enquist K. Evaluation of a theory-based HIV prevention intervention for college students. *AIDS Educ Prevent* 1994; 6:412–424.

187. Chan DKS, Fishbein M. Determinants of college women's intentions to tell their partners to use condoms. *J Appl Soc Psychol* 1993; 23:1455–1470.

188. Jemmott JBI, Jemmott LS, Hacker CI. Predicting intentions to use condoms among African-American adolescents: The theory of planned behavior as a model of HIV risk associated behavior. *J Ethnic Dis* 1992; 2:371–380.

189. Madden TJ, Ellen PS, Ajzen I. A comparison of the theory of planned behavior and the theory of reasoned action. *Personality Soc Psychol Bull* 1992; 18:3–9.

190. Netemeyer RG, Burton S, Johnston M. A comparison of two models for the prediction of volitional and goal-directed behaviors: A confirmatory analysis approach. *Soc Psychol Q* 1991; 54:87–100.

191. Fisher JD, Fisher WA. A general technology for AIDS risk behavior change. Grant submitted to the National Institute of Mental Health (1R01 MH46224) 1991; 31–58.

192. US Department of Health and Human Services. *Understanding AIDS.* HHS-88-8404. Rockville, MD: Centers for Disease Control; 1988.

193. Kelly JA, St. Lawrence JS. *The AIDS Health Crisis: Psychological and Social Interventions.* New York: Plenum Press; 1988.

194. Fisher WA. A theory-based framework for intervention and evaluation in STD/HIV prevention. *Can J Hum Sex* 1997; 6:(2):105–111.

195. Fisher WA. Understanding and preventing adolescent pregnancy and sexually transmissible disease/AIDS. In: Edwards J, Tindale RS, Health L, Posavac EJ, eds. *Social Influence Processes and Prevention.* New York: Plenum Press; 1990:71–101.

196. Hammer JC, Fisher JD, Fitzgerald P, et al. When two heads aren't better than one: AIDS risk behavior in college-age couples. *J Appl Soc Psychol* 1996; 26:375–397.

197. Misovich SJ, Fisher JD, Fisher WA. The perceived AIDS-preventive utility of knowing one's partner well: A public health dictum and individual's risky sexual behaviour. *Can J Hum Sex* 1996; 5:83–90.

198. Williams SS, Kimble D, Covell N, et al. College students use implicit personality theory instead of safer sex. *J Appl Soc Psychol* 1992; 22:921–933.

199. Fisher JD, Fisher WA. The information–motivation–behavioral skills model of AIDS risk behavior change: Empirical support and application. In: Oskamp S, Thompson S, eds. *Understanding and Preventing HIV Risk Behavior*. Thousand Oaks, CA: Sage; 1996:100–127.

200. Carey MP, Carey KB, Kalichman SC. Risk for human immunodeficiency virus (HIV) infection among persons with severe mental illnesses. *Clin Psychol Rev* 1997; 17:271–291.

201. Carey MP, Carey KB, Weinhardt LS, et al. Behavioral risk for HIV infection among adults with a severe and persistent mental illness: Patterns and psychological antecedents. *Community Mental Health J* 1997; 33:(2): 133–142.

202. Byrne D, Kelley K, Fisher WA. Unwanted teenage pregnancies: Incidence, interpretation, intervention. *Appl Prevent Psychol* 1993; 2:101–113.

203. *Program Goals. AIDS Prevention Education Services*. Hartford, CT: Connecticut Department of Public Health; 1997.

204. Misovich SJ, Fisher WA, Fisher JD. A measure of AIDS prevention information, motivation and behavioral skills. In: Davis CM, et al, eds. *Sexuality Related Measures*. Newbury Park, CA: Sage; 1998:328–337.

205. Williams SS, Doyle TM, Pittman LD, et al. Role-played safer sex skills of heterosexual college students influenced by both personal and partner factors. *AIDS Behav* 1998; 2:(3):177–187.

206. Anderson ES, Wagstaff DA, Sikkema KJ, et al. AIDS prevention among low-income, urban African-American and white women: Testing the information–motivation–behavioral skills (IMB) model. Poster presented at the 18th Annual Scientific Sessions of the Society of Behavioral Medicine, San Francisco, CA; April, 1997.

207. DeVroome EM, deWit JB, Sandfort TG, et al. Department of Gay and Lesbian Studies and Department of Social and Organizational Psychology, ed. *Comparing the Information–Motivation–Behavioral Skills-Model and the Theory of Planned Behavior in Explaining Unsafe Sex Among Gay Men*. The Netherlands: Utrecht University; 1996.

208. Bryan AD, Fisher JD, Fisher WA. Translating skills into actions: Tests of the role of safer sex preparatory behavior using the information–motivation–behavioral skills model. Forthcoming.

209. Fisher WA, Williams SS, Fisher JD, et al. Understanding AIDS risk behavior among urban adolescents: An empirical test of the information–motivation–behavioral skills model. *AIDS Behav* 1999; 3:13–23.

210. Carey MP, Maisto SA, Kalichman SC, et al. Enhancing motivation to reduce the risk of HIV infection for economically disadvantaged urban women. *J Consult Clin Psychol* 1997; 65:(4):531–541.

211. Weinhardt LM, Carey MP, Carey KB. HIV risk reduction for the seriously mentally ill: Pilot investigation and call for research. *J Behav Ther Exp Psychol* 1997; 28:1–8.

212. Joseph JG, Montgomery SB, Kirscht J, et al. *Behavioral Risk Reduction in a Cohort of Gay Men: Two-year Follow-Up*. Paper presented at the Third International Conference on AIDS, Washington, DC, June, 1987.

2

Diffusion Theory
A Theoretical Approach to Promote Community-Level Change

EVERETT M. ROGERS

INTRODUCTION

This chapter synthesizes selected applications of diffusion theory to human immunodeficiency virus (HIV) prevention programs in the United States and in other countries. *Diffusion* is the process through which an innovation, defined as an idea perceived as new, spreads via certain communication channels over time among the members of a social system.[1] Diffusion theory is unique in that it deals with new ideas, which necessarily involve uncertainty and risk to the individual who is learning about an innovation.

Over the past six decades since the first investigations of the diffusion process, some 4000 studies have been completed on how innovations spread and are adopted by individuals. These investigations, conducted by sociologists, anthropologists, communication scholars, public health researchers, and other scholars, have yielded a model of the diffusion process, key concepts, and generalizations linking these concepts.

Not surprisingly, when the acquired immunodeficiency syndrome (AIDS) epidemic was detected in 1981, the diffusion model was used in designing HIV prevention programs. Diffusion theory was already widely known by public health professionals who utilized this perspective in family planning programs, preventive health campaigns, and other health improvement interventions (often in connection with social marketing strategies). Tracing the diffusion of an innovation through interpersonal networks in a community after all bears close similarity to epidemiology, and early diffusion models were based in part on epidemiological models of the spread of an infectious disease. Many HIV prevention programs were designed and implemented by epidemiologists working in public health programs, so it is not surprising that these health officials applied diffusion theory in these prevention programs.

A particularly influential HIV prevention program was the Stop AIDS Program in San Francisco in the mid-1980s, in which street outreach workers recruited at-risk individuals to small-group meetings where the prevention message was presented, usually by an influential gay man who was seropositive. Stop AIDS drew directly on diffusion theory for such strategies as (1) the outreach workers being very similar to their target audience, (2) the small-group health educators being respected opinion leaders who were perceived as credible

EVERETT M. ROGERS • Department of Communication and Journalism, University of New Mexico, Albuquerque, New Mexico 87131.

Handbook of HIV Prevention, edited by Peterson and DiClemente.
Kluwer Academic/Plenum Publishers, New York, 2000.

because of their personal involvement with the epidemic, and (3) the use of interpersonal communication from peers.

Here we review the general effectiveness of several of the HIV prevention programs that were based closely on diffusion theory, in order to derive lessons learned about behavior change strategies at the community level. We focus especially on three investigations, each of which deals with a quite different aspect of HIV prevention: (1) a Centers for Disease Control and Prevention (CDC) epidemiological investigation of 40 men who were among the first in the United States to be diagnosed with AIDS,[2] (2) an investigation by the present author and his colleagues of the relative effectiveness of HIV prevention programs in San Francisco,[3,4] and (3) a quasi-experiment on the effects of an entertainment–education radio soap opera on HIV prevention behavior in Tanzania.[5]

Before discussing these three investigations and other studies that deal with the diffusion of HIV prevention behaviors, we present a brief overview of the diffusion model.

THE DIFFUSION MODEL

Diffusion is the process by which an innovation is communicated through certain channels over time among the members of a social system. An innovation is an idea, practice, or object perceived as new by an individual or other unit of adoption (such as an organization). The characteristics of an innovation, as perceived by members of a system, determine the rate of adoption of the innovation. Five attributes of innovations are: (1) *relative advantage*, the degree to which a new idea is perceived as superior to the idea that it replaces; (2) *compatibility*, the degree to which a new idea is perceived as consistent with the existing values, experiences, and needs of potential adopters; (3) *complexity*, defined as the degree to which an innovation is perceived as difficult to understand; (4) *trialability*, the degree to which an innovation may be experimented with on a limited basis; and (5) *observability*, the degree to which the results of an innovation are visible to others.[1]

An innovation that is perceived as having greater relative advantage, compatibility, trialability, and observability, along with less complexity, will be adopted more rapidly than other innovations. HIV prevention is an innovation whose relative advantage is not immediately evident. Preventive innovations are characterized by a relatively slow rate of adoption, defined as the relative speed with which an innovation is adopted by members of a system. A preventive innovation is adopted by an individual in order to avoid the possibility of some unwanted future event. The relative advantage of a preventive innovation is difficult for change agents to demonstrate to their audience because it occurs at some future, unknown time. Furthermore, the unwanted future consequence of nonadoption may not happen with certainty.

A social system is a set of interrelated units that are engaged in joint problem solving to accomplish a common goal. The units in systems of study in research on HIV prevention are typically individuals at risk due to age, gender, sexual orientation, occupation, and other factors. These at-risk communities, like other systems, have a social structure in which certain individuals (opinion leaders) play an especially important role in diffusing new ideas.

A basic notion of diffusion theory is that a new idea is adopted very slowly during the early stages of its diffusion process. Then, if the idea is perceived as relatively advantageous by its early adopters, its rate of adoption takes off as the early adopters share their favorable experiences regarding the innovation with potential adopters. An S-shaped curve of adoption over time is typically formed by the relatively slow initial adoption, which then speeds up when a "critical mass" has occurred, and finally levels off in the rate of adoption as fewer and fewer individuals (or organizations) remain to adopt. Past research shows that the diffusion of innovations is essentially a social process consisting of people talking to others about the new idea as they gradually shape the meaning of the innovation.

In addition to its preventive nature, the innovation of HIV prevention faces difficulties that slow its diffusion because the topic is relatively taboo, defined as the degree to which a topic cannot be discussed with others. The taboo of HIV/AIDS greatly limited who could talk to whom about HIV prevention, although this situation is gradually changing. Discussion of HIV/AIDS implies sexual activity, which is a sensitive topic. In the early stages of the epidemic in the United States, individuals with AIDS were perceived as being intravenous (IV) drug users or gay men, which added to the relative taboo of HIV prevention. These special characteristics of HIV prevention meant that prevention programs had to adapt the diffusion model in important ways in order to identify effective strategies to diffuse the innovation of HIV prevention.

At a certain point in the diffusion of a new idea, usually when about 12 to 15% of the potential adopters have accepted the innovation, a critical mass (defined as the point on the S-shaped diffusion curve after which the rate of adoption becomes self-sustaining) occurs. Until this point, the rate of adoption (measured as the cumulative number of adopters of the innovation per unit of time) is more or less a straight line. After the critical mass point, the rate of adoption begins to increase at an increasing rate, and the cumulative number of adopters per unit of time bends upward. This takeoff in the rate of adoption occurs because an adequate number of satisfied adopters has been achieved, with each individual telling several peers about the innovation. Thus the goal of many diffusion programs is to reach critical mass, after which continuing promotional efforts to diffuse the innovation can be diminished. A main challenge facing HIV prevention programs in the 1980s was to achieve critical mass. This goal may have first been attained in San Francisco in the late 1980s, when the number of newly infected individuals decreased sharply, in large part due to prevention efforts. The "San Francisco model" (as it was then called) was then transferred, with important modifications, to other American communities by the CDC and other government agencies and private organizations. Unfortunately, San Francisco was so unique regarding the AIDS epidemic that other communities faced many difficulties in adapting the San Francisco model to their own conditions.

THE DIFFUSION OF AIDS IN THE UNITED STATES

When the epidemic began in the United States in the early 1980s, the first reported cases were concentrated in San Francisco, Los Angeles, and New York. Individuals diagnosed with AIDS-related symptoms (the epidemic was not yet called AIDS) were young gay men. An immediate question for CDC epidemiologists regarding this strange new illness was to determine the means of transmission. Accordingly, CDC investigators conducted detailed personal interviews with each of the first 40 men diagnosed with AIDS. Data were gathered about each of the respondents' sexual partners.

To the surprise of the epidemiologists, the 19 men who lived in Los Angeles were linked by sexual contacts with the 21 other individuals who resided in San Francisco, New York, and other cities. The 40 men constituted a system of interconnected network links, and the CDC researchers began to call their data set the "cluster study." The 40 individuals with AIDS were very sexually active, averaging 227 different sexual partners per year, with one individual reporting 1560 sexual contacts. One of the 40 men, called "Patient Zero" by the CDC, had played a particularly key role in the diffusion network. Eight of his sexual partners were among the 39 other men. Further, if he were removed from the network, the Los Angeles cluster would no longer be connected with the New York cluster. Patient Zero was named Gaetan Dugas and was a flight attendant who worked for Air Canada. But the CDC investigators could not make much sense out of the dense thicket of network links connecting the 40 men (this problem of information overload frequently occurs with network data).

The CDC researchers called in Professor Alden S. Klovdahl, a noted network scholar at Australian National University, to analyze the network data. He used a special three-dimensional computer program, similar to that used by chemists to visualize molecular structures. On one of the three dimensions Klovdahl plotted the date at which each individual reported the onset of AIDS symptoms. Now the crucial role of Patient Zero became more apparent. While not the first individual diagnosed with AIDS (he was the sixth), once Patient Zero contracted AIDS, many others soon followed. His eight direct sexual contacts in turn linked him to ten other men. So in three steps, Patient Zero infected 26 (63%) of the 39 other individuals with AIDS. Klovdahl's network computer program allowed the CDC researchers to better understand the AIDS network among the 40 men. His results provided the CDC with further evidence that a virus was being transmitted through sexual contact.

Further, the similarities between the diffusion of an innovation and the spread of an epidemic like AIDS became more evident. Both spread through interpersonal networks in a kind of binomial expansion of interpersonal contacts, leading to a takeoff in the rate of diffusion (this point is the critical mass). Disease transmission is a time-ordered process in that an infection cannot travel backward in time.

DIFFUSION STRATEGIES FOR HIV PREVENTION IN SAN FRANCISCO

The issue of AIDS was relatively slow in climbing the national agenda. The first AIDS cases were diagnosed in the United States in 1981, but this issue did not attract much mass media coverage until mid-1985, 4 years later. By that time, more than 10,000 individuals had been diagnosed with AIDS, and about half that number had died. In comparison, the issue of Legionnaire's disease, a mysterious illness that killed more than 100 older men attending a convention in a Philadelphia hotel, jumped immediately to the top of the US media agenda. Neither *The New York Times* nor the White House played their usual role in the agenda-setting process for the issue of AIDS. For example, *The New York Times* published its first page-one story about AIDS on March 25, 1983, a year later than the *Los Angeles Times* and the *Washington Post*, and 21 months after the first AIDS cases were reported by the CDC. The US President saw AIDS as a budget threat and chose to ignore it. President Reagan did not give a talk about AIDS until May 1987, 6 years into the epidemic, a point at which 35,121 people had AIDS.[6,7] Eventually, however, the issue gained media attention, public support, and government funding. HIV prevention activities were launched in many communities.

In the mid-1990s the present author, in collaboration with Professor James W. Dearing at Michigan State University, investigated the relative effectiveness of HIV prevention programs in San Francisco, with funding provided by the US Agency for Health Care Policy and Research.[3,4] We chose San Francisco because of (1) the extensive experience (and relative success) of this city in slowing the rate of the epidemic, and (2) the large number of HIV prevention programs. In 1995, San Francisco had the highest number of HIV-infected persons per capita of any major city in the United States (including 48% of the city's gay and bisexual male population). The San Francisco Department of Public Health estimated that this city of 775,000 had 20,273 deaths due to AIDS by 1997 (1.7% of the population).

We identified 100 community-level HIV prevention programs, operated by 49 organizations, that were intended to inform, persuade, or mobilize a target audience to take preventive actions. The relatively large number of programs, initially a surprise to us when we began our research in 1994, was accompanied by an important characteristic of the programs: They were highly targeted to unique populations of at-risk individuals. (Uniqueness is the degree to which a set of extremely homophilous individuals is different from the larger social system of which it is a part. Homophily is the degree to which individuals who communicate with each other are alike.)

An example of one such highly targeted HIV prevention program was operated by a small, community-based organization of Asian immigrants. This program was aimed at the population of several hundred Thai massage girls in San Francisco, who often were also commercial sex workers. The program, funded in part through the CDC through the city's department of public health, employed several outreach workers who were themselves Thai (and one is a former massage girl). Pamphlets and other message materials were produced in the Thai language and featured culturally appropriate approaches to HIV prevention.

The degree to which each of the 100 HIV-prevention programs were targeted to a unique population was measured by scoring one point for each special characteristic of the intended audience for the program. For instance, one program was targeted to African-American, male, runaway, teenage, low-income, low-education commercial sex workers. This program had a uniqueness score of 7 (for the seven risk factors characterizing the intended audience). Why were the HIV prevention programs in San Francisco so highly targeted? The city is a very culturally diverse metropolis, with a large population of Asian immigrants and also with sizeable populations of African Americans and Hispanics. Many of the programs were operated by community-based organizations, which often represented and served a particular ethnic group.

HIV prevention programs in San Francisco mainly used interpersonal communication channels, including street outreach workers, small-group communication, counseling, and classroom training. One reason for this dependence on interpersonal channels was because mass media channels were more difficult to target to specific audience segments. Further, the program staff members were typically very homophilous with the audience individuals, which gave the program staff a high degree of credibility (defined as the degree to which a source is perceived as expert and trustworthy). Often an HIV prevention program employee or volunteer was seropositive and conveyed this characteristic to their audience individuals. Prevention messages were communicated in a culturally sensitive manner, especially by the relatively more effective HIV prevention programs.

The HIV prevention programs were nonjudgmental in discussing HIV and related matters with their audiences. For example, program staff did not imply that injection drug use, commercial sex work, or promiscuity were undesirable. In some instances, this nonjudgmental quality was conveyed by nuance; for example, program staff used the term "drug *user*" rather than "drug *abuser*" when talking with individuals at-risk for HIV infection, who in many cases were drug users.

Most of the program staff members that we personally interviewed in San Francisco had not heard of the diffusion model (although the pioneering program in the 1980s, Stop AIDS, was based directly on the diffusion model, and certain diffusion strategies had become embedded in most programs in San Francisco). So the HIV prevention programs of study used strategies that were consistent with the diffusion model and in several cases represented a special adaptation or reinvention of diffusion strategies, as we will discuss later in the present chapter.

ENTERTAINMENT EDUCATION FOR HIV PREVENTION IN TANZANIA

Entertainment–education is the intentional incorporation of educational messages into entertainment formats in order to change audience members' behavior.[8] This strategy has been incorporated in radio or television soap operas in a number of developing countries to promote adult literacy, female equality, and family planning. But until the mid-1990s the entertainment–education strategy had not been used for HIV prevention. The present author and his colleagues[5] evaluated the effects of a radio soap opera, "Twende na Wakati" (Let's Go with the Times), which had been broadcast in the East African nation of Tanzania since 1993.

The AIDS epidemic probably spread to Tanzania from neighboring countries in East Africa via long distance truck drivers. They infected commercial sex workers at truck stops along Tanzania's international highways. A 1991 investigation at seven main truck stops found that 28% of the truckers and 56% of the commercial sex workers were HIV positive.[9] The National AIDS Control Programme estimated the number of AIDS cases at about 400,000 (2.6% of the 15 million adults in Tanzania) in 1996. The national program, on the basis of blood donor data, estimated the number of Tanzanians infected with HIV in 1995 at about 8% of all adults.

In 1993, when broadcasts of "Twende na Wakati" began, most Tanzanians already were aware of AIDS, knew about the means of HIV transmission, and had favorable attitudes toward practicing safe sex. However, a nationwide survey in 1992 showed a relatively low level of HIV prevention behavior.[10] Hence, a "KAP-gap" (knowledge–attitude–practice), representing relatively high levels of knowledge and favorable attitudes that were not accompanied by widespread practice (or adoption) of protected sex, existed for HIV prevention (and family planning) in Tanzania in 1993.

The government of Tanzania decided to use the entertainment–education strategy to close these KAP gaps. They knew of a popular radio soap opera promoting family planning that had been broadcast in neighboring Kenya in the late 1980s. The educational themes and the entertainment format for the radio program was planned at a workshop in Dar es Salaam in early 1993, and the broadcasts began in July. The United Nations Population Fund (UNFPA) provided funding for some of the production costs of the radio program and invited communication researchers at the University of New Mexico to conduct evaluation research on the effects of the soap opera. The government radio network, Radio Tanzania, produced and broadcast "Twende na Wakati" with technical assistance from Population Communications International (PCI), a private organization headquartered in New York that played a key role in diffusing the entertainment–education approach to various countries.

The pervasiveness of radio in Tanzania made this medium the most appropriate channel for broadcasting an entertainment–education program. Some 54% of Tanzanian households owned a radio in 1993, and 67% listened regularly. In comparison, only 3% watched television. The educational content of the radio program was organized around 57 statements that were identified at the planning workshop. For instance, one statement said: "It is good that people are educated to understand that mosquitoes cannot spread HIV/AIDS." These goal statements were then implemented by the scriptwriters by designing three types of characters: (1) negative role models, like Mkwaju, a truck driver who is an irresponsible husband and parent, and who contracts HIV by sleeping with commercial sex workers; (2) positive role models, such as a couple who is monogamous; and (3) transitional characters who change from negative to positive behavior regarding the educational value. An example is Tunu, Mkwaju's wife, who changes from a submissive wife who puts up with her husband's promiscuous sexual behavior to divorcing him and becoming economically self-sufficient.

"Twende na Wakati" was very popular in Tanzania, with 55% of the some 3000 adults in our annual surveys reporting that they listened regularly (that is, to at least one of the two episodes broadcast each week). In 1995, of the 67% of adult Tanzanians who listened to radio, some 78% were reached by "Twende na Wakati." Our 1995 survey indicated that 98% had heard of AIDS and 61% believed that they were at risk; these levels of knowledge and attitudes increased only slightly over the first 2 years of the radio broadcasts.

Exposure to "Twende na Wakati" had strong effects in changing HIV prevention behavior. Figure 1 shows that 72% of the listeners said that they adopted a means of HIV prevention because of listening to the radio program. By 1995, after the second year of the

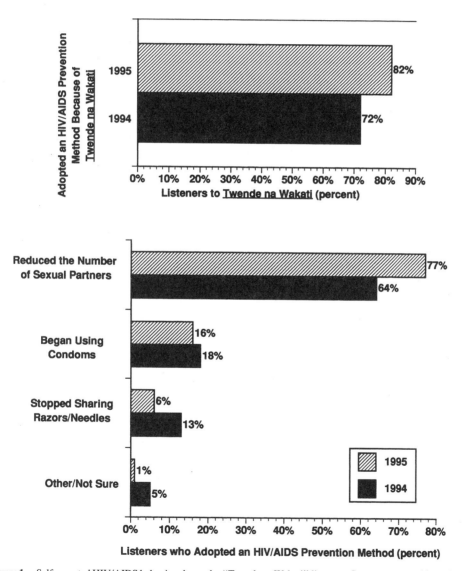

Figure 1. Self-reported HIV/AIDS behavior change by "Twende na Wakati" listeners. SOURCE: personal interviews with 995 listeners in 1994 and 1018 listeners in 1995.

broadcasts, this percentage of self-reported behavior change increased to 82%. The most important behavior change came about through reducing the number of sexual partners: From 2.3 in 1993 to 1.7 in 1994 and 1995, and to 1.6 in 1996 for male respondents; and from 1.9 in 1993 to 1.3 in 1994 to 1.2 in 1995, and to 1.17 in 1996 for female respondents. In the Dodoma region of Tanzania, where the broadcasts of the radio soap opera were blocked from 1993 to 1995, the number of sexual partners also decreased, but only by about half as much. These data are self-reported and might be overestimates of behavior change. We obtained data from the National AIDS Control Programme in Tanzania on the number of condoms distributed. In the areas of Tanzania where the radio program was broadcast, but not in the Dodoma area, a large increase occurred in condom distribution.

How did exposure to the radio soap opera cause the adoption of HIV prevention? Mainly by stimulating interpersonal communication about HIV/AIDS. Listeners who talked with others (61% of the 1018 respondents in our 1995 survey) reported talking to (1) friends, 55%; (2) spouse, 37%; and (3) other individuals, 8%. Listeners who talked with others about the radio program were much more likely to adopt an HIV prevention method (92%) than were listeners who did not talk with other people (69%). We found similar results of the entertainment–education broadcasts for the adoption of family planning methods. As in the case of HIV prevention, listening stimulated interpersonal communication with spouses and peers, which clinched adoption decisions.

The truck driver character, Mkwaju, became the most widely known personality in "Twende na Wakati" to the listeners. Some 49% of our 1996 survey respondents mentioned him spontaneously when asked which characters they remembered from the radio program. Only 3% said that Mkwaju was the best character for them to emulate, while 42% said that he was the character in "Twende na Wakati" least like themselves. Some 69% reported that there was someone like Mkwaju in their village. "Mkwaju" (which means "walking stick" in Swahili and has a sexual connotation) became a part of everyday conversation in Tanzania, as when one man might say to another, "Don't be a Mkwaju or you may get AIDS."

We conclude that an entertainment–education program can have a strong effect in promoting HIV prevention in a nation like Tanzania, where there are relatively few competing media and where high levels of knowledge and perceived risk already exists.

LESSONS LEARNED

What general lessons can be derived from the past studies of the diffusion model and HIV prevention programs?

1. The homophily of change agents with their clients is very important as a basis of trustworthy credibility. Illustrations of this generalization come especially from the HIV prevention programs in San Francisco.
2. An entertainment–education approach, as in the case of the Tanzania radio soap opera, can help close the KAP-gap between knowledge and attitudes on one hand and overt behavior change on the other. The entertainment–education approach involves the audience individuals, which encourages them to identify, both positively and negatively, with the role models provided in the mass medium.
3. Interpersonal communication with spouses and peers, perhaps encouraged and stimulated by an entertainment–education program or by outreach workers, is key to HIV prevention behavior change.

MODIFICATIONS IN DIFFUSION THEORY

What rethinking of the diffusion model is implied by the investigations of its application to HIV prevention programs? An even greater emphasis on interpersonal peer communication is indicated when the innovation is preventive and somewhat taboo, as in the case of HIV prevention. Under these special conditions, change agents must be particularly homophilous with their intended audience members. Change agents must be nonjudgmental when the behavior change involves an issue that may be perceived as ostracizing in the eyes of society. Unique audiences, as in San Francisco, have opinion leaders, although these opinion leaders may be quite different from those in the general population. Much further work is needed to explore the distinctive aspects of the diffusion of innovations when the new idea is preventive and relatively taboo.

REFERENCES

1. Rogers EM. *Diffusion of Innovations*, 4th ed. New York: Free Press; 1995.
2. Klovdahl AS. Social networks and the spread of infectious diseases: The AIDS example. *Soc Sci Med* 1985; 21(11):1203–1216.
3. Dearing JW, Rogers EM, Meyer G, et al. Social marketing and diffusion-based strategies for communicating health with unique populations: HIV prevention in San Francisco. *J Health Communic* 1996;1: 343–363.
4. Rogers EM, Dearing JW, Rao N, et al. Communication and community in a city under siege: The AIDS epidemic in San Francisco. *Community Res* 1995; 22(6):664–678.
5. Rogers EM, Vaughan PW, Swalehe RMA, et al. *Effects of an Entertainment–Education Radio Soap Opera on Family Planning and HIV/AIDS Prevention Behavior in Tanzania.* Albuquerque: University of New Mexico, Department of Communication and Journalism, Report; 1997.
6. Rogers EM, Dearing JW, Chang S. AIDS in the 1980s: The agenda-setting process for a public issue. *Journalism Monographs* 1991; 126:1–86.
7. Dearing JW, Rogers EM. *Agenda-Setting.* Newbury Park, CA: Sage; 1996.
8. Singhal A, Rogers EM. *Entertainment–Education.* Mahwah, NJ: Lawrence Erlbaum Associates; 1999.
9. AMREF. *Tanzania: AIDS Education and Condom Promotion for Transportation Workers: Strengthening STD Services.* Dar es Salaam, Tanzania: African Medical and Research Foundation, Report; 1992.
10. POFLEP. *Preliminary Report on Pre-Production Research.* Arusha, Tanzania: Population/Family Life Education Programme, Report; 1992.

3

Methodological Issues in HIV Behavioral Interventions

DAVID G. OSTROW and SETH KALICHMAN

INTRODUCTION

Human immunodeficiency virus (HIV) behavioral intervention research involves numerous methodological issues that are either unique to the field of HIV research or "cutting edge" in terms of behavioral research in general. The thrust of this chapter will be to review those issues that are either the most important new HIV prevention research issues or the most limiting in the areas of "sensitive" behavioral research (i.e., research on sexual, drug use, and other socially "sensitive" behaviors) in general. With the current trend to integrate HIV research and prevention activities into the larger domains of behavioral prevention and sexually transmitted diseases (STDs) in general, some of the issues and examples discussed in this chapter may go well beyond the purview of HIV intervention research per se. However, they have been selected for discussion here because of their key influence on the directions and opportunities that HIV prevention research are predicted to be going in the next 5–10 years. We have used the schema of an earlier publication, Methodological Issues in AIDS Behavioral Research,[1] in discussing methodological issues by design, sampling and retention, measurement, and analytical/modeling issues and focus on topics that have progressed or changed the most since that book was published in 1993.

EXPERIMENTAL DESIGN ISSUES

Selecting Comparison Conditions

Experimental and quasi-experimental designs compare interventions of interest against some other treatment. In an efficacy study, an experimental intervention is best tested under ideal conditions. Appropriate control groups in such studies are often *no-treatment* conditions, or a delayed treatment (usually referred to as *wait list*) condition. The experimental intervention is therefore tested against no intervention to determine whether the intervention offers any positive outcomes. Because the magnitude for differences in the ideal situation is likely large, efficacy studies provide greater statistical power and therefore may require smaller sample sizes to detect differences between conditions.

DAVID G. OSTROW • Loyola University Medical School, Maywood, Illinois 60153.   *SETH KALICHMAN* • Center for AIDS Intervention Research, Medical College of Wisconsin, Milwaukee, Wisconsin 53202.

Handbook of HIV Prevention, edited by Peterson and DiClemente.
Kluwer Academic / Plenum Publishers, New York, 2000.

Another variation of the no-treatment control group is the use of a time- and contact-matched comparison condition, but where the intervention content does not include relevant STD or HIV prevention information. Examples of non-HIV contact-matched comparison conditions include the use of a dietary nutrition group for women,[2] or a general health information–education intervention for seriously mentally ill adults.[3] Using wait list and non-HIV control groups in HIV prevention studies provides a best-case scenario for testing an experimental intervention.

However, one problem with both designs is the differential experience and demand characteristics of study participation in the respective treatment conditions. Research participants assigned to the experimental HIV prevention intervention know that they are expected to report reduced sexual risk behaviors and increased condom use following their participation in the treatment. In contrast, participants in control groups may wonder why they are being asked so many questions about their sexual behavior after being told that exercise and good eating habits will benefit their health. Thus, studies that compare an HIV prevention intervention to no-treatment, minimal treatment, or other content-unmatched control conditions stack the deck in favor of finding positive outcomes on self-reported measures.

Effectiveness trials, on the other hand, test interventions under conditions closer to actual practice. Control conditions in effectiveness trials consist of interventions that either represent a standard of care or an alternative intervention. For example, an effectiveness study of brief HIV prevention counseling may use existing counseling practices, such as those used in HIV antibody testing, as a comparison condition. Similarly, an effectiveness study of an HIV risk reduction skills training workshop may use a time-matched HIV information and education workshop that is completely void of any skills training. Thus, all participants in such a study would receive equal amounts of AIDS-related prevention activities, but without the potential for differential demand characteristics and outcome expectancies that come with a no-treatment or minimal treatment comparison condition. In addition, content-matched control groups protect against biases that may result from differential incentive payments as well as the negative community relations that can result from only providing some people with AIDS prevention information. An example of a contact-matched control group is provided in a two-group experiment reported by Belcher and colleagues.[4] In this study the same counselors in the same setting randomly assigned women to either a single 2-hour behavioral skills risk reduction counseling session or a 2-hour HIV risk education counseling session. Thus, the study design tested the effectiveness of the skills training intervention against an alternative HIV prevention counseling format. Such an experimental design avoids some of the problems mentioned above, but can require very large numbers of participants, since the differential effect of the two types of HIV risk reduction interventions may be quite small relative to the absolute amount of behavioral change observed in the two groups. Another problem is the inevitable convergence, over time, between the experimental and control intervention especially if both are delivered by the same staff or even within the same community organization. This occurs because counselors will inevitably notice that participants in one group are doing better, clinically or behaviorally, and will begin to incorporate aspects of what they feel is a better treatment into the other condition. This can happen gradually and almost imperceptibly over time and poses a major challenge to such designs. It is therefore still quite controversial whether the two interventions should be delivered by the same staffs or even within the same agencies. However, if separate agencies are used, the problem of a multisite design must be dealt with. Whatever the decision on the design of dual-condition interventions, extreme care must be taken to ensure the integrity of the two interventions, including the observation and reporting back to intervention staff on the content of each intervention condition.

Finally, it is possible to test an intervention using a "quasi-experimental" design, such as comparing the amount of change in the intervention group over time with historical change among persons who were eligible for but did not participate in the intervention and were still willing to take the baseline and follow-up evaluation(s). Given the difficulties of exactly matching the experimental and control conditions in a true experimental design, the addition of quasi-experimental historical "control" groups also can inform even the best study design. For example, following up with men who underwent baseline assessments but did not participate in the controlled intervention trial can provide useful data on the amount of behavioral change taking place in the community over the course of the study, independent of study participation effects.

Randomization

Experimental control requires an unsystematic assignment of research participants to experimental conditions. In some cases, individuals are randomly assigned to conditions, whereas other studies may randomize groups or entire communities to experimental conditions. The appropriate scheme for randomization depends on the level of intervention and the level of outcome analysis, and these factors have a significant impact on sample sizes needed for statistical analysis. There are examples where randomization schemes have indeed broken down and resulted in problems interpreting study outcomes. For example, Peterson and colleagues[5] reported that their groups were not successfully randomized and therefore were unequal at baseline on key outcome variables. In a study that randomized 16 small cities to either experimental or control conditions, Kelly and colleagues[6] reported that variations in seasons across regions where the study took place resulted in systematic differences at baseline. The integrity of randomization cannot be assumed and requires verification through comparisons on preintervention characteristics of samples, particularly on measures used to examine intervention outcomes.

Another innovative approach to this issue has been the "co-opting" of an existing descriptive cohort study (the San Francisco Young Men's Cohort) to assess the impact of a widely disseminated community-based intervention (e.g., the San Francisco Stop AIDS program) on members of the cohort who participated in the intervention versus those who were not exposed to the intervention.[7] This will only be feasible if the intervention has been widely disseminated in the community so that a significant proportion of the descriptive cohort members will have been exposed.

SAMPLING AND RETENTION ISSUES

Sampling Issues

Difficulty of finding "rare" or hidden populations requires innovative approaches that go beyond standard sampling procedures. Snowball sampling and ethnographic-based sampling methods have been used in many studies with varying degrees of success.[8] Generalizability issues always remain with these types of sampling procedures, as they select for a particular subsample rather than employ random selection methods. We are currently trying an innovative technique to combine sampling based on community-level ethnography with sampling based on a household probability sample of men who have sex with men (MSM) in Chicago.[9,10] This will work only if telephone probability samples pick up truly random samples of MSM instead of selecting for more "out" individuals or those men otherwise more willing to talk over the phone. If successful, such hybrid sampling techniques hold the promise of allowing the identification of cohorts based on particular behavioral risk characteristics (in our case drug-using MSM engaging in risky sex) that can be related back to the communities where they live or engage in the behavior of interest. This will allow more generalizable results than has been previously possible.[11]

Retention Issues

Based on need and the epidemic itself, HIV risk reduction interventions target difficult-to-reach-and-retain populations. Loss of intervention participants occurs when people move, die, lose access to a telephone, become displaced, stop engaging in the behavior of interest, or even gain employment. Interventions therefore must build incentives for getting potential participants in the door and then enlisting their participation, oftentimes well beyond the time period of actual intervention delivery. This may becoming more difficult, rather than easier, as HIV and acquired immunodeficiency syndrome (AIDS) increasingly become concentrated among minority and lower socioeconomic status (SES) populations. As researchers focus increasingly on disadvantaged populations, the motivation and stability of targeted persons may become increasingly important limiting factors. Monetary incentives in HIV prevention interventions have been shown to reduce attrition relative to nonmonetary incentives, at least among inner-city substance abusers.[12] Paying participants is relatively unique to funded research studies, however, and may reduce the external validity of intervention implementation in community-based service settings. More ecologically valid incentives may be attached to access to other services, such as employment placement programs, training opportunities, child care, and substance abuse–mental health treatment.

Sample Size and Statistical Power

HIV prevention interventions are deemed successful only when their outcomes show reductions in risk behaviors or increases in protective behaviors. Success is usually measured in terms of meaningful comparisons to behaviors reported at baseline or when compared to a control group. Defining a meaningful difference, however, is often open to debate. In most cases, studies are judged in terms of findings exceeding a statistical probability that such a difference could have occurred by chance. The degree to which a statistical test can detect differences between any given set of conditions is dependant on the size of the observed effect and the sample size; smaller effect sizes require larger sample sizes to achieve adequate power to detect a difference. Effect sizes in the HIV prevention literature vary considerably, depending on the outcome of interest and the characteristics of the study. Multiple factors other than the potency of an intervention influence effect sizes, including measurement error, baseline observations of outcome measures, and the selection of a control condition.

One factor that can seriously threaten power to detect intervention effects in HIV prevention research is the potential for cross contamination of experimental conditions, as mentioned above. Participants in experimental and control conditions can be closely associated when studies sample from a single targeted recruitment site or when they overuse snowball recruitment procedures. Cross contamination can occur when information or prevention techniques are passed on from experimental to control participants. To resolve this issue, many researchers would consider using two recruitment sites or intervention settings and simply use one for delivering the experimental intervention and the other for the control condition. However, this option leads to the potential confounds of linking variations in different sites and samples with experimental conditions. Further, it does not help if the two sites are treated as the unit of randomization because having only two sites provides no power to test for site-level effects. Indeed, it is a common mistake for researchers to treat too few sites as participants in a community-level analysis of interventions.[13]

Cross contamination of experimental conditions can be addressed by (1) recruiting a diverse sample, (2) measuring manipulation checks at multiple postintervention assessments, (3) and evaluating the potential for diffusion of intervention components among comparison group participants. Distributions of behavioral data are invariably nonlinear and how this nonlinearity is managed will influence statistical power as well as meet various assumptions for statistical tests. It is therefore increasingly the case that statistical analyses that are valid for nonlinear data are seen in the behavioral research literature, including nonparametric tests of significance. These methods, in turn, require sophisticated interpretations and education of those applying the research to field conditions on their assumptions and limitations.

MEASUREMENT ISSUES

Outcome Evaluation

Although the goals of HIV prevention interventions are to prevent people from contracting HIV, the impact of a given intervention on HIV infections can rarely be observed.[14] Issues such as low incidence rates of HIV infections in even the highest risk populations, and therefore low statistical power to detect reductions in infection rates, along with small-to-moderate effect sizes for most existing intervention methods, seriously limit our ability to directly measure the impact of interventions on the HIV epidemic. Thus, the field has been left with the question of how to best define prevention-relevant outcomes for a given intervention. Indeed, HIV prevention interventions can have a number of targeted outcomes, including increased risk-related knowledge, sensitization to personal risk, motivation to change, increased self-efficacy, acquisition of risk reduction behavioral skills, reductions in unsafe sexual practices, and increased use of condoms. Interventions may impact on any number of theoretically derived psychological and social correlates of HIV risk, including risk-related knowledge, perceived vulnerability, intentions to change behavior, stages of readiness to change, and self-efficacy.

More proximal to HIV transmission are self-reported enactments of risk-producing as well as risk-reducing behaviors. Along with biological cofactors to HIV transmission, particularly rates of other STDs, self-reported risk and protective behaviors are the closest proxy measure for HIV transmission risk. However, issues of reliability and validity of self-report measures are frequently questioned. The following sections discuss issues of relevance to assessing behavioral outcomes from HIV prevention interventions.

Domains of Outcome Variables

To evaluate the effectiveness of an intervention, investigators typically assess one or more of the following behavioral variables: number of sexual partners; number of protected and unprotected occasions of oral, anal, and vaginal intercourse; percentage of time that condoms are used; and, less often, recently diagnosed STDs. To our knowledge, no study has yet adequately assessed incident HIV infections as an index of change because of low base rates of infection. Even in areas of high HIV seroprevalence, incidence seroconversion rates rarely exceed 2–3%/year of the initially seronegative population, resulting in negligible statistical power for detecting differences with sample sizes in the hundreds. It is therefore assumed that an intervention is effective when it can be demonstrated that participants (1) reduced the number of their sexual partners, the number of occasions of unprotected oral, anal, or vaginal intercourse, and their incidence of more prevalent STDs; and/or (2) increased the number of occasions of protected sexual intercourse as well as the percentage of occasions that condoms were used.

It is also apparent that the same behavior may be safe for one person but risky for the next; for example, unprotected vaginal intercourse is safe in a monogamous relationship with an uninfected partner but not with anonymous or casual partners. Thus, unlike risk assessment associated with smoking or dietary behavior, wherein a person who is smoking or eating high-fat foods is assumed to be at greater risk for pulmonary or vascular disease, risk assessment for HIV infection is inherently idiosyncratic. A participant in an HIV risk reduction program who engages in unprotected intercourse only after knowing their partner has tested HIV negative is at less risk than is the participant who uses condoms with a partner of unknown (i.e., possibly infected) HIV-antibody status; however, the former would be seen as a treatment failure, whereas the latter would be counted as a success.[15] Despite nearly universal recognition of this paradox, investigators typically assume that unprotected sexual activities confer greater risk than do protected ones, due to inherent difficulties in obtaining reliable antibody status for partners.

Because no single index of risk reduction contains all relevant information, most studies collect multiple measures, including self-reported behavior, knowledge, attitudes that support behavior change, and behavioral assessments of skills related to behavior changes. In addition, a few investigators have created composite indexes reflective of overall risk reduction, whereas most authors report each of the measures separately. Composite indexes, which take into account partner type and serostatus as well as the behaviors engaged in with each partner type, can help in incorporating the complexity of dyadic interactions into the assessment of HIV transmission risk. For example, in one of the most widely used composite indexes,[16,17] inconsistent use of condoms with a primary partner during anal sex results in a risk score of "moderate," while inconsistent use of condoms with nonprimary partners results in a risk score of "high." While no single-dimensional composite measure can adequately incorporate all of the dimensions that determine the totality of risk taking in multiple relationships and circumstances, such measures can provide useful and hierarchically valid categorical measures of risk change for use as the dependent outcome measure for multivariate analyses.

Another approach has been to measure actual changes in ability of the person to either use a condom or engage in discussion of safer sex practices with a potential partner.[18] While difficult to measure with acceptable reliability, role-plays of specific safer sex behaviors can provide measures that correlate well with actual safer sex practices while minimizing respondent-related measurement errors.

Truthfulness and Dissembling

Concerns are often raised regarding the reliability of self-report measures of sexual behavior. For example, Brody[19,20] have argued that self-reports of sexual behavior, especially socially disapproved behavior such as anal sex and intravenous drug use, cannot be trusted. They opine that social desirability, demand, and other biases make self-reports unreliable. Numerous other investigators have demonstrated that such assessments are indeed difficult to conduct but can yield reliable information.

A recent example of how question wording can determine the assessed prevalence of unsafe sex is provided by the work of DiFranceisco and colleagues.[21] When these investigators directly asked gay men the number of times they had engaged in unprotected anal sex, they got very low prevalence rates for unsafe sex. However, when they asked the same men to indirectly estimate their prevalence of unsafe sex by first asking how many times they had engaged in any anal sex and then the proportion or number of those times that a condom was used, they got much higher estimates of unsafe sex. Apparently, it is much easier for gay men to admit indirectly to not using condoms a proportion of the times they have had anal sex than to admit right out that they have engaged in unsafe sex. Many investigators use a surrogate measure of such social desirable answering of sensitive questions,[22] but there is very little evidence that the use of a social desirability scale will screen out those respondents giving underestimates of their sexual risk; nor do these investigators provide a practical method for using the social desirability scale to adjust or delete the behavioral data.

The design of some major behavioral studies allows for the use of multiple forms of behavioral data collection in order to detect or eliminate these biases in self-reported risk taking. For example, one of us (DGO) was able to compare the face-to-face interview data from participants in the Chicago Multicenter AIDS Cohort Study with self-administered take-home questionnaire data from the parallel Coping and Change Study to validate the findings in a case–control study of predictors of seroincidence in the cohort.[23] Fortunately, that study was able to confirm that the same behavioral risk factors for seroconversion (namely, unprotected receptive anal sex and drug use) were associated with seroconversion across time and with both sets of behavioral data. Since most investigations do not have the luxury of asking similarly sensitive questions using parallel but different questionnaire modes or question wordings, it is important that each investigation include, at a minimum, some combination of checks on the validity of self-report data (see above on the use of surrogate measures including role-play and STD testing data).

Assessment Administration Format

The two most widely used formats for collecting HIV-related sexual history data are self-administered questionnaires and face-to-face interviews. Self-administered surveys afford respondents privacy, which is particularly important when study participants provide sensitive information about potentially stigmatized behaviors. Studies show that increased privacy when responding to sex surveys corresponds to reduced measurement error.[24] A limitation of self-administered questionnaires, however, is their reliance on reading ability and adequate comprehension of item response formats. Because reading ability can pose a barrier to assessing low-income populations, interviews provide a viable alternative administration format. Structured and standardized interviews can assure that respondents comprehend instructions and items. Face-to-face interviews elicit higher frequencies of self-reported risk behavior than questionnaires and minimize refusal rates.[25] These findings support the validity of face-to-face interview assessments. Nevertheless, face-to-face interviews are limited by potential response biases invoked by the interpersonal context of the interview as well as the potential for interviewer biases.[26] However, studies that compare responses obtained from telephone and face-to-face interviews find few differences between formats despite socio-demographic differences of women completing each.[27,28] Studies comparing audiotape versus written modes of questionnaire administration also find more similarities than differences between these formats.[29] It is possible to blend the privacy of self-administered questionnaires with standardized interpersonal instruction by using overhead projected facsimiles of instruments where assessors read items aloud and explain instructions to groups of respondents, page by page, item by item, with participants marking responses privately on their own questionnaires. This method has been used with considerable success in HIV prevention research with inner-city low-income populations.[2,30–32] Additional methods for collecting self-report risk behavior data include the use of audio-assisted computerized assessments,[33] real-time coded behavioral records,[34,35] and partner-verified reports. Recent methodological studies comparing audio-assisted computer self-interviewing (ACASI) with standard interview techniques have shown considerably higher rates of risky sex when ACASI was employed.[36]

REACTIVITY

There are potential reactive effects of self-reported sexual behaviors that have not been tested among HIV-vulnerable populations. Reactivity is of particular importance to intervention outcome evaluations, especially brief interventions that could feasibly be overshadowed by reactivity and sensitization produced by in-depth assessments of HIV risk behavior history. Self-report behavioral assessments can influence subsequent behavior (reactivity), as may occur for measures of smoking, weight reduction, and alcohol use.[37,38] Assessments of sexual behavior have shown less evidence of reactivity, with most effects being small, evaluated among people of high literacy and assessed over relatively long periods of time.[39–41] For example, Halpern et al.[42] found that repeated assessments of adolescents did not significantly affect behavior change. However, this study used archival data from four samples of adolescents who completed either one, two, three, or five assessments over 2 years. Thus, participants were not randomly assigned to assessment conditions and short-term reactivity was not tested. There also are no data available on the differential reactive effects attributable to instrument depth and administration formats. Use of nonreactive measures, such as a reduced incidence of diagnosed STDs following an intervention, provides a useful supplement to self-report measures but may be less sensitive to intervention effects due to relatively low base rates of STDs. In addition, some common STDs, such as hepatitis B or C, may be transmissible through routes commonly thought to be low risk for HIV transmission.[43] Other creative evaluation strategies, such as monitoring condom acquisition, also provide an indirect and corroborative measure of treatment effectiveness. For example, HIV prevention intervention studies have used opportunities to redeem coupons or vouchers for condoms as proxy measures of condom use. In addition, use of multiple measures, such as knowledge, attitudes, and self-reported behavior with converging evidence of successful outcomes support conclusions of intervention effectiveness to a greater degree than do single outcomes. However, when multiple outcome measures do not converge, as was recently observed in the National Institute of Mental Health multisite trial,[44] researchers are left speculating on why one dimension such as behavioral risk may have changed, while another such as STD rates did not change.

Almost all HIV prevention interventions have reported behavioral changes immediately following the intervention. Many studies also report additional follow-up assessments of behavior change 3, 6, and/or 12 months after the last intervention session. However, some studies report follow-ups relative to the baseline assessment. For example, Rotheram-Borus and colleagues[45] reported 3-month follow-up data relative to the baseline assessment point. Thus, participants who received 20 sessions of intervention completed their follow-ups at least one month closer to their last intervention session than did those participants who completed zero to nine sessions. This assessment schedule complicates the interpretation of findings. Relapse to baseline following behavioral interventions is common in the literature, including programs that target substance use and smoking cessation. Maintenance is therefore a likely problem in HIV prevention interventions. However, most studies do not report assessments that are delayed long enough to assess maintenance of intervention effects. In one case, Kelly et al.[46] collected 16-month follow-up assessments from 68 gay and bisexual men who had completed their HIV prevention intervention. They found that 41 (60%) of the men maintained safer sexual practices. Baseline assessments, taken 16 months earlier, showed that risk behavior, younger age, and substance use with sex best predicted high-risk practices at follow-up. Most studies, however, do not provide long-term behavioral data and cannot examine factors that predict risk behavior relapse. Therefore, little information is available about the durability of behavioral changes resulting from interventions. While there is a trend toward longer-term follow-up of behavioral risk reduction interventions, precisely because of the problem of relapse it is often very difficult to locate the highest-risk study participants after the initial intervention and postintervention assessment. Therefore, it is important to balance the need for long-term follow-up information against the increased attrition rates inherent in such extended follow-up studies. Innovative approaches to this problem include the use of community-based follow-up sampling, as discussed above.

The Need to Develop Hierarchical Measures of Multifactorial Risk

The history of development of HIV risk measures began with the assumption that singular behaviors, such as unprotected intercourse and needle sharing, were the only outcome measures of interest. The limitations of such outcome measures for use with nongay populations or populations with both sexual and drug use risk were soon shown to be readily apparent. For example, we still do not have a good idea of the relative risk of unprotected oral versus anal sex among gay men due to the obviously lower efficiency of oral HIV transmission and the assumption that any unprotected anal intercourse is obviously the route of infection.[23,47] Even if we could develop ideal HIV risk measures, we would still have the problem that we might be losing the richness of the original outcome measure data and/or might be missing a particular factor related to one subgroup that makes the risk typology measure nonlinear for that subgroup. One approach has been to count all intercourse occasions, multiply each type by a risk level indicator, and sum the total for an overall risk score.[48]

ANALYSIS AND MODELING ISSUES

Handling Dropouts and Attrition

Intervention study participants are typically lost due to dropout during the intervention or incomplete follow-up assessments. As would be expected, studies with the least amount of attrition are those that have the shortest-term follow-up. For example, St. Lawrence and colleagues[49] reported no attrition immediately following the intervention; Kalichman and colleagues[32] lost 15% of participants 1 month after the intervention, whereas Valdiserri and colleagues[50] reported 50% attrition at 12 months follow-up. There are, however, exceptions to this rule, with St. Lawrence and colleagues[49] reporting only 8.5% attrition at 12-months follow-up and Kelly and colleagues[2] reporting over 50% attrition at 3 months.

Studies also vary with respect to how attrition is handled in outcome analyses. It is most common for intervention outcomes to be based on those participants who completed all aspects of the study. In most cases, dropouts and noncompleters are compared to participants who completed the intervention on relevant measures collected at baseline. Methods for analyzing data from all enrolled participants usually fall under the rubric of intent to treat and data imputation models. These methods involve replacing missing values with estimates derived from existing values in the data set. There are a number of methods for analytically dealing with attrition, and all are controversial. For example, Kelly and colleagues[2] used a multiple imputation procedure to replace missing assessments with data from retained participants matched on key demographic characteristics, including age, education, and sexually transmitted disease history. This method increased the within-subject variability, and therefore increased the error term in the analyses, yielding a conservative test of intervention effects. Imputing data also can involve using regression models to estimate values or other means of modeling lost data. For example, we recently used a novel procedure to replace missing data in an analysis of long-term predictors of sexual safety/relapse over a 12-year period.[51] This method involved determining the percentage split between safe and unsafe anal behaviors among the men with data for any particular semiannual assessment and replacing missing data for men not assessed at that time point randomly but in proportion to the split between safe and unsafe behavior among the men assessed. Such procedures, however, pose problems as well, including the difficulties inherent in interpreting findings from values that were not originally observed outcomes.

Modeling Complex Causal Relationships

The use of multidimensional models of influence to model complexly determined behaviors is perhaps the cutting edge of behavioral research analyses. Most health behavior models that have been used to model sexual or drug use behavioral change focus on a small set of behavioral determinants or determinants of "anticipated" behavior. While it is oftentimes necessary to focus on a particular behavioral situation, such as first-time dating with a member of the opposite sex among college students (cf Lynn Cooper's work[52]), we and others have observed that most episodes of unsafe behavior among MSMs are related to specific and unique situational factors, such as substance use, lack of a condom, or particular affective states.[53,54] For analysis of complex causal relationships between multiple potential determinants of multiple potential behavioral outcomes, it is necessary to first create a multidimensional model that is valid for the multiple levels of input to the behavior and then study enough individuals and situations such that path analysis or multideterminant logistic regression analysis can be used. Two recently adapted multipath models of human behavior are the Awareness Intervention for Men (AIM) model of sexual behavior outcomes[55] and the triadic influence model of Flay and colleagues.[56] While these models allow investigators to test multiple paths of influence, both in the present and past state, and include both transient "state" and characterological "trait" measures, they require relatively large sample sizes and complicated assessments in order to provide sufficient detail and size for the path or multivariate analyses. In a time of limited resources for assessment and analysis of large cohorts, there is a need for collaborative investigations that use standardized assessment and sampling procedures. Such multisite collaboration will permit investigation of both site-specific and more universal determinants of complex behaviors that lie at the heart of HIV prevention.

The use of "nonreferent" analytical models (such as the theory of triadic influence), which do not require any particular group to be treated as the "normal" group in contrast to the "other" or "deviant" labeled group(s), is also important. Such models allow examination of the multiple paths of influence on individual's behavior, however, and are not clear in how they can be used to model group differences. Instead, they are important whenever groups are being analyzed for within-group rather than between-group influences, as would be the case when studying women separately from men or African Americans separately from whites.[57]

In summary, there has been much progress recently in developing the types of models urgently needed in HIV prevention research. What is needed is to start applying these new models of multiple paths of influence to HIV prevention research data; to devise experimental designs that take advantage of multipath determinant models and nonreferent models; and to educate reviewers of grant applications and publications about the usefulness of these models.

Integrating Qualitative with Quantitative Survey Responses

For many years, multimethod research (e.g., the concurrent or sequential use of qualitative and quantitative data collection techniques) has been used to describe and understand various social phenomena, including drug use.[58–60] Researchers investigating HIV-related behaviors among injection drug users have been able to successfully apply multimethod techniques to locate and identify the risk behaviors of previously hidden populations[61] and to evaluate behavioral change.[62] This suggests that these techniques could be successfully applied to evaluate HIV prevention program clients among other populations.

Increasingly, intervention researchers are finding that quantitative assessments alone do not capture the richness of the experience of participants in intervention studies, nor do they allow for full interpretation of the differences found between experimental and control groups. For example, it is difficult to impossible to assess the degree to which there has been crossover between two interventions on the basis of quantitative data alone. We have combined qualitative and quantitative data collection procedures to monitor this phenomenon in the AIM intervention project in Chicago,[63] by combining behavioral skill checklists with in-depth interviews focusing on the strategies and skills that participants have used during discrete sexual events. The checklists contain behavioral skills that are unique both to each intervention condition as well as those that are shared. This information then can be used to evaluate the skills depicted within the participants' sexual event narratives. A crossover effect would be detected if a pattern of newly acquired skills were identified among participants that fulfilled the two following conditions. First, participants from one intervention would need to select behavioral skills items that were unique to the other intervention condition. Second, their utilization of those skills, as depicted in their sexual event narratives, would need to be indistinguishable from those of participants who had received specific training in those skills in the other intervention condition. Combining these two types of data allows us to validate that the skills participants have identified as helpful are actually being used and to determine whether specific training in those skills makes a difference in how they are executed.

SUMMARY AND NEW RESEARCH SUGGESTIONS

We believe that several important areas for education and future research have been suggested. The first is that progress in methodological research can only be made if journal editors, reviewers, and granting agencies and their reviewers are sensitized to these issues. For example, when attempting to develop or advance methodology, it is often impossible to guarantee results or satisfy reviewer expectations based on traditional methodology. There has to be more willingness to take risks when new methodology is proposed or reported in the scientific literature. To some extent, the new guidelines for the National Institutes of Health grant reviews emphasize innovative methodology over detailed descriptions of measurement or analytical strategies, but these guidelines are only used to the extent that scientific review groups are educated and sensitized to the new guidelines. Many innovative studies may appear to be the most "risky" in terms of striking out into new methodological territory. How can funding agencies better support these "emerging" methodologies so that behavioral research can move forward in some of the most vexing areas related to "sensitive" behaviors, generalizability of findings, and translations that work in the field? The remainder of this volume provides examples of where this has been done successfully and the barriers that have been faced in attempting to bring new research methodologies to the field of HIV prevention research.

While researchers and community agencies move forward in applying what is already known about interventions that work, there remains a need for long-term support of preintervention studies to provide data on long-term influences on HIV risk behavior and temporal trends in risky behaviors. There is an absolute need that has been discussed frequently, yet is rarely reflected in the time lines and priorities of granting agencies. Ten or more years is not an unusual time line for a prospective study of behavioral change and stability over time when it comes to lifetime behaviors such as sexuality and drug use. Yet behavioral researchers are rarely provided the flexibility to work over such time periods when the "intervention du jour" is the one that everyone is running to try out, basically ignoring the longer time periods over which HIV risk and infection invariably play out. As HIV moves from an acute series of epidemics toward a chronic disease similar to diabetes, the need to balance "newness" with stability in long-term research methodologies and to chart the long time lines of this infection will be a major challenge for the future of biomedical research in HIV and other chronic illnesses.

REFERENCES

1. Ostrow DG, Kessler RC. *Methodological Issues in AIDS Behavioral Research*. New York: Plenum Press; 1993.
2. Kelly JA, Murphy DA, Washington CD, et al. The effects of HIV/AIDS intervention groups for high risk women in urban clinics. *Am J Public Health* 1994; 84:1918–1922.
3. Otto-Salaj L, Kelly J, Stevenson L, et al. Outcomes of a randomized small-group HIV prevention intervention trial for people with serious mental illness. Submitted for publication; 1998.
4. Belcher L, Kalichman SC, Topping M, et al. Randomized trial of a brief HIV risk reduction counseling intervention for women. *J Consult Clin Psychol* 1998; 66:856–861.
5. Peterson JL, Coates T, Catania J, et al. Evaluation of an HIV risk reduction intervention among African-American gay and bisexual men. *AIDS* 1996; 10:319–325.
6. Kelly JA, Murphy D, Sikkema K, et al. Outcomes of a randomized controlled community-level HIV prevention intervention: Effects on behavior among at-risk gay men in small US cities. *Lancet* 1997; 350:1500–1505.
7. Stall RD, Paul JP, Barrett DC, et al. An outcome evaluation to measure change in sexual risk-taking among gay men undergoing substance use disorder treatment. *J Studies Alcohol* 1999; in press.
8. Martin JL. The impact of AIDS on sexual behavior patterns in New York City. *Am J Public Health* 1987; 77: 578–581.
9. Binson D, Moskowitz J, Mills T, et al. Sampling men who have sex with men: Strategies for a telephone survey in urban areas in the United States. *Proc Am Stat Assoc* 1996; 68–72.
10. Catania JA, Binson D, Canchola J, et al. *Urban Men's Health Study: A Probability Survey of MSMs in Four Large Urban Centers*. Paper presented at the American Public Health Association Convention, Washington, DC; 1998.
11. Kalton G. Sampling considerations in research on HIV risk and illness. In: Ostrow DG, Kessler RC, eds. *Methodological Issues in AIDS Behavioral Research*. New York: Plenum Press; 1993:53–75.
12. Deren S, Stephens R, Davis WR, et al. The impact of providing incentives for attendance at AIDS prevention sessions. *Public Health Rep* 1994; 109:548–554.

13. Fishbein M. Editorial: Great expectations, or do we ask too much from community-level interventions? *Am J Public Health* 1996; 86:1075–1076.
14. National Institutes of Health. *Consensus Conference on HIV Prevention.* Washington, DC: USDHHS, Government Printing Office; 1997.
15. Kippax S. A commentary on negotiated safety. *Venereology* 1996; 96–98.
16. Ostrow DG. Risk reduction for transmission of human immunodeficiency virus in high-risk communities. *Psychiatric Med* 1989 7:79–96.
17. Joseph JG, Montgomery SB, Ostrow DG, et al. Assessing the costs and benefits of an increased sense of vulnerability to AIDS in a cohort of gay men. In: Temoshok K, Baum A, eds. *Psychosocial Perspectives on AIDS. Etiology, Prevention and Treatment.* Hillsdale, NJ: Lawrence Erlbaum Associates; 1990:65–79.
18. Somlai AM, Kelly JA, McAuliffe TI, et al. Role play assessments of sexual assertiveness skills: Relationships with HIV/AIDS sexual risk behavior practices. *AIDS Behav* 1998; 4:319–328.
19. Brody S. Patients misrepresenting their risk factors for AIDS. *Int J STD AIDS* 1995; 6:392–398.
20. Brody S. Heterosexual transmission of HIV. *N Engl J Med* 1995; 331:1718.
21. DiFrancesico W, McAuliffe TL, Sikkema KJ. Influences of survey instrument format and social desirability on the reliability of self-reported high risk sexual behavior. *AIDS Behav* 1998; 4:329–337.
22. Crowne D, Marlowe D. A new scale of social desirability independent of psychopathology. *J Consult Clin Psychol* 1960; 24:349–354.
23. Ostrow DG, DiFrancesico WJ, Chmiel JS, et al. A case–control study of human immunodeficiency virus type 1 seroconversion and risk-related behaviors in the Chicago MACS/CCS cohort, 1984–1992. *Am J Epidemiol* 1995; 142:875–883.
24. Catania JA, Gibson D, Chitwood D, Coates TJ. Methodological problems in AIDS behavioral research: Influences on measurement error and participation bias in studies of sexual behavior. *Psychol Bull* 1990; 108:339–362.
25. James NJ, Bignell CJ, Gillies PA. The reliability of self reported sexual behavior. *AIDS* 1991; 5:333–336.
26. Bradburn N, Sudman S. *Improving Interview Method and Questionnaire Design.* San Francisco: Jossey Bass; 1979.
27. Analysis of sexual behaviour in France. A comparison between two modes of investigation: Telephone survey and face-to-face survey. *AIDS* 1992; 6:315–323.
28. Nebot M, Celentano DD, Burwell L, et al. AIDS and behavioural risk factors in women in inner city Baltimore: A comparison of telephone and face-to-face surveys. *J Epidemiol Community Health* 1994; 48:412–418.
29. Boekeloo B, Schiavo L, Rabin DL, et al. Self-reports of HIV risk factors by patients at a sexually transmitted disease clinic: audio vs. written questionnaires. *Am J Public Health* 1994; 84:754–760.
30. Carey MP, Maisto SA, Kalichman SC, et al. Enhancing motivation to reduce risk for HIV infection for economically disadvantaged urban women. *J Consult Clin Psychol* 1997; 65:531–541.
31. Hobfoll SE, Jackson AP, Lavin J, et al. Reducing inner city women's AIDS risk activities: A study of single, pregnant women. *Health Psychol* 1994; 13:397–403.
32. Kalichman SC, Sikkema KJ, Kelly JA, Bulto M. Use of a brief behavioral skills intervention to prevent HIV infection among chronic mentally ill adults. *Psychiatric Services* 1995; 46:275–280.
33. Turner CF, Ku L, Rogers SM, et al. Adolescent sexual behavior, drug use, and violence: Increased reporting with computer survey technology. *Science* 1998; 280:867–873.
34. Midanik L, Hines A, Barrett D, et al. Self-reports of alcohol use, drug use and sexual behavior: Expanding the timeline follow-back technique. *J Stud Alcohol* 1998; 59:681–689.
35. Coxon APM. *Between the Sheets: Sexual Diaries and Gay Men's Sex in the Era of AIDS.* London: Casswell Press; 1996.
36. Metzger DS, Koblin B, Turner C, et al. A randomized controlled trial of audio-assisted computer self-interviewing: Impact, feasibility, and acceptability. 1999, in preparation.
37. McFall RM. Effects of self monitoring on normal smoking behavior. *J Consult Clin Psychol* 1970; 35:135–142.
38. Webb GR, Redman S, Gibberd RW, et al. The reliability and stability of a quantity frequency method and a diary method of measuring alcohol consumption. *Drug Alcohol Depend* 1991; 27:223–231.
39. Persky H, Strauss D, Lief HI, et al. Effects of the research process on human sexual behavior. *J Psychiatry Res* 1981; 16:41–52.
40. Reading AE. A comparison of the accuracy and reactivity of methods of monitoring male sexual behavior. *J Behav Assess* 1983; 5:11–23.
41. Fujita BN, Wagner NN, Perthous N, Pion RJ. The effects of an interview on attitudes and behavior. *J Sex Res* 1971; 7:138–152.
42. Halpern CT, Udry JR, Suchindran C. Effects of repeated questionnaire administration in longitudinal studies of adolescent males' sexual behavior. *Arch Sex Behav* 1994; 23:41–57.

43. Ostrow DG, Vanable PA, McKirnan DJ, Brown L. Hepatitis and HIV risk among DU-MSMs: Demonstration of Hart's law of inverse access and application to HIV. *Journal of Gay & Lesbian Medical Association* 1999; 4: 127–135.

44. The National Institute of Mental Health (NIMH) Multisite HIV Prevention Trial Group. The NIMH Multisite HIV Prevention Trial: Reducing HIV sexual risk behavior. *Science* 1998; 280:1889–1894.

45. Rotheram-Borus MJ, Koopman C, Haignere C. Reducing HIV sexual risk behaviors among runaway adolescents. *JAMA* 1991; 266:1237–1241.

46. Kelly JA, St. Lawrence JS, Brasfield TL. Predictors of vulnerability to AIDS risk behavior relapse. *J Consult Clin Psychol* 1991; 59:163–166.

47. Samuel MC, Hessol N, Shiboski S, et al. Factors associated with human immunodeficiency virus seroconversion in homosexual men in three San Francisco cohort studies, 1984–1989. *J Acquir Immune Defic Syndr* 1993; 6: 303–312.

48. McAuliffe T, Kelly JA. The measurement of HIV risk exposure based on sexual behavior pattern: A summary HIV risk index score. In: *XI International Conference on AIDS*. Vancouver, BC, July 1996.

49. St. Lawrence JS, Eldridge G, Shelby M, et al. HIV risk reduction for incarcerated women: A comparison of brief interventions based on two theoretical models. *J Consult Clin Psychol* 1997; 65:504–509.

50. Valdiserri RO, Lyter D, Leviton L, et al. AIDS prevention in homosexual and bisexual men: Results of a randomized trial evaluating two risk reduction interventions. *AIDS* 1989; 3:21–26.

51. DiFranceisco W, Ostrow DG, Adib DS, et al. Predictors of long-term maintenance of safer sex and lapse/relapse: A nine-year follow-up of the Chicago CCS/MACS cohort. *AIDS Behav* 1999; 3:325–334.

52. Cooper MI. Alcohol and human sexuality: Review and integration. *Alcohol Health Res World* 1992; 16:64–72.

53. Gold RS, Skinner MJ, Grant PJ, Plummer DC. Situational factors and thought processes associated with unprotected intercourse in gay men. *Psychol Health* 1991; 5:259–278.

54. McKirnan DJ, Ostrow DG, Hope B. Sex, drugs, and escape: A psychological model of HIV-risk behaviors. *AIDS Care* 1996; 8:655–669.

55. Ostrow DJ, McKirnan D. Prevention of substance-related high-risk sexual behavior among gay men: Critical Review of the literature and proposed harm reduction approach. *J Gay Lesbian Med Assoc* 1997; 1:97–110.

56. Flay B, Petraitis J. The theory of triadic influence: A new theory of health behavior with implications for preventive interventions. *Adv Med Sociol* 1994; 4:19–44.

57. Betancourt H, Lopez SR. The study of culture, ethnicity, and race in American psychology. *Am Psychol* 1993; 48:629–637.

58. Agar M, MacDonald J. Focus groups and ethnography. *Human Organ* 1995; 54:78–86.

59. Denzin N. *The Research Act*, 2nd ed. New York: McGraw-Hill; 1978.

60. Jick T. Mixing qualitative and quantitative methods: Triangulation in action. In: VanMaanen J, ed. *Qualitative Methodology*. London: Sage; 1983.

61. Blumenthal R, Watters J. Multimethod research from targeted sampling to HIV risk environments. In: Lambert R, Ashery RS, Needle R, eds. *Qualitative Methods in Drug Abuse and HIV Research*. NIDA Research Monograph #157. DHHS Pub. No. 95-4025. Washington, DC: Superintendent of Documents; 1995.

62. Booth R, Koester S, Reichardt C, Brewster J. Quantitative and qualitative methods to assess behavioral change among injection drug users. *Drugs Soc* 1993; 7:161–183.

63. Bell B, McKirnan D, Ostrow DG, et al. Drug use in context and its relationship to sex among gay/bisexual men: Qualitative analysis of the formative AIM Project data. 1999; manuscript submitted.

Applications to Behavioral Interventions

School-Based Interventions to Prevent Unprotected Sex and HIV among Adolescents

DOUGLAS KIRBY

INTRODUCTION

Throughout history some adolescents have engaged in sexual intercourse and contracted a sexually transmitted disease (STD) or become pregnant. However, during the last century and especially during the last few decades, the average ages of menarche and spermarche have decreased and the average age of marriage has substantially increased, producing a gap between puberty and marriage of about 12 years for both males and females.[1] With the increase in the puberty–marriage gap, and also with the advent of more reliable contraceptives and with changes in beliefs about premarital sex, an increasingly large percentage of adolescents have decided to engage in sex prior to marriage. They have begun having sex at an increasingly early age. With an increasing number of years of sexual activity prior to marriage, their number of sexual partners also have increased. All these trends have led to greater possible exposure to STDs.

Sexual intercourse is rare among very young teenagers, but the proportion of teens who have had sexual intercourse increases rapidly with age. Among students in grades 9–12 across the United States in 1997, 48% reported ever having had sexual intercourse; this included 38% of the 9th graders and 61% of the 12th graders who reported having sex.[2]

The percentage of youth who had ever had sex by any given age increased steadily until about 1990, but then stabilized and even declined slightly.[1–3] This indicates that it is possible to reverse the continual decrease in age at first intercourse that occurred during previous decades.

Most teenagers do not have sexual intercourse with more than one sexual partner during any given period of time; that is, they most commonly practice serial monogamy.[1] However, their numbers of sexual partners accumulate over time. Among high school students in 1997, about 16% of students previously had had sexual intercourse with four or more sexual partners.[2]

Most sexually experienced teenagers use contraception, and condoms are the method of contraception most commonly used during first intercourse and among younger sexually experienced youth. In 1997, among 9th graders who had sex in the three preceding months, 59% reported using a condom the last time they had sex.[2] However, the use of condoms

DOUGLAS KIRBY • ETR Associates, Santa Cruz, California 95061.

Handbook of HIV Prevention, edited by Peterson and DiClemente.
Kluwer Academic/Plenum Publishers, New York, 2000.

declines somewhat with age and with sexual experience, and the use of oral contraceptives increases. Among seniors in high school in 1997, the use of condoms was only 52%.[2] Condoms are used disproportionately with casual partners and less commonly with more regular sexual partners. Although teen use of condoms decreases as individual teens become older, teen use of condoms has increased over the years, reflecting in part the advent of AIDS.[1,2]

According to some measures, teenagers use condoms or oral contraceptives as effectively as never-married females in their 20s.[1] However, like adults, many teenagers do not consistently use contraceptives properly, thereby exposing themselves to risks of STDs or pregnancy. For example, among females relying on condoms as their primary method of contraception, only 35% of 15- to 17-year-olds and 31% of 18- to 19-year-olds used a condom during every act of intercourse.

When adolescents are asked why they did not use contraception when they had sex, one of the most frequent responses is that they did not expect or plan to have sex, and thus were not prepared.[4,5] Adolescents say far less frequently that they cannot afford condoms or contraception, do not know where to get them, cannot get them, or do not know how to use them.

Because they have unprotected sex with multiple partners, about 3 million teenagers acquire an STD every year.[6] This represents roughly one in eight young people between the ages of 13 and 19 and about one in four of those who have ever had sexual intercourse. In addition, about 25% of all young people have become infected by an STD by age 21.[7] Sexually active adolescents have the highest age-specific rates for some STDs, for example, chlamydia.[8]

Between July 1997 and June 1998, 15% of all new HIV cases were among young people ages 13 to 24.[9] Notably, of these cases, 63% were among African-American youth and another 20% were among Hispanic youth. About half of these new cases were among females,[9] and about half of their infections were transmitted heterosexually.[10]

ANTECEDENTS OF ADOLESCENT SEXUAL AND CONTRACEPTIVE BEHAVIORS

During the last three decades many researchers have studied the antecedents of these adolescent sexual behaviors, in part to inform the development of effective programs. These studies have been summarized in numerous reports.[11–15]

The results of the research in this area demonstrate that there are a multitude of antecedents that are related to sexual behavior (age of initiation of sex, frequency of sex, or number of sexual partners) and use of condoms or other kinds of contraception. These antecedents include characteristics of the adolescents themselves, their peers, romantic partners, families, schools, communities and states.[11,12] No single one antecedent is highly related to behavior; rather, each of many antecedents is weakly (or occasionally moderately) related to behavior.

The antecedents can be divided roughly into three groups. The first group includes some of the antecedents that are most strongly related to sexual behaviors—the biological antecedents, for example, gender,[1] age,[1] testosterone level,[16,17] and pubertal timing.[18] They are both causally and moderately related to adolescent sexual behavior. However, for all practical purposes, these cannot be modified by social programs.

The second group includes various beliefs, attitudes, and norms directly related to sexual behavior, for example, permissive attitudes toward premarital sex,[19] perceptions that friends have sex,[20] norms toward number of sexual partners,[21] knowledge about acquired immunodeficiency syndrome (AIDS),[22] attitudes toward condoms,[23] embarrassment getting condoms,[24] self-efficacy in using condoms,[25] peer norms about condom use,[25] perceived costs of using condoms,[25] perceived efficacy in using condoms,[25] and perceived susceptibility to STD and human immunodeficiency virus (HIV).[25] Concern about pregnancy—especially perceived male responsibility for the prevention of pregnancy—was also related to condom use.[26] Although the results differ with the study, most of these antecedents are weakly or moderately related to actual sexual and contraceptive behaviors. These are the antecedents that are most commonly addressed by sexuality and HIV education programs.

Finally, the third group includes a remarkably large proportion of the remaining risk factors: those involving some aspect or manifestation of social disorganization at the community, family, or individual level. For example, at the community level, youths at greatest risk of initiating sex early, having multiple partners, or having unprotected sex are more likely to live in communities with high residential turnover,[27] low levels of education,[27] high poverty rates,[28] high divorce rates,[27] and high rates of adolescent nonmarital births.[27] Similarly, the parents of these youth have lower levels of education,[14] are poorer,[27,29] are more likely to have experienced a divorce or separation or to be single,[29,30] and their mothers are more likely to have given birth as adolescents.[31] In addition, their parents' child-rearing practices are poorer,[32,33] and the adolescents receive less support or supervision from their parents.[34] The youths themselves invest less effort in school,[35] do more poorly in school,[27,35,36] and have lower expectations for their future.[37] They are more likely to use alcohol and drugs excessively, and to engage in other unconventional and unhealthful behaviors.[36–40] They experience sexual pressure or even abuse.[41,42] Depending on the study and level of analysis, some of these antecedents are strongly related to sexual behavior, while others are only weakly related.

SCHOOL-BASED PROGRAMS

Numerous school-based programs have been developed to address these antecedents, especially the second group of antecedents. These programs have included sexuality education and HIV education programs, school-based clinics, school condom availability programs, and other more comprehensive programs to reduce adolescent sexual risk-taking behavior.

For a variety of reasons, schools have the potential for playing an important role in reducing sexual risk taking behaviors among adolescents. Schools are the one institution in our society regularly attended by most young people; nearly 95% of all youth aged 5–17 years are enrolled in elementary or secondary schools.[43] Moreover, virtually all youth are attending schools before they initiate sexual risk-taking behaviors, and a majority are enrolled at the time they initiate intercourse. Additionally, schools are especially well suited to educate youth, particularly about topic areas such as sexuality in which different concepts should be taught during different developmental stages. They are also well designed to involve youth in programs that may motivate them to delay early childbearing. Finally, schools are capable of identifying at-risk youth and then either providing health and social services directly or referring them for these services.

For decades there has been and continues to be widespread support for sexuality and HIV education in schools. For example, in 1988, a Harris poll indicated that 85% of adults approved of sexuality education in schools.[44] Further, a 1999 Hickman–Brown national opinion poll found that 93% of adults supported sexuality education in schools and 90% thought condoms should be covered.[45]

The approval for sexuality and HIV education also is manifested in state policy: 23 states require that sexuality education be taught in schools, while an additional 15 states require that schools offer STD/HIV education.[46,47] In addition, 47 states either recommend or require the teaching of sexuality education, while all 50 states recommend or require AIDS education programs.[48,49] Thus, the controversies surrounding sexuality and HIV education programs do not focus on whether these programs should be offered in school but rather on what topics should be taught. Some groups believe that only abstinence until marriage should be emphasized, whereas other groups believe that contraception and other topics related to sexuality should be covered.

There also has been considerable support for the provision of condoms or contraceptives through school condom availability programs and school-based health centers. For example, a 1991 Roper poll indicated that 64% of American adults favored making condoms available in high schools,[50] and a 1999 poll found that 53% of adults thought school personnel should make condoms available for sexually active young people.[45]

Given the need for effective educational programs and public support for such programs, schools have responded. A vast majority of junior and senior high schools have implemented programs aimed to reduce unprotected sexual intercourse, either by delaying the onset of intercourse or by increasing the use of protection against HIV, other STDs, and pregnancy. By far the most common programs are sexuality education and HIV prevention programs. Indeed, according to a 1994 national study by the Centers for Disease Control and Prevention (CDC), approximately 86% of all schools surveyed required instruction on HIV prevention and 80% required instruction on human sexuality.[51] Additionally, some schools have school-based or school-linked health centers, some of which provide contraceptives. Other schools have implemented school condom availability programs to increase youth access to condoms. Still others have implemented multicomponent programs, which typically include an educational component and a component aimed to increase access to condoms or other contraceptives.

STUDIES UNDER REVIEW

This chapter reviews the published research on these school-based programs, focusing primarily on their impact on sexual and contraceptive behaviors. A total of 40 studies are included, which represent the studies known by the author that meet the following five conditions: (1) they focused on school-based programs (or curriculum-based programs that could be implemented in schools); (2) they employed experimental or quasi-experimental designs; (3) they measured program impact on sexual or contraceptive behavior or pregnancy rates; (4) they had a sample size of at least 90; and (5) they have been published as major reports or have been published in peer-reviewed journals or volumes.

Not surprisingly, the quality of the research methods employed and the strength of the resulting evidence for the impact of the programs vary greatly from study to study. For example, to minimize selection biases, some studies used random assignment of youth to the intervention or comparison conditions, whereas others did not. Some studies involved large sample sizes to ensure adequate statistical power in detecting statistically significant results, while others used relatively small samples, reducing the chance for finding programmatically significant differences. Some measured program effects for only 3 months, while others measured longer-term impact up to 24 months. And finally, some used more rigorous statistical analyses, while others failed to control statistically for design limitations. Because of this variation in quality, the strength of the evidence from each study should be considered when reviewing the results. Additionally, the strengths of any conclusions about the impact of programs are confined by the limitations both of individual studies and of all the studies as a group.

CURRICULUM-BASED SEX AND HIV EDUCATION PROGRAMS

Most adolescents in this country know a considerable amount about the risks of un-protected sexual intercourse and methods of preventing those risks. For example, nearly all youth know that unprotected sexual intercourse can lead to pregnancy or STD, and most know that condoms can be obtained at stores and provide protection against pregnancy and STD. They learn this and other information through a variety of sources, such as their school sex and HIV education programs, the media, their parents and other adults, their peers, and others. Indeed, innumerable studies have demonstrated that sex and HIV/AIDS education programs do increase knowledge. Unfortunately, research suggests that despite this knowledge, youth continue to practice behaviors that put them at risk for pregnancy, HIV, and other STDs.

As a result of the increasing body of research on the effectiveness of curriculum-based programs, it is now possible to formulate preliminary conclusions regarding their impact on sexual risk behaviors and to analyze characteristics that distinguish effective from ineffective programs.

Abstinence-Only Programs

Abstinence-only programs focus on the importance of abstinence from sexual inter-course, typically abstinence until marriage. Either these programs do not discuss contraception or they briefly discuss contraceptive failure to provide complete protection against pregnancy and STD. To date, six studies of abstinence programs have been published.[52–57]

Five of the studies measured impact on initiation of sex, none found both a consistent and significant impact on delaying the onset of intercourse, and at least one study provided strong evidence that the program did not delay the onset of intercourse.[52–56] Thus, the weight of the evidence indicates that these abstinence programs do not delay the onset of intercourse.

On the other hand, this evidence is not strong, because all but one of these evaluations had significant methodological limitations that could have obscured program impact. For example, two of the studies measured the impact of the program for only 6 weeks after the end of the program, and during that brief period of time too few youth in the comparison group initiated sex in order for the program group to have had significantly fewer youth initiate sex.[52,55] Other studies included as few as 91 study participants.[53] Given these limitations, there is too little evidence to determine whether or not different types of abstinence programs can delay the onset of intercourse.

Sex and HIV Education Programs That Include Both Abstinence and Contraception

These programs differ from the abstinence-only programs in that they discuss both condoms and other methods of contraception as methods of providing protection against STDs or pregnancy. This group includes a wide variety of programs, ranging from sex or AIDS education programs taught during school classes, to those taught on school campuses but after school, to programs implemented in community settings. Because some of the programs originally evaluated in community settings are now taught in classroom settings, they also are included in this review, even though their original evaluations were not school based. Twenty-five studies meet the criteria above.

Although this chapter will focus primarily on the impact of programs on behavior, it should be noted that nearly all evaluations of programs have demonstrated that programs do increase students' knowledge about different aspects of sexuality and contraception. Although this knowledge may or may not lead to behavior change, it does help build a foundation for better decision-making.

Impact on Sexual Activity

The studies of these programs strongly support the conclusion that sexuality and HIV education curricula do not increase sexual intercourse, either by hastening the onset of intercourse or by increasing the frequency of intercourse. Of the 21 evaluations of middle school, high school, or community sexuality or HIV education programs that measured the impact of the programs on the initiation of intercourse, none found that their respective programs significantly hastened the onset of intercourse.[58–75]

Similarly, none of the 14 studies that examined the impact of programs upon the frequency of intercourse found a significant increase.[58,61,63–69,72,76–78] Thus, these data strongly indicate that sex and HIV education programs do not significantly increase sexual activity as some people have feared.

Furthermore, these studies indicate that some but not all of these programs reduced sexual behavior, either by delaying the onset of intercourse or reducing the frequency of intercourse. Seven of the 21 studies that examined the impact of programs on the initiation of intercourse found evidence that their respective programs significantly delayed the onset of intercourse.[60–62,64,66,70,72] Similarly, 7 of the 14 studies that measured program impact on frequency of intercourse found evidence that their programs reduced the frequency of intercourse.[61,63,64,68,72,78]

Impact on Number of Partners

Consistent with the results regarding impact on the initiation and frequency of sexual activity, none of the ten studies that examined impact on number of sexual partners found a significant increase.[58,63,67–69,72,76,79,80] To the contrary, three of the studies that measured impact on the number of sexual partners found that programs decreased the number of partners.[63,69,72]

Impact on Use of Condoms and Other Contraception

These studies suggest that some but not all of the programs increased condom use or contraceptive use more generally. Nine of the 15 studies that examined program impact on condom use found that the programs did increase some measure of condom use.[7,58,63,64,66–69,72,75–77,79,80] Similarly, 5 of the 11 studies that examined program impact on the use of contraception more generally found significant positive results.[58,59,62,65–67,70,73,74,78,81] In combination, these results are quite positive, indicating that some sex and HIV education programs can significantly increase condom or contraceptive use, while other programs do not.

A disproportionate number of the programs that significantly increased condom or contraceptive use were AIDS education programs. Eight of the eleven AIDS education programs found significant effects on condom use, while only 5 out of the 11 sex education programs found significant effects. It cannot yet be determined whether AIDS education programs are inherently more effective than sex education programs that cover pregnancy, STD, HIV, and other topics, or whether AIDS education programs simply have been better funded, had better training, had studies with larger sample sizes, targeted youth who voluntarily participated, or had some other advantage that might improve measured results.

The data also suggest that these sex and AIDS education programs may be more effective with African Americans than with other ethnic groups. The only curricula for middle school-aged youth that have presented positive results are Postponing Sexual Involvement, Healthy Oakland Teens, and the Jemmotts' curricula. Notably, all achieved positive results when implemented among African-American youth. When Postponing Sexual Involvement was implemented among many different ethnic groups in California, no impact was found. In addition, both Be Proud Be Responsible and Be a Responsible Teen, two of the four curricula with the strongest evidence for effectiveness, were implemented among African-American youth. Because HIV is more prevalent among heterosexual African Americans than among heterosexual whites or Hispanics, African Americans may be more receptive to the messages of these AIDS curricula.

It also may be the case that curricula are simply more effective with high-risk youth, regardless of their ethnicity. This may be partly programmatic and partly statistical. When large percentages of youth initiate sex within short periods of time or fail to use condoms consistently, it is easier both programmatically and certainly statistically for the intervention group to do statistically better than the control group. For example, if only 10% of the control group initiates sex within a year, then the intervention must have a very large proportional effect or the sample size must be very large in order for the program impact to be statistically significant. In contrast, if 40% of the control group initiates sex within a year, then either the intervention does not have to have such a large proportional impact or the sample size can be smaller in order for the impact to be significant.

Effective Curricula and Their Common Characteristics

These studies of educational programs raise important questions: What curricula are the most effective at changing sexual risk-taking behaviors, either by delaying or reducing sexual activity or by increasing use of condoms? What are their characteristics?

There are four curricula with particularly strong evidence demonstrating that they reduce adolescent sexual risk taking in some manner. One of these has been evaluated twice by independent research teams in different states and found to be effective,[82] while the remaining three employed very strong experimental designs.[83–86] Two of these three were actually implemented in a community setting and are discussed in the preceding chapter.[85,86] However, both of them are curriculum based and both can be (and are) implemented in school settings.

When these four curricula and other curricula with less strong evidence of success are compared with curricula without positive behavioral results, the effective curricula share several characteristics, which may be linked to their success, while the ineffective curricula lack one or more of these characteristics. These characteristics were first published by a panel of experts selected by CDC[87] and subsequently updated by the author. Some of them have also been identified in other reviews of impact studies.[11,88,89] These characteristics reflect different aspects of effective pedagogy. In addition, they are similar to the characteristics of educational programs found to be effective at reducing substance abuse.[90]

The ten characteristics are as follows:

1. *Effective programs focused on reducing one or more sexual behaviors that lead to unintended pregnancy or HIV/STD infection.* These programs focused narrowly on a small number of specific behavioral goals, such as delaying the initiation of intercourse or using condoms or other forms of contraception; relatively little time was spent addressing other

sexuality issues, such as gender roles, dating, and/or parenthood. Nearly every activity was directed toward these behavioral goals.

Few studies evaluated the impact of a focused and potentially effective curriculum unit that was embedded in a larger more comprehensive sexuality education program. Such units may or may not be as effective. Their effectiveness cannot be known until additional research is completed.

2. *Effective programs were based on theoretical approaches that have been demonstrated to be effective in influencing other health-related risky behaviors*, for example, social cognitive theory,[91] social influence theory,[92] social inoculation theory,[93] cognitive behavioral theory,[76,91] and the theory of reasoned action.[94] These theories address many of the individual sexuality-related antecedents of sexual behavior. Thus, these programs strive to go far beyond the cognitive level; they focus on recognizing social influences, changing individual values, changing group norms, and building social skills.

These theories specified the particular antecedents that the interventions strived to change. Because interventions cannot directly change adolescent sexual behavior, they tried to change the antecedents of sexual behavior—the beliefs, attitudes, norms, self-efficacies, and skills—so that changes in these antecedents would lead to voluntary change in sexual or contraceptive behavior. Thus, each activity was designed to change one or more antecedents specified by the particular theoretical model for the curriculum, and every important antecedent in the theoretical model was addressed by one or more activities.

3. *Effective programs gave a clear message by continually reinforcing a clear stance on these behaviors*. This particular characteristic appeared to be one of the most important criteria that distinguished effective from ineffective curricula. Effective curricula did not simply lay out the pros and cons of different sexual choices and implicitly let the students decide which was right for them; rather, most of the curriculum activities were directed toward convincing the students that abstaining from sex, using condoms, or using other forms of contraception was the right choice. To the extent possible, they tried to use group activities to change group norms about what was the expected behavior.

4. *Effective programs provided basic, accurate information about the risks of unprotected intercourse and methods of avoiding unprotected intercourse*. Although increasing knowledge was not the primary goal of these programs, effective programs provided basic information that students needed to assess risks and avoid unprotected sex. Typically, this information was not unnecessarily detailed or comprehensive. For example, the curricula did not provide detailed information about all methods of contraception or different types of STD. Instead, they provided a foundation; they emphasized the basic facts needed to make behaviorally relevant decisions and they provided information that would lead to changes in beliefs, attitudes, and perceptions of peer norms. Some curricula also provided more detailed information about how to use condoms correctly.

5. *Effective programs included activities that address social pressures on sexual behaviors*. These activities took a variety of forms. For example, several curricula discussed situations that might lead to sex. Most of the curricula discussed "lines" that are typically used to get someone to have sex and some discussed how to overcome social barriers to using condoms (e.g., embarrassment about buying condoms). Some also addressed peer norms about having sex or using condoms. For example, some curricula provided data showing that many youth do not have sex or do use condoms, or they had students engage in activities in which they concluded that students should abstain from sex or use condoms and then expressed those beliefs to other students.

6. *Effective programs provided modeling and practice of communication, negotiation, and refusal skills.* Typically, the programs provided information about skills, modeled effective use of skills, and then provided some type of skill rehearsal and practice (e.g., verbal role-playing and written practice). Some curricula taught different ways to say no to sex or unprotected sex, how to insist on the use of condoms, how to use body language that reenforced the verbal message, how to repeatedly refuse sex or insist on condom use, how to use condoms in a more erotic manner, how to suggest alternative activities, and how to help build the relationship while refusing unprotected sex.

7. *Effective programs employed a variety of teaching methods designed to involve the participants and have them personalize the information.* Instructors reached students through active learning methods of instruction, not through didactic instruction. Students were involved in numerous experiential classroom and homework activities: small-group discussions, games, or simulations; brainstorming; behavioral rehearsal (role-playing); written rehearsal; verbal feedback and coaching; locating contraception in local drugstores; visiting or telephoning family planning clinics; and interviewing parents. In addition to these experiential activities, a few effective curricula used peer educators or videos with characters (either real or acted) who resembled the students and with whom the students could identify. All these activities kept the students more involved in the program, got them to think about the issues, and helped them personalize the information, that is, to apply it to their own lives.

8. *Effective programs incorporated behavioral goals, teaching methods, and materials that were appropriate to the age, sexual experience, and culture of the students.* For example, programs for younger youth, few of whom had engaged in intercourse, focused on delaying the onset of intercourse. Programs designed for high school students, some of whom had engaged in intercourse, emphasized that students should avoid unprotected intercourse, either by not having sex or by using contraception if they did have sex. Programs for higher-risk youth, most of whom were already sexually active, emphasized the importance of using condoms and avoiding high-risk situations. Some of the curricula were designed for specific racial or ethnic groups and emphasized statistics, values, and approaches that were tailored to those groups.

9. *Effective programs lasted a sufficient length of time to complete important activities adequately.* In general, it requires considerable time and multiple activities to change the multiple antecedents of sexual risk-taking behavior. Thus, the short programs that lasted only a couple of hours did not appear to be effective, while longer programs that implemented multiple activities had a greater effect. More specifically, effective programs tended to fall into two categories: those that lasted 14 or more hours and those that lasted a fewer number of hours but were implemented in small-group settings with a leader for each group. The latter type may have been able to involve the youth more completely, to tailor the material to each group, and to cover more material and more concerns more quickly in each group.

10. *Effective programs selected teachers or peers who believed in the program they were implementing and then provided training for those individuals.* The training ranged from approximately 6 hours to 3 days. In general, the training was designed to give teachers and peers information on the program as well as practice using the teaching strategies included in the curricula (e.g., conducting role-playing exercises and leading group discussions). Some of the teachers in these effective programs also received coaching and/or follow-up training to improve the effectiveness of their teaching.

Despite these commonalities, there is little evidence regarding which factor or combinations of factors contribute most to the overall success of the programs. For example, simply increasing knowledge is not likely to change behavior. However, to assume that the positive behavioral effects resulted from just the skill practice or the instruction on social influences would be premature.

In summary, the data from abstinence, sex education, and HIV prevention programs indicate that education programs do not increase sexual intercourse, either by hastening the onset of intercourse, increasing the frequency of intercourse, or increasing the number of sexual partners. The data also indicate that some but not all programs may either reduce one or more measures of sexual activity or increase use of condoms or other forms of contraception. However, there are severe limitations to these studies.

SCHOOL-BASED AND SCHOOL-LINKED HEALTH CENTERS

School-based health centers are clinics located in schools that offer services to students in their respective schools; school-linked clinics are adolescent clinics located near schools that provide many of the same services and can be integrated into the schools. These clinics typically provide basic primary health care services; some of them also dispense contraceptives. When these clinics are well staffed and well run and dispense contraceptives, they have many of the characteristics of ideal reproductive health programs, for example, their location is convenient to the students, they can reach both females and males, they provide comprehensive health services, they are confidential, their staff is selected and trained to work with adolescents, they can easily conduct follow-up, their services are cost-free, and they can integrate education, counseling, and medical services. On the other hand, they may not easily reach older males, the males who are most likely to father children born to adolescent females.

School-based and school-linked clinics do provide contraceptives to substantial percentages of sexually experienced youth. For example, in a study of four clinics that provided prescriptions or actually dispensed contraceptives, the proportion of sexually experienced females who obtained contraceptives through the clinic varied from 23 to 40%.[95]

Six studies have examined the impact of these health centers.[95–100] Five of these studies examined programs in three or more schools. The outcomes they measured and their quasi-experimental designs varied considerably. In general, the quasi-experimental designs were not strong. For example, some did not collect baseline data and some did not have equivalent comparison groups or comparison groups at all. In addition, these studies measured population effects. That is, they measured the effects on the entire school population and not just on those students who actually used the clinics for family planning services. Consequently, inferences should be drawn cautiously from these studies.

Three of these studies measured the impact of school-based clinics and school-linked clinics on sexual and contraceptive behaviors.[95,98,100] They evaluated the impact of 6 clinics, 19 clinics, and 1 clinic, respectively. The Kirby et al.[95] study found that the presence of the clinic did not affect the onset of sexual intercourse either positively or negatively. In contrast, both the Kisker et al.[98] study and the Zabin et al.[100] study found some data indicating that the clinic and its educational programs may have delayed the onset of intercourse. The Kirby et al.[95] study and the Kisker et al.[98] study also found that clinic presence was not associated with greater frequency of intercourse. In combination, these studies indicate that providing contraceptives on campus does not hasten the onset of intercourse or increase its frequency, as some people have feared.

Regarding contraceptive use, the Kisker et al.[98] study produced the most negative results:

clinic presence was associated with lower rates of contraceptive use. It is not clear what produced this anomalous result, but it should be noted that this study did have important limitations, for example, baseline data could not be collected.

The results of the Kirby et al.[95] study were more mixed. At one site where the clinic focused on high-risk youths, emphasized pregnancy prevention, and dispensed oral contraceptives, there was a significantly greater use of oral contraceptives among females than among females in the comparison school; there was no significant difference in condom use. At two other sites that dispensed both condoms and oral contraceptives but did not have strong educational components, no significant differences were found between the clinic and comparison schools in use of condoms by male students or use of oral contraceptives by female students. At these schools there clearly were substitution effects; even though many sexually experienced students obtained contraception from the clinics, most of those students would have obtained them elsewhere if the clinics had not been there. The Zabin et al.[100] study found that clinic presence was associated with greater use of contraception.

In sum, these data consistently demonstrate that providing contraceptives in school-based or school-linked clinics does not hasten or increase student sexual activity. Data also indicate that these clinics do provide contraceptives to substantial numbers of sexually experienced students in their schools. Other results are more mixed. Although one study did report increased contraceptive use after a clinic was opened, the weight of the evidence suggests that these clinics do not increase schoolwide contraceptive use significantly. To the contrary, the data indicate that there is a large substitution effect, although not all students who obtained contraceptives from the clinics would have obtained them elsewhere.

SCHOOL CONDOM AVAILABILITY PROGRAMS

Given the threat of AIDS, as well as the threat of other STDs and pregnancy, more than 300 schools without school-based clinics have begun making condoms available through school counselors, nurses, teachers, vending machines, or baskets.[101] These schools are in addition to the 92 schools that make condoms available to students through school-based clinics.

The number of condoms obtained by students from schools varies greatly from program to program; in some schools students obtain very few condoms from the school, while in other schools, they obtain large numbers.[101] In general, students in smaller alternative schools obtain many more condoms per student than students in larger schools or students in mainstream schools. In addition, when schools make condoms available in baskets (a barrier-free method), students obtain many more condoms than when they must obtain condoms from school personnel or from vending machines. Finally, if schools have clinics, students obtain many more condoms than when schools do not have clinics.

Thus far, four studies have presented results on the effects on behavior of school condom availability. The study with the strongest evaluation design evaluated the effects of making condoms available through vending machines in five Seattle schools without school-based clinics and through vending machines and baskets in five additional Seattle schools with preexisting school-based clinics. Schoolwide data were collected both before condoms were made available in the schools and then again 2 years later. In neither group of schools was there an increase in either sexual activity or use of condoms during last intercourse.[102] Notably, these schools had an educational intervention, but because it existed prior to the baseline data collection, the effect of the educational component was not measured.

A second study measured the impact of making condoms available in baskets in nine Philadelphia schools.[103] Students in those schools could receive reproductive health information, condoms, and general health referrals. Both before and after the centers were opened, youths were randomly selected for personal interviews from census tracts surrounding these nine schools and other comparison schools. Results revealed that in the schools with centers, changes over time on four measures of sexual behavior or condom use were not significantly different from the changes over time in the schools without centers. However, the authors noted that there were nonsignificant differences in the trends over time in the desired directions (i.e., students in schools with centers reduced their sexual activity and increased their condom use more than students in schools without centers). Relatively small samples may have limited the ability to detect programmatically meaningful results.

The third study evaluated a New York program. The school district implemented a comprehensive AIDS prevention program in the city high schools. It included additional instruction about AIDS, schoolwide activities, and condom availability. Because baseline data could not be collected in New York, analyses compared students in New York schools with a matched sample from Chicago schools. Results indicated that students in the New York schools were not more likely to have initiated intercourse but were more likely to have used a condom the last time they had sex than were Chicago students.[104]

Finally, the fourth study measured the impact of making condoms available in baskets in a single high school in Los Angeles.[105] Schoolwide data were collected both before and after the condoms were made available. A change in school policy, however, required a change from passive parental consent to active parental consent, and thus a much smaller percentage of the students completed the posttest survey than the pretest survey. Comparison of the pretest and posttest surveys indicated that there was not a significant change in the percent of students who had ever had sex or in the frequency of sexual activity. However, among males sexually active during the year, there was an increase in the percent who used a condom every time they had sex, and among males who recently had initiated intercourse there was an increase in the percent who used a condom the first time they had sex. There were no significant changes, however, among females.

In summary, the results from these studies are similar to those of school-based clinics; they confirm that making condoms available on school campuses does not increase sexual activity, but their impact on use of condoms is mixed. It is unclear why results suggest that school condom availability may have increased condom use in New York and Los Angeles, but not in Seattle.

MULTICOMPONENT PROGRAMS

One program included multiple components, some of which were implemented in the schools. It was designed to reduce pregnancy in a small rural South Carolina community.[106,107] Teachers, administrators, and community leaders were given training in sexuality education; sex education was integrated into all grades in the schools; peer counselors were trained; the school nurse counseled students, provided male students with condoms, and took female students to a nearby family planning clinic; and finally, local media, churches, and other community organizations highlighted special events and reinforced the messages of avoiding unintended pregnancy. After the program was implemented, the pregnancy rate for 14- to 17-year-olds declined significantly for several years. After parts of the program ended (for example, the school nurse resigned, linkages to contraceptives were terminated, and some teachers left the school), the pregnancy rates returned to preprogram levels.

Although this program and its evaluation focused on pregnancy, not STD or HIV, it is informative for several reasons. It indicates that it is possible to (1) implement larger, more comprehensive programs addressing adolescent sexual behavior, (2) include condom availability in such programs, and (3) have a sufficiently large impact on adolescent sexual activity and contraceptive use that pregnancy rates apparently declined.

YOUTH DEVELOPMENT PROGRAMS

Youth development programs represent an alternative way for schools (and communities) to reduce adolescent sexual risk-taking behavior. Youth development programs do not focus primarily on sexuality, as do traditional sex and HIV education programs. Instead, they are more holistic and strive to improve adolescents' life skills and belief in their future more generally. In one sense, they address some of the third group of antecedents discussed above: those involving various manifestations of poverty and social disorganization. Some programs embodying a youth development framework strive to provide mechanisms for youth to fulfill their basic needs, including a sense of safety and structure, a sense of belonging and group membership, a sense of self-worth and contribution, a sense of independence and control over one's life, a sense of closeness and relationships with peers and nurturing adults, and a sense of competence. Fulfilling these needs cannot be done quickly or sporadically; thus, some youth development programs strive to change multiple facets of adolescents' lives over a continuous and prolonged period of time.

Thus far, there are no studies that have examined the impact of youth development programs on adolescent sexual behavior, condom use, or STD rates. However, there are four studies that have examined the impact of these programs on pregnancy or birth rates and found that they significantly reduced these rates. These include the Youth Incentive Entitlement Pilot Projects (YIEPP),[108] the Teen Outreach Program,[109,110] the Quantum Opportunities Project (QOP),[111] and the American Conservation and Youth Service Corps.[112]

Notably these programs varied considerably. One focused primarily on employment (YIEPP). Another provided volunteer community service with ongoing discussions with a caring adult (TOP). A third, Quantum Opportunities, was much more comprehensive and included educational activities (e.g., tutoring, computer-based instruction, homework assistance); service activities (e.g., community service projects, assistance at public events, regular jobs); and development activities (curriculum on life and family skills, and college and job planning). The fourth, the American Youth and Conservation Corps, provided remedial, vocational, and academic education coupled with work experience and community service.

Because studies have not yet examined the impact of these programs on sexual behavior, condom use, and STD rates, they should be viewed cautiously as a partial solution to unprotected sex and STD. On the other hand, because some of them did reduce pregnancy or childbearing, it is certainly plausible that they reduced sexual behavior that would have placed them at risk of STD and HIV. In addition, some youth development programs have reduced substance use and other risk taking behaviors that are associated with sexual risk-taking, and they increased other educational and social behaviors that are associated with lower levels of sexual risk-taking. Thus, their possible role in preventing STD and HIV warrants further examination.

SUMMARY AND CONCLUSIONS

Although this chapter has reviewed many studies, several factors limit the conclusions that can be drawn from these studies. First, given the complexity of adolescent sexual behavior and the diversity of programs addressing this behavior, there are simply too few studies evaluating the effectiveness of each of the different approaches. This research challenge is increased by the fact that programs are implemented in different settings with different target groups, and their success may vary with setting and target population.

Second, some but not all of these studies were limited by methodological problems or constraints. Some studies did not use experimental designs, and thus suffered from self-selection effects, had sample sizes that were too small, and thus failed to detect programmatically important outcomes or may have produced anomalous results; or did not use proper analytic techniques. Thus, the results that are published are undoubtedly biased in unknown ways.

Third, there are very few replications of evaluations. When they have occurred, the subsequent studies sometimes found the same success in reducing risk-taking behavior and other times failed to replicate the previous positive results.

Given these important caveats about the evaluations of programs, conclusions about the impact of programs must be expressed somewhat cautiously. Nevertheless, there do exist several conclusions well supported by these studies:

1. The overwhelming weight of the evidence demonstrates that programs that focus on sexuality, including sex and AIDS education programs, school-based clinics, and condom availability programs, do not cause harm, as some people fear. None of the evaluations of any program found significant results indicating that any of them increased any measure of sexual activity.

2. Nearly all sex and AIDS education programs that have been evaluated have produced some outcome deemed socially desirable by our society, for example, an increase in knowledge. Studies of some programs have produced credible evidence that their respective programs reduced sexual risk-taking behavior either by delaying sex, reducing the frequency of sex, reducing the number of sexual partners, or increasing the use of either condoms or other forms of contraception. Studies of other sex and AIDS education programs have failed to find positive effects on behavior. The ten characteristics discussed above may distinguish effective from ineffective programs.

3. Even though abstinence-only programs may be appropriate for many youth, especially middle-school youth, currently there does not exist any evidence that they have actually delayed the onset of sexual intercourse or reduced any other measure of sexual intercourse. At this point, their impact on sexual behavior is simply unknown. Because abstinence-only programs are very heterogeneous, it is too early to reach any conclusions about their impact on sexual or contraceptive behavior.

4. Substantial percentages of sexually experienced female students in schools with school-based or school-linked clinics obtain contraceptives from those clinics; nonetheless, the weight of the evidence indicates that these clinics typically do not increase significantly the schoolwide proportion of students using contraception, nor do they decrease the schoolwide pregnancy and birth rates significantly.

5. There are few studies of school condom availability programs, and those studies provide inconsistent results. If schools provide condoms in a manner that reduces barriers to obtaining condoms (e.g., through baskets in clinic bathrooms), then students obtain large numbers of condoms from that source. However, studies have produced mixed results regarding the impact of school condom availability on actual condom use.

6. Studies of some youth development programs that address the multitude of non-sexual risk factors associated with adolescent unprotected sexual behavior indicate

that those programs have reduced unprotected sex sufficiently to reduce pregnancy or birth rates. These results are very encouraging, but the impact of these programs on condom use and STD needs to be evaluated.

In conclusion, these studies demonstrate that reducing adolescent sexual risk-taking behavior and STDs, including HIV, is challenging. Sex and HIV education programs, and even programs that provide condoms or contraceptives in schools are not likely to have a dramatic impact upon STD and HIV transmission, given the existing knowledge base of youth and the relatively widespread availability of condoms in stores. Clearly, these programs are not a complete solution to reducing unprotected sexual intercourse.

On the other hand, studies also indicate that some programs can have some success and can modestly reduce one or more sexual behaviors. Some programs may have a somewhat larger impact on high-risk youth, a particularly important group. Thus, sex and HIV education programs may be an important component in a larger more comprehensive initiative to reduce adolescent sexual risk-taking behavior, STD, and HIV.

ACKNOWLEDGMENT. This chapter has been adapted from *No Easy Answers: Research Findings on Programs to Reduce Teen Pregnancy*. Washington, DC: The National Campaign to Prevent Teenage Pregnancy in Washington, DC, 1997.

REFERENCES

1. Alan Guttmacher Institute. *Sex and America's Teenagers*. New York: Alan Guttmacher Institute; 1994.
2. Centers for Disease Control. Trends in sexual risk behaviors among high school students—United States, 1991–1997. *Morb Mortal Wkly Rep* 1998; 47(36):749–752.
3. Centers for Disease Control and Prevention. *Pregnancy, Sexually Transmitted Diseases, and Related Risk Behaviors among US Adolescents*. Atlanta: Centers for Disease Control and Prevention; 1995.
4. Kirby D, Waszak C, Ziegler J. *An Assessment of Six School-Based Clinics: Services, Impact and Potential*. Washington DC: Center for Population Options; 1989.
5. Princeton Survey Research Associates. *Kaiser Family Foundation Survey on Teens and Sex: What They Say Teens Today Need to Know, And Who They Listen To*. Menlo Park, CA: Kaiser Family Foundation; 1996.
6. Office of National AIDS Policy. *Youth and HIV/AIDS: An American Agenda*. Washington DC: Office of National AIDS Policy; March 1996.
7. Alan Guttmacher Institute. *Sex and America's Teenagers*. New York: Alan Guttmacher Institute; 1994:38.
8. Centers for Disease Control. *Sexually Transmitted Disease Surveillance 1997*. Atlanta: CDC, 1998.
9. Centers for Disease Control. *Young People at Risk: Epidemic Shifts Further Toward Young Women and Minorities*. Atlanta: CDC, 1998.
10. Office of National AIDS Policy. *Youth and HIV/AIDS: An American Agenda*. Washington DC: Office of National AIDS Policy; March 1996.
11. Kirby D. *No Easy Answers: Research Findings on Programs to Reduce Teen Pregnancy*. Washington, DC: National Campaign to Prevent Teen Pregnancy; 1997.
12. Kirby D. Looking for reasons why: The antecedents of adolescent sexual risk-taking, pregnancy, and childbearing. Washington, DC: National Campaign to Prevent Teen Pregnancy; 1999.
13. Miller BC. Risk factors for adolescent non-marital childbearing. In: *Report to Congress on Out-of-Wedlock Childbearing*. Washington, DC: Dept of Health and Human Services; 1995: 217–227, DHHS Pub. No. (PHS) 95-1257.
14. Moore KA, Sugland BW, Blumenthal C, et al. *Adolescent Pregnancy Prevention Programs: Interventions and Evaluations*. Washington, DC: Child Trends, Inc.; 1995.
15. Santelli JS, Beilenson P. Risk factors for adolescent sexual behavior, fertility, and sexually transmitted diseases. *J School Health* 1992; 62(7):271–279.

16. Halpern CT, Udry JR, Campbell B, Suchindran C. Testosterone and pubertal development as predictors of sexual activity: A panel analysis of adolescent males. *Psychosom Med* 1993; 55:436–447.

17. Udry JR. Biological predispositions and social control in adolescent sexual behavior. *Am Soc Rev* 1988; 53: 709–722.

18. Flannery D, Rowe D, Gulley B. Impact of pubertal status, timing and age on adolescent sexual experience and delinquency. *J Adolesc Res* 1993; 8(1):21–40.

19. Miller BC, McCoy JK, Olson TD. Dating age and stage as correlates of adolescent sexual attitudes and behavior. *J Adolesc Res* 1986; 1:361–371.

20. East PL. The younger sisters of childbearing adolescents: Their sexual and childbearing attitudes, expectations, and behaviors. Paper presented at the Society of Research on Adolescence; February 1994.

21. Basen-Engquist K, Parcel G. Attitudes, norms and self-efficacy: A model of adolescents' HIV-related sexual risk behavior. *Health Educ Q* 1992; 19(2):263–277.

22. Ku LC, Sonenstein FL, Pleck JH. The association of AIDS education and sex education with sexual behavior and condom use among teenage men. *Fam Plann Perspec* 1992; 24(3):100–106.

23. Hingson RW, Strunin L, Berlin BM, Heeren T. Beliefs about AIDS, use of alcohol, drugs and unprotected sex among Massachusetts adolescents. *Am J Public Health* 1990; 80:295–299.

24. McAnarney ER, Schreider C. *Identifying Social and Psychological Antecedents of Adolescent Pregnancy: The Contribution of Research to Concepts of Prevention.* New York: William T. Grant Foundation; 1984.

25. DiClemente RJ. Psychosocial determinants of condom use among adolescents. In: DiClemente R, ed. *Adolescents and AIDS: A Generation in Jeopardy.* Newbury Park: Sage; 1992:159–180.

26. Pleck JH, Sonenstein FL, Ku LC. Adolescent males' condom use: Relationships between perceived cost-benefits and consistency. *J Marriage Fam* 1991; 53:733–745.

27. Brewster KL, Billy JOG, Grady WR. Social context and adolescent behavior: The impact of community on the transition to sexual activity. *Soc Forces* 1993; 71:713–740.

28. Brewster K. Race differences in sexual activity among adolescent women: The role of neighborhood characteristics. *Am Soc Rev* 1994; 59:408–424.

29. Miller BC, Norton MC, Curtis T, et al. The timing of sexual intercourse among adolescents: Family, peer, and other antecedents. Paper presented at the Society for Research on Adolescence; February 1994.

30. Wu LL, Martinson BB. Family structure and the risk of a premarital birth. *Am Soc Rev* 1993; 58:210–232.

31. Sonenstein FL, Pleck JH, Ku LC. Cost and opportunity factors associated with pregnancy risk among adolescent males. Paper presented at the Annual Meeting of Population Association of America, Denver, Colorado; April 30, 1992.

32. Feldman S, Brown N. Family influences on adolescent male sexuality: The mediational role of self-restraint. *Soc Dev* 1993; 2(1):15–35.

33. Jaccard J, Dittus PJ, Gordon VV. Maternal correlates of adolescent sexual and contraceptive behavior. *Fam Plann Perspec* 1996; 28(4):159–165,185.

34. Esminger ME. Sexual activity and problem behaviors among black, urban adolescents. *Child Dev* 1990; 61:2032–2046.

35. Ohannessian C, Crockett L. A longitudinal investigation of the relationship between educational investment and adolescent sexual activity. *J Adolesc Res* 1993; 8(2):167–182.

36. Robbins C, Kaplan HB, Martin SS. Antecedents of pregnancy among unmarried adolescents. *J Marriage Fam* 1985; 47:567–583.

37. Whitley BE, Schofield JW. A meta-analysis of research on adolescent contraceptive use. *Pop Environ* 1986: 173–203.

38. Costa FM, Jessor R, Donovan JE, Fortenberry JD. Early initiation of sexual intercourse: The influence of psychosocial unconventionality. *J Res Adolesc* 1995; 5:91–121.

39. Hercog-Baron R, Harris KM, Armstrong K, et al. Factors differentiating effective use of contraception among adolescents. In: *Advances in Adolescent Mental Health*, vol. 4. Jessica Kingsley Publishers, Inc.; 1990.

40. Serbin LA, Peters PL, McAffer VJ, Schwartzman AE. Childhood aggression and withdrawal as predictors of adolescent pregnancy, early parenthood, and environmental risk for the next generation. *Can J Behav Sci* 1991; 23(3):318–331.

41. Boyer D, Fine D. Sexual abuse as a factor in adolescent pregnancy and child maltreatment. *Fam Plann Perspect* 1992; 24:4–11.

42. Miller BC, Monson BH, Norton MC. The effects of forced sexual intercourse on white female adolescents. *Child Abuse Neglect* 1995; 19(10):1289–1301.

43. National Center for Education Statistics. *Digest of Education Statistics, 1993.* Washington, DC: US Department of Education, Office of Educational Research and Improvement; 1993.

44. Louis Harris and Associates: Public Attitudes toward Teenage Pregnancy, Sex Education and Birth Control. Poll conducted for the Planned Parenthood Federation of America, New York; May 1988.

45. Haffner D, Wagoner J. Vast majority of Americans support sexuality education. *SIECUS Rep* 1999; 27(6): 22–23.

46. The NARAL Foundation. *Sexuality Education in American: A State-by-State Review*. Washington, DC: The NARAL Foundation; 1995.

47. The NARAL Foundation. *Who Decides? A State-by-State Review of Abortion and Reproductive Rights*. Washington, DC: The NARAL Foundation; 1997.

48. DeMauro D. Sexuality education 1990: A review of state sexuality and AIDS curricula. *SIECUS Rep* 1990; 18(2):1–9.

49. Gambrell AE, Haffner D. *Unfinished Business: A SIECUS Assessment of State Sexuality Education Programs*. New York: SIECUS; 1993.

50. Roper Organization, Inc. *AIDS: Public Attitudes and Education Needs*. New York: Gay Men's Health Crisis; 1991.

51. Collins JL, Leavy Small M, Kann L., et al. School health education. *J School Health* 1995; 65(8):302–311.

52. Christopher FS, Roosa MW. An evaluation of an adolescent pregnancy prevention program: Is "just say no" enough? *Fam Relations* 1990; 39:68–72.

53. Jorgensen SR, Potts V, Camp B. Project taking charge: Six-month follow-up of a pregnancy prevention program for early adolescents. *Fam Relations* 1993; 42:401–406.

54. Kirby D, Korpi M, Barth R, Cagampang H. *Evaluation of Education Now and Babies Later (ENABL): Final Report*. Berkeley: University of California, School of Social Welfare, Family Welfare Research Group; 1995.

55. Roosa M, Christopher S. Evaluation of an abstinence-only adolescent pregnancy prevention program: A replication. *Fam Relations* 1990; 39:363–367.

56. St. Pierre TL, Mark MM, Kaltreider DL, Aikin KJ. A 27-month evaluation of a sexual activity prevention program in Boys & Girls Clubs across the nation. *Fam Relations* 1995; 44:69–77.

57. Young M, Core-Gebhart P, Marx D. Abstinence-oriented sexuality education: Initial field tests of the Living Smart curriculum. *Fam Life Educ* 1992; 10(4):4–8.

58. Coyle KK, Basen-Enquist KM, Kirby DB, et al. Short-term impact Safer Choices: A multi-component school-based HIV, other STD and pregnancy prevention program. *J School Health* 1999; 69(5):181–188.

59. Eisen M, Zellman GL, McAlister AL. Evaluating the impact of a theory-based sexuality and contraceptive education program. *Fam Plann Perspect* 1990; 22:(6):261–271.

60. Ekstrand ML, Siegel DS, Nido V, et al. Peer-led AIDS prevention delays onset of sexual activity and changes peer norms among urban junior high school students. Presented at the XI International Conference on AIDS, Vancouver, Canada; July 1996.

61. Howard M, McCabe J. Helping teenagers postpone sexual involvement. *Fam Plann Perspec* 1990; 22:21–26.

62. Hubbard BM, Giese ML, Rainey J. A replication of Reducing the Risk, a theory-based sexuality curriculum for adolescents. *J School Health* 1998; 68(6):243–247.

63. Jemmott III JB, Jemmott LS, Fong GT. Reductions in HIV risk-associated sexual behaviors among black male adolescents: Effects of an AIDS prevention intervention. *Am J Public Health* 1992; 82(3):372–377.

64. Jemmott JB, Jemmott LS, Fong GT. Abstinence and safer sex: A randomized trial of HIV sexual risk-reduction interventions for young African-American adolescents. *JAMA* 1998; 279:(10):1529–1536.

65. Kirby D. *Sexuality Education: An Evaluation of Programs and Their Effects*. Santa Cruz, CA: Network Publications; 1984.

66. Kirby D, Barth R, Leland N, Fetro J. Reducing the risk: A new curriculum to prevent sexual risk-taking. *Fam Plann Perspec* 1991; 23(6):253–263.

67. Kirby D, Korpi M, Adivi C, Weissman J. An impact evaluation of SNAPP, a pregnancy- and AIDS-prevention middle school curriculum. *AIDS Prevent Educ* 1997; 9(suppl A):44–67.

68. Levy SR, Perhats C, Weeks K, et al. Impact of a school-based AIDS prevention program on risk and protective behavior for newly sexually active students. *J School Health* 1995; 65(4):145–151.

69. Main DS, Iverson DC, McGloin J, et al. Preventing HIV infection among adolescents: Evaluation of a school-based education program. *Prevent Med* 1994; 23:409–417.

70. Moberg DP, Piper DL. An outcome evaluation of project model health: A middle school health promotion program. *Health Educ Q* 1990; 17(1):37–51.

71. Nicholson HJ, Postrado LT. *Girls Incorporated Preventing Adolescent Pregnancy: A Program Development and Research Project*. New York: Girls Incorporated; 1991.

72. St. Lawrence JS, Jefferson KW, Alleyne E, Brasfield TL. Comparison of education versus behavioral skills training interventions in lowering sexual HIV risk behavior of substance dependent adolescents. *J Consult Clin Psychol* 1995; 63(2):221–237.

73. Thomas B, Mitchell A, Devlin M, et al. Small group sex education at school: The McMaster teen program. In: Miller B, Card J, Paikoff R, Peterson J, ed. *Preventing Adolescent Pregnancy*. Newbury Park, CA: Sage; 1992: 28–52.

74. Walker G, Vilella-Velez F. *Anatomy of a Demonstration*. Philadelphia, PA: Public/Private Ventures; 1992.

75. Walter HJ, Vaughn RD. AIDS risk reduction among a multi-ethnic sample of urban high school students. *JAMA* 1993; 270(6):725–730. Warren WK, King AJC. *Development and Evaluation of an AIDS/STD/Sexuality Program for Grade 9 Students*. Kingston, Ontario: Social Program Evaluation Group; 1994.

76. Kipke MD, Boyer C, Hein K. An evaluation of an AIDS risk reduction education and skills training (ARREST) program. *J Adolesc Health* 1993; 14:533–539.

77. Rotheram-Borus MJ, Koopman C, Haigners C, Davies M. Reducing HIV sexual risk behaviors among runaway adolescents. *JAMA* 1991; 266(9):1237–1241.

78. Smith MAB. Teen incentives program: Evaluation of a health promotion model for adolescent pregnancy prevention. *J Health Educ* 1994; 25(1):24–29.

79. Gillmore MR, Morrison DM, Richey CA, et al. Effects of a skill-based intervention to encourage condom use among high-risk heterosexually active adolescents. *AIDS Prevent Educ* 1997; 9(suppl A):44–67.

80. Magura S, Kang S, Shapiro JL. Outcomes of intensive AIDS education for male adolescent drug users in jail. *J Adolesc Health* 1994; 15:457–463.

81. Schinke S, Blythe B, Gilchrist L. Cognitive–behavioral prevention of adolescent pregnancy. *J Counsel Psychol* 1981; 28:451–454.

82. Barth RP. *Reducing the Risk*, 3rd ed. Santa Cruz, CA: ETR Publications; 1996.

83. Coyle KK, Fetro JV. *Safer Choices: Preventing HIV, Other STD and Pregnancy: Level 2*. Santa Cruz, CA: ETR Associate; 1998.

84. Fetro JV, Barth RB, Coyle KK. *Safer Choices: Preventing HIV, Other STD and Pregnancy: Level 1*. Santa Cruz, CA: ETR Associate; 1998.

85. Jemmott LS, Jemmott III JB, McCaffree KA. *Be Proud! Be Responsible!* New York: Select Media; 1994.

86. St. Lawrence JS. *Becoming a Responsible Teen: An HIV Risk Reduction Intervention for African-American Adolescents*. Jackson, MS: Jackson State University; 1994.

87. Kirby D, Short L, Collins J, et al. School-based programs to reduce sexual risk behaviors: A review of effectiveness. *Public Health Rep* 1994; 109(3):339–360.

88. Frost JJ, Forrest JD. Understanding the impact of effective teenage pregnancy prevention programs. *Fam Plann Perspec* 1995; 27(5):188–195.

89. Miller BC, Paikoff RL. Comparing adolescent pregnancy prevention programs: Methods and Results. In: Miller BC, Card JJ, Paikoff RL, Peterson JL, eds. *Preventing Adolescent Pregnancy*. Newbury Park, CA: Sage Publications; 1992.

90. Dusenbury L, Falco M. Eleven components of effective drug abuse prevention curricula. *J School Health* 1995; 65(10):420–425.

91. Bandura A. *Social Foundations of Thought and Action*. Englewood Cliffs, NJ: Prentice Hall; 1986.

92. McGuire W. Social Psychology. In: Dodwell PC, ed. *New Horizons in Psychology*. Middlesex, England: Penguin Books; 1972.

93. Homans GC. Group factors in worker productivity. In: Proshansky H, Seidenbert L, eds. *Basic Studies in Social Psychology*. New York: Holt, Reinhart & Winston; 1965.

94. Fishbein M, Ajzen I. *Belief, Attitude, Intention, and Behavior*. Reading MA: Addison-Wesley; 1975.

95. Kirby D, Waszak C, Ziegler J. Six school-based clinics: Their reproductive health services and impact on sexual behavior. *Family Plann Perspec* 1991; 23:6–16.

96. Edwards L, Steinman M, Arnold K, Hakanson E. Adolescent pregnancy prevention services in high school clinics. *Fam Plann Perspec* 1980; 12(1):6–14.

97. Kirby D, Resnick MD, Downes B, et al. The effects of school-based health clinics in St. Paul upon school-wide birth rates. *Fam Plann Perspec* 1993; 25(12):12–16.

98. Kisker EE, Brown RS, Hill J. *Health Caring: Outcomes of the Robert Wood Johnson Foundation's School-based Adolescent Health Care Program*. Princeton: Robert Wood Johnson Foundation; 1994.

99. Newcomer S, Duggan A. Do school-based clinics influence adolescent birth rates? Paper presented at the annual meetings of the Population Association of America. New Orleans; May 9, 1996.

100. Zabin LS, Hirsch MB, Streett R, et al. The Baltimore pregnancy prevention program for urban teenagers: How did it work? *Fam Plann Perspec* 1988; 20(4):182–187.

101. Kirby D, Brown N. School condom availability programs in the United States. *Fam Plann Perspec* 1996; 28(5): 196–202.

102. Kirby D, Brener ND, Brown NL, et al. The impact of condom distribution in Seattle schools on sexual behavior and condom use. *Am J Public Health* 1999; 89(2):182–187.

103. Furstenberg FF, Geitz LM, Teitler JO, Weiss CC. Does condom availability make a difference? An evaluation of Philadelphia's health resource centers. *Fam Plann Perspec* 1997; 29(3):123–127.

104. Guttmacher S, Lieberman L, Ward D, et al. Condom availability in New York City public high schools: Relationships to condom use and sexual behaviors. *Am J Public Health* 1997; 87(9):1427–1433.

105. Schuster MA, Bell RM, Berry SH, Kanouse DE. Impact of a high school condom availability program on sexual attitudes and behaviors. *Fam Plann Perspec* 1998; 30(2):67–72,88.

106. Koo HP, Dunteman GH, George C, et al. Reducing adolescent pregnancy through a school- and community-based intervention: Denmark, SC, revisited. *Fam Plann Perspec* 1994; (26):206–211,217.

107. Vincent M, Clearie A, Schluchter M. Reducing adolescent pregnancy through school and community-based education. *JAMA* 1987; 257(24):3382–3386.

108. Olsen R, Farkas G. The effects of economic opportunity and family background on adolescent cohabitation and childbearing among low-income blacks. *J Labor Econ* 1990; 8:341–362.

109. Allen JP, Philliber S, Hoggson N. School-based prevention of teen-age pregnancy and school dropout: Process evaluation of the national replication of the Teen Outreach Program. *Am J Community Psychol* 1990; 18(4): 505–524.

110. Allen JP, Philliber S, Herrling S, Kupermine GP. Preventing teen pregnancy and academic failure: Experimental evaluation of a developmentally-based approach. *Child Dev* 1997; 64(4):729–742.

111. Hahn A, Leavitt T, Aaron P. *Evaluation of the Quantum Opportunities Program (QOP): Did the Program Work?* Waltham, MA: Center for Human Resources, Brandeis University; 1994.

112. Jastrzab J, Masker J, Blomquist J, Orr L. *Youth Corps: Promising Strategies for Young People and Their Communities.* Cambridge, MA: Abt Associates Inc; 1997.

5

HIV Behavioral Interventions for Adolescents in Community Settings

JOHN B. JEMMOTT, III,
and LORETTA SWEET JEMMOTT

INTRODUCTION

Adolescence is a period of the life cycle characterized by biological, psychological, and social changes and transitions. There is growing concern that for many young people it is also a time of risks associated with sexual involvement. Adolescent pregnancy is a national concern, and far too many adolescents contract sexually transmitted infections, including infection with the human immunodeficiency virus (HIV)—the cause of acquired immunodeficiency syndrome (AIDS). In this chapter, we review research aimed at identifying effective interventions to reduce the risk of sexually transmitted HIV infections among adolescents in community settings.

THE RISK OF SEXUALLY TRANSMITTED HIV INFECTION AMONG ADOLESCENTS

That adolescents are at risk of sexually transmitted HIV infection is suggested by evidence from several sources. To be sure, adolescents represent less than 1% of the cumulative total reported AIDS cases[1] in the United States. However, about 18% of reported AIDS cases have involved young adults 20 to 29 years of age. Many of them were infected during adolescence, because about 10 to 12 years typically elapse between the time a person is infected with HIV and the appearance of the clinical signs sufficient to warrant a diagnosis of AIDS. Data on newly diagnosed cases of HIV infection from the 27 states requiring confidential reporting of persons with HIV infection suggest a high risk of HIV infection among adolescents. About 18% of the cumulative HIV infections reported through December 1997 occurred in young people 13 to 24 years of age.[1]

Rates of unintended pregnancy and sexually transmitted diseases (STDs) also suggest an elevated risk of HIV infection among adolescents. Despite recent reports that birth rates for adolescents have dropped,[2] adolescent pregnancy remains a national concern. Adolescent pregnancy rates in the United States remain among the highest in industrialized countries.[3]

JOHN B. JEMMOTT, III • Annenberg School for Communication, University of Pennsylvania, Philadelphia, Pennsylvania 19104.   *LORETTA SWEET JEMMOTT* • School of Nursing, University of Pennsylvania, Philadelphia, Pennsylvania 19104.

Handbook of HIV Prevention, edited by Peterson and DiClemente.
Kluwer Academic/Plenum Publishers, New York, 2000.

Rates of STDs, including syphilis, gonorrhea, and chlamydia, have been highest among adolescents.[4–5] Each year an STD is contracted by one in four sexually active adolescents—3 million adolescents.[3,6] This is astonishing when juxtaposed with the fact that not all adolescents are sexually experienced, and many who are sexually experienced have sexual intercourse infrequently.

These statistics on STDs and unintended pregnancy are consistent with data on adolescent sexual behavior. About 56% of adolescent women and 73% of adolescent men report having had sexual intercourse by the time they are 18 years of age.[3] The use of latex condoms[7–9] can reduce substantially the risk of STD, including HIV. Although condom use among adolescents has risen considerably since 1979,[10] far too many sexually active adolescents still fail to use condoms consistently.[10–13] The 1997 Youth Risk Behavior Survey revealed that only 57% of high school students reported using a condom the last time they had sexual intercourse.[14] Failure to use condoms is especially likely among adolescents who have been sexually active during early adolescence.[15–17]

The risk of sexually transmitted HIV infection is particularly great among African-American and Latino adolescents. These adolescents tend to be residents of low-income disenfranchised communities in inner-city neighborhoods, with poor access to health care of good quality.[18] African Americans comprise 15% of the US adolescent population 13 to 19 years of age, but 47% of AIDS cases in this population reported through December 1997 involved African Americans.[1] Latinos comprise 13% of the US adolescent population but 19% of adolescents with AIDS.

There also are important gender differences in the risk of HIV infection among adolescents.[1] Among adults, approximately 15% of people with AIDS are women. Among adolescents, there also is a gender difference in AIDS cases, but it is smaller. About 37% of reported adolescent AIDS cases have been among female adolescents. Moreover, gender and ethnicity interact to affect the prevalence of AIDS. The gender difference in the number of reported adolescent AIDS cases is much greater among white adolescents than among African-American or Latino adolescents.

FACTORS ASSOCIATED WITH ADOLESCENTS' HIV RISK-ASSOCIATED SEXUAL BEHAVIOR

The identification of the correlates and predictors of HIV risk-associated sexual behaviors is central to efforts to develop and implement effective interventions to change such behaviors. In this section, we will briefly summarize research on the factors associated with whether or not adolescents engage in HIV risk-associated sexual behaviors. Interventions that are based on a systematic understanding of the causes of behavior they seek to change are most likely to be effective. Systematic understanding of the causes of behavior flows from a theoretical model of behavior and empirical tests of theory-based hypotheses. Several theories have been applied to HIV risk-associated behavior, including the health belief model,[19] the theory of reasoned action,[20,21] the theory of planned behavior,[22–24] social cognitive theory,[25–27] protection motivation theory,[28] and the information–motivation–behavioral skills model.[29] There is considerable overlap in the constructs used in these theories, though sometimes seemingly similar constructs have different names in different theories.

We will organize the literature on correlates and predictors of HIV risk-associated sexual behavior in terms of the theory of planned behavior. The theory is illustrated in the Figure 1. According to the theory, behavior is the result of a psychological mediation process involving

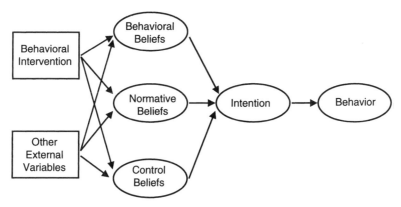

Figure 1. The theory of planned behavior.

intentions, beliefs, and external variables. Intentions are the sole direct determinant of behavior. Behavioral beliefs, normative beliefs, and self-efficacy beliefs influence intentions and, by so doing, indirectly influence behavior. Variables that are external to the theory have indirect effects on intentions and behavior by influencing the three classes of beliefs. In the language of the theory, a behavioral intervention would be one such external variable. Beliefs and consequentially intentions are mutable. They are potential targets of interventions designed to motivate reductions in HIV risk-associated behavior. Let us consider research bearing on intentions and the three classes of beliefs and then turn to research on several external variables.

Behavioral Intentions

Several studies provide evidence that intentions are strong predictors of sexual behavior, including condom use.[30–35] For instance, Adler and colleagues[30] found that intentions to use condoms significantly predicted condom use 12 months later. Stanton and colleagues[32] found that intentions regarding sexual intercourse in the next 6 months were predictive of subsequent self-reported sexual intercourse among African-American adolescents living in urban public housing. Evidence suggests that self-efficacy beliefs, behavioral beliefs, and normative beliefs are related to intentions.

Self-Efficacy Beliefs

Self-efficacy beliefs[25–27,36] concern individuals' perceptions of whether they can perform a specific behavior. Bandura[25–27] introduced this construct as part of his social cognitive theory, and it has subsequently been incorporated in other theoretical frameworks. Considerable evidence suggests a positive relation between adolescents' self-efficacy beliefs and their intentions to use condoms. For instance, Pendergrast et al.[37] found that confidence in the ability to use condoms was associated with greater intentions to use condoms in urban male adolescents. Basen-Engquist and Parcel[33] reported that self-efficacy was correlated with increased intentions to use condoms among 9th graders. Jemmott et al.[38] found that self-efficacy added a significant increment to the prediction of intentions among African-American and Latino adolescents.

Four types of self-efficacy beliefs have been distinguished. Availability beliefs concern adolescents' confidence that they can have condoms available when needed. Negotiation beliefs, which concern adolescents' confidence that they can persuade their sexual partners to use condoms, are perhaps most emphasized in HIV prevention research. Impulse control beliefs concern adolescents' confidence that they can control themselves enough to use condoms when sexually excited. A longitudinal study[39] has revealed that impulse control and self-efficacy predicted subsequent condom use among African-American adolescents in public housing. Technical skill beliefs concern adolescents' perceived ability to use condoms with facility and without ruining the mood. There is evidence that beliefs regarding technical skills to use condoms were related to stronger intentions to use condoms in African-American and Latino adolescents.[38]

Behavioral Beliefs

Behavioral beliefs concern individuals' perceptions of the consequences of engaging in a specific behavior. Behavioral beliefs are similar to the social cognitive theory construct of outcome expectancies and the health belief model constructs of response efficacy and costs and benefits of an act. Several studies have found that adolescents who believe that condom use is associated with negative consequences are less likely to report using condoms.[12,40-42]

Some studies distinguish between conceptually distinct types of behavioral beliefs. Hedonistic beliefs[43] are beliefs about the consequences of sexual activities for sexual enjoyment. Several studies have tied such beliefs to condom use or intentions to use condoms.[12,40,44-46] Prevention beliefs concern the perception that the use of condoms can reduce the risks of pregnancy and STD, including HIV infection. Such beliefs have been associated with condom use in several studies. For example, specific knowledge about the behaviors that cause pregnancy or STD is associated with a lower frequency of such behaviors among adolescents.[11-13] Perceptions of "condom efficacy" have been associated with more consistent condom use among adolescents.[41]

Normative Beliefs

Normative beliefs reflect the influence of other people as mediated through the individuals' perceptions of their opinions and desires. Normative beliefs concern individuals' perceptions of whether important referents would approve or disapprove of their engaging in the behavior. This would include perceived peer pressure or social support. Basen-Engquist and Parcel[33] reported that adolescents who perceived more normative support for condom use expressed stronger intentions to use condoms than did those who perceived less normative support for condom use. In addition, several studies suggest that perceived norms and the perceived approval of important referents are related to self-reported condom use.[12,39,42,47]

Given that HIV risk-associated sexual behaviors require at least a modicum of cooperation from another person, sexual partners should be important referents. Consistent with this, several studies have found that adolescents who perceived that their sexual partner would approve of the use of condoms expressed stronger intentions to use condoms than did other adolescents.[37,38,44] Longitudinal studies have tied perceived sexual partner approval of condom use to subsequent self-reported condom use among adolescents.[45,48]

Other significant referents who may affect adolescents' risky sexual behavior include friends or peers and family members.[49-51] Jemmott et al.[38] found that normative beliefs regarding mother's approval of condom use were associated with higher intentions to use condoms. Although Jemmott et al.[38] found that perceived approval of friends was not related to intentions to use condoms, some studies[47] reveal more consistent condom use among adolescents who perceive peer norms supporting condom use.

External Variables

Variables that are not a part of the theory of planned behavior but that may affect adolescents' HIV risk-associated sexual behavior are external variables. The notion is similar to the use of modifying factors in the health belief model. External variables and modifying factors can be demographic and psychosocial variables that are not mutable. They may be important for several reasons. External variables help identify adolescents who are more likely to engage in HIV risk-associated sexual behavior. They may be important antecedents of self-efficacy, behavioral, or normative beliefs. They may determine the relative influence on intentions of different beliefs. Consider ethnicity, for instance. Different ethnic groups might vary in how strongly they hold particular beliefs and in the strength of the relation between such beliefs and intentions.[52] In this view, behavioral beliefs may be more important predictors than normative beliefs for one ethnic group, whereas normative beliefs may be more important predictors than behavioral beliefs in another ethnic group.

Among the potentially important external variables in the prediction of HIV risk-associated sexual behavior are age and a close correlate of age, sexual experience. Older adolescents are more likely to report having had sexual intercourse than are younger adolescents.[14] Older adolescents have higher rates of STD and pregnancy.[5,14,53] In addition, several studies reveal that older adolescents and those who have more sexual experience are less likely to use condoms than are younger or less sexually experienced adolescents.[11–13,39,45,54] There also is evidence of a negative relation between the age of an adolescent's sexual partner and condom use.[55] Reduced condom use among older more experienced adolescents is accompanied by an increased use of birth control pills as a method of contraception.[13,42,45,54] The decreased use of condoms and increased use of birth control pills associated with age may reflect a greater concern among adolescents with pregnancy prevention rather than STD prevention.

Race and ethnicity also are important external variables. Adolescent pregnancy rates and STD rates are substantially higher among African Americans and Latinos than among whites.[5,14,53] National surveys of adolescents[10,14,56] have consistently indicated that a greater proportion of African-American adolescents compared with whites or Latinos report sexual experience. However, differences in sexual behavior cannot entirely explain the racial gap in STD rates. Although the percentage of high school students who reported having sexual intercourse during their lifetime with four or more partners was higher among African-American adolescents than among white or Latino adolescents, African-American high school students were more likely to report that either they or their partner used a condom during most recent sexual intercourse than were white or Latino high school students. Other possible explanations for racial and ethnic differences in STD rates include socioeconomic status, access to and utilization of health care, and varying risk of STDs among sexual networks.[6]

Gender also is significantly related to HIV risk-associated sexual behavior. Male adolescents are more likely to report ever having sexual intercourse and a larger number of sexual partners than are female adolescents.[14] On the other hand, several studies have found that adolescent males reported higher rates of condom use than did adolescent females.[14,57] For instance, in the 1997 Youth Risk Behavior Survey, 62% of males but only 51% of females reported that they or their sexual partner used a condom during their most recent sexual intercourse.[14] This is a somewhat puzzling finding. If it is assumed that the male and female adolescents in the sample were part of the same sexual network, why do they not report similar rates of condom use?

One possible explanation for the sex difference is that males are responding in a socially desirable fashion. The trouble with this explanation is that there is no reason to believe that adolescent males are more prone to socially desirable responding than are adolescent females. Indeed, one could easily argue the opposite, that female adolescents are more keen to seek social approbation. Moreover, male adolescents do not report greater use of other forms of contraception than do female adolescents. For instance, in the 1997 Youth Risk Behavior Survey, 20% of adolescent females but only 13% of adolescent males reported that birth control pills were used before their most recent sexual intercourse.[14] We would argue that another possible reason for the sex difference in reported condom use is sex differences in responsibility for condom use. To the extent that male adolescents are more likely than are their female sexual partners to buy condoms or otherwise acquire condoms, carry condoms, put condoms on, and remove condoms, they may more likely to remember that condoms were used. Condom use, then, may be an "event" for males but less of an event for females.

Another potentially important external variable is involvement in a steady romantic relationship. Adolescents perceive that they are at low risk and that it is unnecessary to use condoms for protection from disease. Consistent with this, studies have found that adolescent females reported less consistent use of condoms with steady sexual partners than with casual partners.[58] In addition, there is evidence that as the duration of adolescents' relationship increases, their self-reported use of condoms decreases.[48]

Alcohol and drug use also are related to sexual behavior among adolescents. Several studies have found that adolescents who use alcohol or illicit drugs are more likely to report having sexual intercourse, less likely to report using condoms, and more likely to report a large number of sexual partners.[12,59–61] Alcohol and drug use may impair adolescents' judgment during sexual encounters, which increases the likelihood that they engage in high-risk behavior. On the other hand, it may be that adolescents who engage in one problem behavior (i.e., substance use) are likely to engage in another problem behavior (i.e., sexual intercourse).

One of the most frequently considered potential predictors of HIV risk-associated behavior is knowledge. Although it is often stated that knowledge is not sufficient to induce health-promoting behavior, this is somewhat of an overstatement. "Knowledge" can be in many different domains that may vary in relevance to risk behavior. The knowledge that one is unlikely to contract HIV by hugging a person who has AIDS is irrelevant to risk of HIV infection. In contrast, knowledge about the correct way to use condoms is relevant to risk reduction.

A number of studies have examined the relation of perceived vulnerability to HIV risk-associated behavior.[6,62] The results have been inconsistent. Some studies have found that adolescents who perceive themselves to be at higher risk of infection are more likely to use condoms. Other studies find that those who perceive themselves to be at lower risk are more likely to use condoms. Still other studies have found no relationship. There is the added complexity that although perceived risk is seen as a predictor of behavior according to some theoretical frameworks (e.g., health belief model), it also may be a consequence of behavior.[62] In other words, adolescents who engage in high-risk behavior may consequently perceive themselves to be at higher risk of infection.

In summary, then, a host of variables have been considered as possible correlates and predictors of HIV risk-associated sexual behaviors. The theory of planned behavior provides a theoretical framework that can incorporate all of these variables. Many of the variables are mutable and, as we shall see, have been targeted by interventions as potential mediators of behavior change. Others have been examined as moderators of intervention effects.

BEHAVIORAL INTERVENTIONS TO REDUCE THE RISK OF SEXUALLY TRANSMITTED HIV INFECTION: KEY CHARACTERISTICS OF STUDIES

In this section, we review studies that tested behavioral interventions to curb HIV risk-associated sexual behavior among adolescents in community settings. Studies were included in the review if they had a sample whose mean age was between 10 and 21 years, compared an intervention group with a comparison group, and reported results for at least one behavioral outcome. An article by Gillmore and colleagues[63] reported data on two different samples, and therefore each sample was treated as a study. The characteristics of the studies are summarized in Table 1.

Study Designs

A total of 21 independent studies are represented in Table 1. As the table shows, 12 of the 21 studies were randomized, controlled trials in which individual adolescents were randomly assigned to conditions. Four were randomized trials in which groups of adolescents were randomly assigned to conditions. Five were nonrandomized intervention studies that included a control group. The follow-up data collection periods ranged from 1 month to 24 months postintervention. The most common follow-ups reported were 6-months postintervention (52%) and 3-months postintervention (48%). Six studies (29%) reported follow-ups of 12 or more months postintervention, including two studies with 24-month follow-ups.

Sample Characteristics

The samples included a wide range of ages within adolescence. Adolescence is traditionally divided into three developmental stages: early adolescence (11–13 years of age), middle adolescence (14–16 years of age), and late adolescence (17 years of age to early 20s). The youngest mean age in any study was 11.4 years; the oldest was 20.1 years. Several studies were conducted with the adolescents in each of these stages, but the majority of studies (53%) were conducted with youth in late adolescence.

African Americans and Latinos are at disproportionate risk of HIV infection. Although African Americans are well represented in these intervention studies, there is a paucity of studies on Latino adolescents. One half of the studies included no Latino participants; only one study had a majority of Latino participants. Participants in these studies were recruited from a wide range of settings, including clinics, college campuses, juvenile detention facilities, community-based organizations, schools, recreational centers in public housing developments, and homeless shelters.

Sample Sizes

The initial sample sizes in the 21 studies ranged from 43 to 659. A total of 18 studies provided data on participant attrition. Among these studies, attrition was relatively low. For example, attrition at short-term follow-up, defined as 6 months or less postintervention, ranged from 3 to 46%, with a mean of 20%. Two thirds of the studies had less than 25% attrition. Some

Table 1. Characteristics of 21 HIV Intervention Studies Conducted with Adolescents in Community Settings

Author (year)	N (% women)	Race-ethnicity	Source	Conditions
Randomized controlled trials—individuals as the unit				
Ricket et al.[91] (1990)	75 (100%), age range = 13–21	53% African American, 47% white	Clinic	1. 40-min AIDS lecture and video 2. 15-min AIDS lecture only 3. No-treatment control
St. Lawrence et al.[72] (1995)	246 (72%), mean age = 15.3	100% African American	Clinic	1. 8-session, 18-hour AIDS intervention 2. 1-session, 2-hour education-only control
Orr et al.[96] (1996)	209 (100%), mean age = 17.4	55% African American, 45% white	Clinic	1. 1-session, 20-min AIDS intervention 2. No-treatment control
Bryan et al.[34] (1996)	198 (100%), mean age = 18.6	3% African American, 5% Asian, 8% Latino, 79% white, 4% American Indian	College campus	1. 45-min condom motivation 2. 45-min exercise control
Sanderson and Jemmott[79] (1996)	136 (64%), mean age = 19.8		College campus	1. AIDS communication skills 2. AIDS technical skills 3. Waiting-list control
Sikkema et al.[83] (1995)	43 (100%), mean age = 20.1	5% African American, 95% white	College campus	1. 4-session, 5.5 hour AIDS intervention 2. 1-session, 1.5 hour education-only control
Stone et al.[65] (1994)	72 (56%), mean age = 19.2	21% Asian, 9% Latino, 70% white	College campus	1. Dissonance-arousing AIDS intervention 2. Commitment-only control 3. Mindful-only control 4. Information-only control
Rotheram-Borus et al.[86] (1998)	151 (58%), mean age = 18.1	53% African American, 39% Latino	Community	1. 7-session, 10-hour AIDS intervention 2. 3-session, 10-hour AIDS intervention 3. No-treatment control
Kirby et al.[75] (1997; community sample)	554 (58%), mean age = 12.8	9% African American, 13% Asian, 30% Latino, 39% white	Community	1. 5-session, 4.5-hour abstinence intervention 2. No-treatment control
Jemmott et al.[80] (1992)	157 (0%), mean age = 14.6	100% African American	School/community	1. 1-session, 5-hour AIDS intervention 2. 1-session, 5-hour career opportunities control

Study	Sample	Race/ethnicity	Setting	Intervention conditions
Jemmott et al.[70] (in press)	496 (54%), mean age = 13.2	100% African American	School	1. 1-session, 5-hour AIDS intervention 2. 1-session, 5-hour general health promotion control
Jemmott et al.[69] (1998)	659 (53%), mean age = 11.8	100% African American	School	1. 2-session, 8-hour safer sex AIDS intervention 2. 2-session, 8-hour abstinence-based AIDS intervention 3. 2-session, 8-hour general health promotion control
Randomized controlled trials—Groups as the unit				
Gillmore et al.[63] (1997, clinic sample)	168 (58%), mean age = 17.1	46% African American, 54% white	Clinic	1. 27-min AIDS video 2. 16-page comic book control
Gillmore et al.[63] (1997, juvenile detention sample)	228 (46%), mean age = 15.7	52% African American, 48% white	Juvenile detention	1. 2-session, 8-hour AIDS intervention 2. 27-min AIDS video 3. 16-page comic book control
Fisher et al.[90] (1996)	134 (51), median age = 20.0	3% African American, 4% Asian, 3% Latino, 88% white	College	1. 3-session, 6-hour AIDS intervention 2. No-treatment control
Stanton et al.[76] (1996)	383 (44%), mean age = 11.4	100% African American	Community	1. 8-session, 18-hour AIDS intervention in friendship groups 2. 8-session, 18 hour AIDS intervention not theory based, not in friendship groups
Nonramdomized control group trials				
O'Leary et al.[82] (1996)	347 (66%), mean age = 18.6	23% African American, 15% Asian, 13% Latino, 44% white	College campus	1. AIDS intervention 2. No-treatment control
Rotheram-Borus et al.[71] (1991)	197 (64%), mean age = 15.5	64% African American, 22% Latino, 8% white	Community	1. 20-session, 35-hour AIDS intervention 2. No-treatment control
Sellers et al.[73] (1994)	586 (48%), age range = 14–20	100% Latino	Community	1. AIDS intervention 2. No-treatment control
St. Pierre et al.[74] (1995)	359 (25%), mean age = 13.6	42% African American, 14% Latino, 45% white	Community	1. 3-session, 4.5 hours abstinence-only intervention 2. No-treatment control
Magura et al.[101] (1994)	238 (0%), mean age = 17.8	65% African American, 33% Latino, 2% white	Juvenile detention	1. 4-session, 4-hour AIDS intervention 2. Waiting list control

analyses were performed on subsets of the samples. For example, analyses of condom use were performed only on the subset of participants who had had sexual intercourse during the time period referenced. Because sexual activity among adolescents, particularly young adolescents, is sporadic, this subset was often relatively small. In analyses of condom use in which the investigator desires to control for baseline condom use, the sample size can be especially small. To be included in such an analysis, a participant would have to have had sex both in the period before the intervention and in the period after the intervention.

Interventions

The interventions in these studies varied considerably in the dose of content to which participants were exposed. Although the median number of intervention sessions was 2 and the mode was 1, the total number of intervention sessions ranged from 1 to 20. The number of contact hours of intervention ranged from about 0.3 hours to 35 hours, with a median of 4.5 hours.

Theoretical Frameworks

Efforts to dissuade adolescents from engaging in HIV risk-associated behavior may be most effective if they have a solid theoretical foundation. Theory is important in the identification of effective intervention strategies. By measuring the theoretical mediators of intervention-induced behavior change, a better conceptual understanding of risk behavior can emerge. If an intervention is ineffective, assessment of theoretical mediators can inform the analysis of why it is ineffective. The studies in this review used a variety of theoretical frameworks. The most common theoretical frameworks were cognitive behavioral theory, social cognitive theory, the theory of reasoned action, the health belief model, and theories that build on them, including the theory of planned behavior, the information–motivation–behavior model, and protection motivation theory. A theoretical framework could not be discerned for two of the studies. Some studies relied on more than one theoretical framework. A common combination was the social cognitive theory and the theory of reasoned action. Cognitive behavioral models in general and the social cognitive theory, theory of reasoned action, and health belief model have been used successfully in a variety of health behavior domains. One study used a theoretical framework that is seldom applied to health behavior—dissonance theory,[64]—which formed the theoretical foundation for an intervention by Stone and colleagues.[65]

Behavioral Outcomes

For a complete picture of behavior change, it would be optimal to measure behavioral outcomes and putative mediators of behavioral change. Both types of variables would have to be measured in a study to provide the best evidence regarding the mediation of intervention effects. All the studies except two measured at least one mediator variable. Although the overwhelming majority of studies measured behavioral outcomes and mediators, they varied in the specific behavioral outcomes and mediators they assessed. The most frequently used behavioral outcomes in the studies reviewed were frequency of condom use (62%) and number of sexual partners (52%). Other behavioral outcomes included condom acquisition, frequency of unprotected sexual intercourse, abstinence, frequency of sexual intercourse, number of sexual partners, and frequency of anal intercourse.

Mediator Variables

The most common mediators were self-efficacy, which was assessed in 62% of the studies, attitudes and intentions assessed in 48% of the studies, knowledge and hedonistic beliefs assessed in 43% of the studies, and perceived vulnerability assessed in 34% of the studies. Although skill development is an important component of several interventions, only three studies (14%) reported data on behavioral skill assessment. This may reflect the logistical difficulties in obtaining measures of skill acquisition as opposed to self-reported behavior.

EFFECTS OF INTERVENTIONS ON BEHAVIORAL OUTCOMES

We used meta-analytic techniques[66,67] to estimate intervention effect sizes. A strength of this approach is that it allows for an estimate of the magnitude and direction of the intervention effect on each outcome. This estimate is based on the results of all studies that included the outcome independent of sample size or statistical power[68] in any single study.

To estimate effect size, we computed Cohen's *d*, a standardized mean difference statistic for comparing differences between means.[68] It is the mean of one group (e.g., the intervention group) minus the mean of a second group (e.g., the control group), all divided by their pooled standard deviation. We followed the convention of assigning a plus sign to effect size estimates that are in the predicted direction (e.g., the HIV intervention is better than the control) and a minus sign to effect size estimates that are in the unpredicted direction (e.g., the HIV intervention is worse than the control). For example, an effect size of 0.25 would indicate that an intervention group scored one quarter of 1 standard deviation (SD) higher on the outcome variable than did the control group with which it is compared. We computed effect sizes using the formula presented by Cohen[68] when means and SDs were available or using the formulas presented by Rosenthal[66] when only a *t*, χ^2, or *F* statistic or *P* value was available. In most cases, this involved calculating a correlation coefficient based on a test statistic or *P* value and the total population size or degrees of freedom and then converting it to *d*. If results were simply reported as nonsignificant without a numerical test statistic or p value, we assigned a *d* of 0.0.

Some studies included multiple follow-up sessions. A majority (86%) included at least one short-term follow-up, defined as 6 months or less postintervention. In calculating estimated effect size, we used the short-term follow-up. We averaged the effect sizes from short-term follow-ups for the six studies that reported more than one short-term follow-up.[34,63,69–72] We used the shortest follow-up period to estimate effect size for the three studies[73–75] where all the follow-ups were more than 6 months postintervention.

For each study, we averaged the effect sizes calculated for each behavioral outcome to assess the overall impact of the study on the behaviors measured. In addition, we examined the effect sizes for each of the outcomes considered separately. Table 2 presents the mean effect sizes for the averaged behavioral outcome and the specific behavioral outcomes. It presents mean weighted effect sizes, which were calculated by multiplying each effect size by the reciprocal of its variance[67] before calculating the mean. Effect sizes weighted in this manner give extra importance to studies with larger samples and therefore more reliable results. The table also presents 95% confidence intervals, *t* test statistics, and one-tailed significance probabilities.

Considered as a group, the studies reveal that the interventions significantly reduced HIV

Table 2.   Mean Effect Size (d), 95% Confidence Interval (CI),
and Significance Probabilities for Behavioral Outcomes
in HIV Intervention Studies on Adolescents in Community Settings

Behavioral outcome	k	Mean (d)	Mean (d)	Lower	Upper	t	P
Average behavioral outcome	21	0.23	0.20	0.12	0.27	5.54	0.00001
Condom use	14	0.38	0.38	0.25	0.50	6.54	0.000009
Condom acquisition	5	0.38	0.33	0.13	0.53	4.53	0.0053
Unprotected sexual intercourse	7	0.21	0.14	0.01	0.27	2.69	0.0181
Number of sexual partners	10	0.12	0.11	0.00	0.22	2.36	0.0213
Frequency of sexual intercourse	5	0.11	0.06	−0.10	0.23	1.05	0.1745
Abstinence	6	0.13	0.11	−0.03	0.25	2.00	0.0509

NOTE. k is the number of studies on which the mean effect size is based. The weighted effect sizes were calculated by multiplying each effect size by the reciprocal of its variance.

risk-associated behavior. As shown in Table 2, the mean averaged effect size was statistically significant. In addition, the effect sizes for several specific behavioral outcomes, including condom acquisition, condom use, frequency of unprotected sexual intercourse, and number of sexually partners, were statistically significant. The effect size for abstinence was marginally significant, whereas the effect size for frequency of sexual intercourse was nonsignificant. The magnitude of effects suggests that interventions have had the greatest impact on condom use and on condom acquisition. Effects of the interventions on frequency of sexual intercourse, abstinence, and number of sexual partners were considerably smaller.

Long-term Follow-up

An important question is whether the effects of the interventions are sustained at long-term follow-up. Only a few studies examined the long-term effects of interventions on behavioral outcomes beyond 6-month follow-up. Some of these studies tested interventions that taught adolescents to reduce their risk by abstaining from sexual intercourse or by using condoms if they have sexual intercourse, whereas other studies taught abstinence without providing skills to use condoms. The studies that emphasized both abstinence and condom use were more likely to have long-term effects than were those that emphasized abstinence only. For example, St. Pierre et al.[74] found no main effect for an abstinence intervention at 12-month or 24-month follow-up. Kirby et al.[75] found no significant effects for an abstinence intervention at 17-month follow-up. In contrast, St. Lawrence et al.[72] reported significant effects on unprotected sexual intercourse at 12-month follow-up. Sellers et al.[73] found significant effects on condom acquisition at 18-month follow-up. However, they found no differences on frequency of intercourse, abstinence, or number of sexual partners. Stanton and colleagues[76] found significant intervention effects at 6-month but not at 12-month follow-up. They implemented a booster intervention 15 months after the initial intervention and observed significant treatment effects at 18-month but not at 24-month follow-up.[77] Jemmott et al.[69] examined the effects of both abstinence and safer sex interventions. They found that at 3-month follow-up, the abstinence intervention reduced the percentage of adolescents who engaged in sexual intercourse and the safer sex intervention increased the frequency of condom use. However, at 12-month follow-up, the effects of the abstinence intervention were no longer significant, whereas the effects of the safer sex intervention were significant.

EFFECTS OF INTERVENTIONS ON MEDIATOR VARIABLES

The mean effect sizes in Table 3 reveal that, for the most part, the HIV interventions caused positive changes on the putative mediators of HIV risk-associated sexual behavior, particularly condom use. The effect sizes for behavioral skill assessment, HIV risk reduction knowledge, perceived vulnerability, self-efficacy, behavioral intention, attitude, prevention beliefs, and hedonistic beliefs were statistically significant. The mean effect size for perceived norm was small and nonsignificant. Effect sizes for perceived severity were positive if the HIV intervention caused increases in perceived severity of HIV compared with the control group. As shown in Table 3, the mean effect on perceived severity in three studies was not significant and was negative.

The best evidence for mediation of intervention effects on behavior would come from studies that demonstrate three criteria of mediation.[78] First, the intervention must affect the behavior. Second, the intervention must affect the putative mediator. Third, the effect of the intervention on the behavior must be reduced when the mediator is statistically controlled. For the most part, studies have investigated whether interventions affected behavior and mediator variables, the first two criteria of mediation. Only two studies considered all criteria of mediation. Mediational analyses performed by Sanderson and Jemmott[79] suggested that intentions to use condoms mediated the effects of HIV interventions on college students' condom use. After demonstrating that postintervention condom use intentions predicted condom use at 6-month follow-up, Bryan and colleagues[34] found that increased intentions were mediated by condom use self-efficacy and attitudes toward condoms and condom users. We turn now to an examination of the potential moderators of the effects of the interventions.

POTENTIAL MODERATORS OF INTERVENTION EFFECTS

Moderators are variables that interact with the interventions to affect outcomes.[78] A focus on moderators can highlight characteristics of interventions or the characteristics of partici-pants that influence the magnitude and direction of intervention effects. In this connection, it is

Table 3. Mean Effect Size (d), 95% Confidence Interval (CI), and Significance Probabilities for Theory-Based Mediator Variables in HIV Intervention Studies on Adolescents in Community Settings

Mediator	k	Mean (d)	Mean (d)	Lower	Upper	t	P
Behavioral skill assessment	3	0.82	0.42	0.05	0.78	4.88	0.0197
HIV knowledge	9	0.54	0.47	0.38	0.57	10.99	0.000002
Self-efficacy	13	0.38	0.27	0.19	0.34	7.55	0.000003
Behavioral intention	10	0.37	0.31	0.02	0.41	7.67	0.00002
Attitude toward risk behavior	9	0.29	0.30	0.18	0.42	5.94	0.0002
Prevention beliefs	6	0.38	0.32	0.19	0.45	6.43	0.0007
Hedonistic beliefs	9	0.18	0.20	0.10	0.30	4.78	0.0007
Perceived risk/vulnerability	6	0.17	0.15	0.01	0.30	2.66	0.0225
Perceived norms	6	0.02	0.04	−0.09	0.16	0.82	0.2251
Perceived severity	3	−0.11	−0.03	−0.36	0.31	−0.33	0.6126

NOTE. k is the number of studies on which the mean effect size is based. The weighted effect sizes were calculated by multiplying each effect size by the reciprocal of its variance.

often argued that it is important to match the characteristics of facilitators and participants to enhance the effectiveness of HIV risk reduction interventions. However, despite the compelling intuitive nature of the matching hypothesis, several studies have not supported it. One study[80] randomly assigned African-American male adolescents to an African-American male facilitator or an African-American female facilitator, but found no consistent effect of the gender of the facilitator. Male facilitators were more effective in increasing HIV knowledge among the participants; however, female facilitators were more effective in changing self-reported sexual behavior. Another randomized controlled trial[70] on African-American seventh and eighth grade students found that the effects of an HIV risk reduction intervention did not significantly vary depending on whether the facilitator was male or female, whether the facilitator was African American or white, or whether the intervention group was all male, all female, or mixed gender. A third randomized controlled trial[69] also found that matching the gender of facilitators and participants did not enhance the effects of safer sex or abstinence interventions with African-American sixth and seventh graders. In addition, the study revealed that the effects of the interventions did not differ with adult facilitators compared with peer cofacilitators.

At first blush, the lack of empirical support for the matching hypothesis may seem puzzling. After all, both the social psychological literature on the importance of similarity in attitude change and persuasion[81] and real-world casual observations on the nature of social interaction and trust among individuals of different as opposed to the same gender and ethnicity can be marshaled to support the matching hypothesis. So why did we find no support for such an intuitively obvious notion in the studies we reviewed? One possible explanation revolves around the nature of the interventions used in the studies.[70] First, the interventions were designed to be culturally sensitive. Second, the activities were highly structured and the training of the facilitators emphasized the importance of implementing the interventions according to the protocol. This would have minimized the importance of differences between facilitators with different characteristics. Third, the fact that all facilitators trained together would have helped them to calibrate their facilitation styles so that they were more similar to each other than they might have been otherwise. Perhaps in the absence of such training, if culturally inappropriate materials had been used and if the intervention had been less highly structured, differences in facilitator behavior by race and gender might have emerged.

Another potential moderator that has been considered is characteristics of the participants. Two studies revealed different effects for gender of participants. One study found that gender did not moderate effects of an HIV intervention among African-American adolescents.[70] In contrast, the other study found evidence of moderation by gender in their study on college students.[82] Male students at a campus where an HIV intervention was implemented reported fewer unprotected sexual acts than did those at a control campus, but female students at the intervention and control campuses did not differ significantly.

Two studies that analyzed whether sexual experience moderated intervention effects revealed mixed results. St. Pierre and colleagues[74] found that sexually experienced adolescents who received an abstinence intervention reported less frequent sexual intercourse than did their counterparts in the control condition, whereas virgins in the intervention and control groups did not differ. In sharp contrast, Jemmott and colleagues[69] found that an abstinence intervention was less effective with sexually experienced adolescents than with virgins. On the other hand, Jemmott and colleagues[69] found that a safer sex intervention was more effective with sexually experienced adolescents as compared with virgins.

Relationship status affects condom use.[48,58] Because of this some studies of adolescents have excluded potential participants who are involved in a steady romantic relationship. A randomized controlled trial by Sanderson and Jemmott[79] found that relationship status moderated the effects of HIV interventions with college students. Among students who were not in a steady relationship, those who received an HIV risk reduction intervention reported less HIV risk-associated sexual behavior than did those in the waiting list control condition. However, among those in a steady relationship, there was no difference among conditions.

In summary, the 21 studies we reviewed provide clear evidence that behavioral interventions can curb HIV risk-associated sexual behavior among adolescents in community settings. These effects were evident on the aggregate index of sexual behavior outcomes and on specific sexual behaviors, including condom use, frequency of unprotected sexual intercourse, and number sexual partners—behaviors that have well-established ties to risk of STD. The studies also revealed that the interventions had ameliorative effects on many of the predictors and correlates of risk behavior, including self-efficacy, intentions, and attitudes. In the next section, we will consider the important issue of what characteristics of HIV interventions are key to stronger intervention effects.

CHARACTERISTICS OF EFFECTIVE INTERVENTIONS

Dose of Intervention

One characteristic that often has been suggested as key to the effectiveness of interventions is the dose of intervention content. It might be argued, for instance, that brief interventions are inadequate to provide the motivation and skill to change behaviors. Moreover, multiple-session interventions allow for practice between sessions, which can be followed up by corrective feedback. In single-session interventions this is not possible. Evidence from studies demonstrating that longer HIV interventions are more effective than are shorter interventions is consonant with this line of argument. In a prototypical study, a multiple-session cognitive behavioral HIV risk-reduction intervention is a contrasted with a single-session HIV education-only control group and found to be more effective.[72,83] However, the researchers have typically attributed the effectiveness of the multiple-session intervention to the content of the intervention (i.e., a focus on skill acquisition and cognitive behavioral mediators) rather than to its length.

Also relevant is a study showing that as the number of intervention sessions attended increased, runaway adolescents' reports of consistent condom use increased significantly and their reports of engaging in a high-risk pattern of sexual behavior decreased significantly.[71] However, this study does not provide compelling evidence that intervention dose is important, because self-selection might explain this correlation. The more highly motivated adolescents may have chosen to attend more sessions than did the less highly motivated adolescents. Thus, none of the studies we reviewed provided solid evidence on whether longer interventions are more effective than shorter interventions covering the same basic content.

Another approach to this question is to compare findings in different studies via meta-analysis. Did studies testing longer interventions reveal larger effect sizes than did those testing shorter interventions? We performed such an analysis on the relations of the number of hours of intervention to the averaged behavioral outcomes and the two most common behavioral outcomes: condom use and number of sexual partners. These analyses did not support the hypothesis that dose affects intervention outcomes. We found no significant relationship between number of hours of intervention and the effect size for the averaged behavioral outcomes ($r = .12$, $N = 19$, $P = .638$). There was a positive but small and nonsignificant relation between the number of hours of intervention and the effect size for condom use ($r = .33$, $N = 14$, $P = .253$). There was a small nonsignificant and negative relation between the number of hours of intervention and the effect size for number of sexual partners ($r = -.08$, $N = 8$, $P = .857$). Analyses on number of intervention sessions revealed similar results. Moreover, consistent with the present meta-analysis, a meta-analysis by Kalichman et al.[84] also did not find a significant relation between intervention dose and the magnitude of intervention effects on behavioral outcomes. Similarly, Kim and co-workers'[85] meta-analysis found that although intervention dose was associated with increased effect size for number sexual partners, it was unrelated to effect size for condom use, abstinence, intentions, attitude, and knowledge. Thus, neither the present meta-analysis nor other recent meta-analyses provides cogent evidence of a relation between the duration of interventions and the magnitude of intervention effects.

Spacing of Intervention Sessions

A related issue is the spacing of intervention session. One study has examined whether an intervention is more effective if the content is presented over a longer period.[86] African-American and Latino adolescents were randomly assigned to a no-intervention control group or one of two 10.5-hour HIV interventions: an intervention that involved seven 1.5-hour sessions or an intervention that involved three 3.5-hour sessions. At 3-month follow-up, the adolescents who received the seven-session intervention reported fewer unprotected risk acts and fewer sexual partners than did those in the other two conditions, which would suggest that presenting the content over a longer period is more effective. On the other hand, another potential explanation is that differences in the dose of intervention the participants actually received may account for the differential results. The participants in the seven-session intervention attended a mean of 5.4 sessions, which means they received 77% of the intervention content or 8.1 hours. The participants in the three-session intervention attended a mean of 1.4 sessions, which means they received only 47% of the intervention content or 4.9 hours. Thus, the possibility that the greater dose of intervention (i.e., 3.2 hours), rather than the spacing of intervention content, accounts for the greater impact of the seven-session intervention cannot be excluded.

Theoretical Mediators of Behavior Change

It is often asserted that theory-based interventions are likely to be more effective than are atheoretical interventions. Consonant with this assertion, a review by Kim and colleagues[85] found that studies that cited a theoretical framework were more likely to show positive intervention effects with adolescents. We found that the overwhelming majority of the studies we reviewed cited an explicit theoretical basis of the intervention and measured putative theoretical mediator variables. However, some studies achieved behavior change, whereas others did not. In this connection, it might be argued that if theory is indeed important to interventions, then interventions that cause bigger changes on theoretical mediator variables should have bigger effects on risk behavior.

We found support of this view. The interventions that had larger effects on hedonistic beliefs had larger effects on averaged behavioral outcome ($r = .81$, $N = 9$, $P = .008$), condom use ($r = .98$, $N = 6$, $P = .0004$), and number of sexual partners ($r = .86$, $N = 7$, $P = .02$). Effect sizes on intentions were positively related to effect sizes for averaged behavioral outcomes ($r = .43$, $N = 10$, $P = .22$) and condom use ($r = .43$, $N = 9$, $P = .25$), but these relations were not statistically significant. However, the effect sizes for intentions were significantly related to effect size for number of partners ($r = .99$, $N = 4$, $P = .01$). Surprisingly, effect sizes for self-efficacy were unrelated to the effect sizes for averaged behavioral outcomes ($r = .04$, $N = 13$, $P = .89$), condom use ($r = .12$, $N = 9$, $P = .76$), or number of sexual partners ($r = .45$, $N = 7$, $P = .31$).

SUMMARY AND CONCLUSIONS

There is ample evidence that adolescents are at high risk of sexually transmitted HIV infection. In this light, the results of this body of research are encouraging: They suggest that theory-based interventions can curb HIV risk-associated sexual behavior among adolescents in a variety of community settings. Reductions in HIV risk-associated sexual behaviors were demonstrated across several populations of adolescents: male and female adolescents, young and older adolescents, and African-American and white adolescents. They were demonstrated across different facilitator characteristics: male and female facilitators, African-American and white facilitators, adult facilitators and peer cofacilitators. They were demonstrated in single- and mixed-gender intervention groups. Moreover, the findings cannot be explained as a simple result of Hawthorne effects among the adolescents who received the HIV risk-reduction interventions.[87] Several studies included comparison groups that provided controls for Hawthorne effects so that the effects of the HIV interventions could not be attributed to special attention or group interaction. These studies[69,70,80] also demonstrated that participants in HIV risk reduction interventions reported less HIV risk-associated sexual behaviors than did those in structurally similar interventions that concerned other issues.

Adolescents were typically paid to participate in the studies we reviewed. Consequently, questions might be raised regarding the implications for generalizability of such incentives. An advantage of incentives is that they can increase the likelihood that adolescents will participate in interventions. In addition, when incentives are used, a more diverse population may be enrolled. The study might include people who are participating because they have an intrinsic interest in the topics (these are people who would be involved without the incentives) as well as those who are involved because of the incentives (people who might not participate without an incentive). In this way, the use of incentives might permit a test of the intervention with a larger sample of a broader population and might permit generalizations beyond people who have an intrinsic interest in the topic. The use of incentives also can increase generalizability by reducing attrition.

Although incentives are not limited to money, it might be argued that the likely end users of HIV prevention interventions, including poorly funded community-based organizations, may not have the resources to provide strong incentives for potential participants. Would HIV risk reduction interventions that proved to be effective using monetary incentives also be effective without monetary incentives? First, we would argue that community-based organizations may be able to provide participants with relatively inexpensive nonmonetary incentives, tokens that would be valuable to the population. For example, community-based organizations might use appropriately designed T-shirts and key chains. The Urban League of metropolitan Trenton's HIV prevention program uses this approach.[44] Second, we would argue that if an intervention is effective with the use of monetary incentives, it is also likely to be effective when such incentives are not used. This is because the use of monetary incentives may provide a more stringent test of HIV risk reduction interventions. It may be easier to change the sexual behavior of a population of adolescents who have a specific interest in a behavior change intervention (those willing to participate without monetary incentives) than to change the behavior of a population of adolescents with a mix of motives for participating. Third, recent economic analyses are consistent with the view that HIV risk reduction interventions with adolescents in community settings can be cost-effective in averting HIV infections even if the participants are paid.

A common objection to HIV education programs for adolescents is the fear that exposing adolescents to information about sexual risk reduction would encourage them to engage in sexual activity. The results of the present review, however, provide clear evidence against this view. None of the effect sizes for behavioral outcomes were negative. Thus, the interventions did not have adverse effects on any of the behavioral outcomes considered. Indeed, the interventions had positive impact across several behavioral outcomes. The adolescents who received the interventions were less likely to have sexual intercourse, and those who did have sexual intercourse were more likely to use condoms and had sex with fewer partners. Thus, the fear that providing adolescents with information about reducing their risk of sexually transmitted HIV infection will result in greater sexual activity is perhaps simply a fear.

One important challenge of HIV sexual risk reduction research has been the fact that, by its very nature, risky sexual behavior is private behavior and consequently must be assessed with self-report measures. Thus, these studies examined not risky sexual behaviors but self-reports of risky sexual behaviors. There is the possibility that the participants' reports of their sexual practices might have been unintentionally or intentionally inaccurate. On several grounds, however, confidence about the accuracy of the self-reports in the studies is warranted. To reduce problems in memory, researchers have typically asked adolescents to recall their sexual behaviors over a relatively brief period, which would enhance their ability to recall their behavior.[88] It is more difficult to recall accurately behavior over a 12-month period as compared with the 2- or 3-month period typically used in studies of adolescents. To increase further the accuracy of recall, studies have provided participants calendars with the dates clearly marked. This makes salient to respondents the dates that are included when they are asked to recall their behavior over a specific temporal interval.

Researchers employed several techniques to make it less likely that participants would minimize or exaggerate reports of their sexual experiences. In some studies, demand characteristics were reduced because the facilitators who implemented the interventions were not involved in any way in the data collection.[69,70,80] Participants have been told that their responses would be used to help improve HIV prevention programs for other youths like themselves and that optimum programs would be created only if they answered the questions truthfully. Here, the attempt is to arouse the "social responsibility motive" to counteract any possible social desirability motive.[69] In addition, participants have been assured that their responses would be kept confidential. Such assurances have been shown to increase frank responses to sensitive questions among adolescents.[89]

Another approach was to use other indirect measures of sexual behavior that do not share the same problems as self-report measures. For example, measures of condom acquisition[64,90,91] have been used as a measure of protected sexual behavior (or at least behavior that would seem to emanate from intentions to practice safer sex). In many of these studies, the participants acquired their condoms outside of the intervention setting, where there is less demand for socially desirable responses. In addition, the participants would have to expend greater effort to make a socially desirable response. Another nonreactive measure is behavioral skill acquisition. Many HIV risk reduction interventions are designed to increase adolescents' skills at negotiating safer sex or using condoms. Some studies have assessed behavioral skill acquisition through role-playing scenarios or condom demonstrations.[72] In addition, some studies employed objective tests of whether the adolescents acquired the knowledge to perform safer behavior, for example, knowledge of how to use a condom.[69]

Researchers also have addressed the issue of socially desirable responding statistically by testing hypotheses about its impact. If participants' concern about how they would be viewed by others influenced their reports of their sexual behavior, the effects of HIV risk reduction interventions should be stronger among participants who were higher in the need for social approval than among other participants. However, three studies[69,70,80] examining this issue have found that the changes in reported behavior were unrelated to social desirability response bias.[92] Confidence in adolescents' self-reported behavior also is based on studies demonstrating significant relations between self-reports of sexual involvement or condom use and the incidence of clinically documented sexually transmitted infections.[93,94]

A strength of the studies we reviewed is that they assessed both behavioral outcomes and potential mediators. However, there was considerable variation in the particular mediators and behavioral outcomes assessed. Reviews of this literature could draw stronger conclusions if there were greater consistency in measures across studies. Accordingly, we would offer the following recommendation. All HIV intervention studies on adolescents should include measures of at least the following sexual behaviors: frequency of unprotected sexual intercourse, frequency of condom use, frequency of sexual intercourse, and number of sexual partners. In addition, we would recommend that all such studies assess mediators, including intentions, self-efficacy, hedonistic beliefs, perceived norms, and behavioral skill.

The chief focus of the studies we reviewed was testing whether HIV risk reduction interventions were effective. There has not been a comparable interest in statistically testing the nature of the mediation process that accounts for any observed behavior change or for a lack of behavior change. Yet, to devise more effective interventions, data on why interventions are effective or ineffective are essential. Many studies have shown that the interventions had significant effects on mediators, but only two studies[34,79] actually performed an analysis to test whether the putative mediators explained the intervention effects on behavior. Although our meta-analysis suggested that interventions that caused larger positive changes on mediators had greater impact on condom use, this does not explain mediation at the individual level of analysis. The best way to address the mediation issue is with individual studies that report mediational analyses.

Most of the research, particularly the studies showing the strongest results, has used a cognitive behavioral framework and small-group interventions. In future research, there should be greater effort to examine other theoretical approaches that also might be effective with adolescents. One potentially valuable approach is the diffusion model. For example, Kelly and colleagues[95] have identified opinion leaders in gay bars, trained them in behavior change methods, and encouraged them to intervene with bar patrons to endorse safer sex practices. This approach has been successful in inducing reduced HIV risk-associated sexual behavior among men who have sex with men. One can imagine interventions in which opinion leaders are identified in schools or public housing developments, trained in behavior change techniques, and then encouraged to intervene with their peers. Another theoretical framework that would seem to merit wider application is the theory of cognitive dissonance. Stone and colleagues[64] showed that an intervention based on dissonance theory caused increased condom acquisition and condom use among college students. The magnitude of behavior change induced by this simple, brief intervention was comparable to the behavior change induced by much longer interventions that would seem to be much more expensive to implement. More research is needed to evaluate whether the results replicate in other populations besides college students.

Additional research is also needed into interventions that stress abstinence from sexual intercourse. Although the correct and consistent use of latex condoms can sharply reduce the risk of HIV infection, abstinence is the only way to eliminate the chance of sexually transmitted HIV infection. Abstinence is a reasonable risk reduction strategy for adolescents, especially young adolescents, who may not have the capacity to negotiate condom use or to grapple with the adverse consequences of unprotected sexual intercourse. There is a considerable body of research demonstrating that interventions emphasizing abstinence and condom use if adolescents choose to have sex can reduce HIV risk-associated behavior. There is far less evidence on the effectiveness of interventions stressing abstinence only, and most of the evidence comes from studies designed to prevent pregnancy. To our knowledge, only one HIV intervention study has tested an abstinence intervention.[69] It found that the abstinence intervention was effective at 3-month follow-up but not at 12-month follow-up. We need a better understanding of what kinds of interventions are most effective in encouraging abstinence.

There also is a need for research on the effects of behavioral interventions on health outcomes. We now know that behavioral interventions can influence sexual risk behaviors and mediators of such behaviors. The next generation of research must establish whether changes in self-reported sexual behavior translate into changes in health outcomes such as the incidence of sexually transmitted infections. To our knowledge, only two controlled studies on adolescent populations that included clinically documented STDs as an outcome have been published. One study[96] was included in this review but the other[97] was not because it did not report data on behavioral outcomes. Both studies reported that the interventions did not significantly reduce the incidence of STDs among adolescent women.

In the past, the drawback of biological outcomes was the logistics of data collection. Data collection was typically feasible only in a clinic population. However, with the relatively recent availability of DNA amplification techniques[98–100] that can detect STDs in urine specimens, it is now possible to screen for STDs in a noninvasive manner in a broad range of nonclinical settings. More studies have to be conducted to test the hypothesis that behavioral interventions reduce the incidence of STDs. At the same time, it should be recognized that reducing the incidence of STDs may not be a reasonable goal for every study. It is unlikely that the incidence of STDs will be changed in a short-term study conducted in a population with little sexual activity or in a community with a low prevalence of STDs. Populations with a high degree of sexual activity and a high prevalence of STDs are ideal for studying the effects of behavioral interventions on STD incidence. Such studies should be conducted with samples that are large enough and follow-ups that are long enough to provide excellent statistical power.

The argument here is not that STD incidence should replace the assessment of self-reported sexual risk behavior. Rather, STD incidence should complement self-reports of behavior. This is because the relation between unprotected sexual intercourse and STDs is not perfect. The presence of STD suggests that the person has engaged in unprotected sexual activity, but the absence of a STD does not necessarily mean the person has practiced abstinence or safer sex. The test could be negative not because of the person practiced abstinence or used condoms, but because the person had unprotected sex with a partner who was not infected. A potential secondary advantage of testing for STDs should be noted. Such testing may encourage the adolescents to report their sexual behavior more accurately.

Another area in which more research is needed is the effectiveness of interventions with Latino adolescents. Despite the high risk of sexually transmitted HIV infection among Latino adolescents, few controlled intervention studies have been conducted with this population. Although our review suggests that behavioral interventions have been effective in reducing the HIV risk-associated sexual behavior among adolescents, the evidence on the effectiveness of such interventions among Latinos is meager. Indeed, as the HIV epidemic approaches the 20-year mark in the United States, we could identify only four published controlled intervention studies[73,75,86,101] that had sizable proportions (25% or more of the sample) of Latino adolescents. Latinos constituted the majority of participants in only one study.[73] Moreover, there have been no controlled trials of interventions conducted with Latino adolescents who are monolingual in Spanish.

Future research in this area must ensure that hypotheses are tested with adequate statistical power. Sample size, effect size, and the alpha level or significance criterion affect statistical power.[68] By convention, statistical power of at least 0.80 is considered appropriate, just as the .05 alpha level is commonly used. In the present meta-analysis, the mean weighted effect size for averaged behavioral outcomes was 0.20. To have 0.80 statistical power to detect an effect of this magnitude at a probability level of .05, two-tailed, a total sample of about 786 participants must be included in the analysis.[68] To have 0.80 statistical power to detect an effect size of 0.38—the estimated effect size on condom use in this review—a total sample size of 218 participants must be included in the analysis. By these standards, the set of HIV intervention studies we reviewed had insufficient statistical power. The initial sample sizes ranged from 43 to 659 participants; hence, none of the studies had as much as 0.80 statistical power to detect effect sizes as small as 0.20. The effective sample sizes for analyses were further reduced by attrition, which averaged 20%, and by analyses performed on the subset of adolescents who were sexually active in particular periods (e.g., condom use). This raises the possibility that the set of studies reviewed in this chapter may have underestimated the effectiveness of HIV risk reduction interventions in changing adolescents' behavior due to relatively low statistical power.

As we identify HIV interventions that are effective in curbing HIV risk-associated sexual behavior among adolescents, an important concern arises: Will those interventions be disseminated to likely end users, including teachers in classrooms, health educators in clinics, and facilitators in community-based organizations? There is always the possibility that successful interventions will remain buried in the pages of scientific and public health journals, unavailable to those who might be in the best position to apply them. However, there has been progress along these lines. A fine example is the curriculum dissemination project of the Division of Adolescent and School Health of the Centers for Disease Control and Prevention, entitled "Research to Classrooms: Programs that Work." The project identifies HIV prevention curricula that have credible evidence of effectiveness in changing the behavior of youth and that are *user-friendly* and then brings them to the attention of educators and others concerned with the welfare of youth. The interventions evaluated by Jemmott and colleagues,[80,102] St. Lawrence and colleagues,[72] and Stanton and colleagues[76] are among the five curricula that have been selected thus far.

In conclusion, although adolescence is usually thought of as a period of good health, many adolescents are at high risk of sexually transmitted HIV infection. The studies reviewed in this chapter demonstrate that behavioral interventions can significantly influence HIV risk-associated sexual behavior, including condom acquisition, condom use, frequency of unprotected sexual intercourse, and number of sexual partners. Future research must extend these findings by exploring intervention effects among Latino adolescents. It is also essential that future studies include appropriately large samples to achieve adequate statistical power, that a core set of mediators and behavioral outcomes be assessed, and that objective outcomes such as STD incidence be included in the mix. Although the expense of such studies may be considerable, the alternative is to continue to conduct studies that despite great cost and effort are not fully capable of answering some of the questions that are now of central interest to the field. By conducting research along these lines, it may be possible to identify the most effective strategies to curb the further spread of sexually transmitted HIV infection among adolescents in community settings.

ACKNOWLEDGMENTS.   Preparation of this chapter was supported in part by National Institute of Mental Health grants R01-MH52035, R01-MH55442, and R01-MH55742 and National Institute of Child Health and Human Development grant U01-HD30145.

REFERENCES

1. Centers for Disease Control and Prevention. *HIV/AIDS Surveillance Rep* 1997; 9(No. 2):1–44.
2. Centers for Disease Control and Prevention. State-specific birth rates of teenagers—United States 1990–1996. *Morb Mortal Wkly Rep* 1997; 46(36):837–842.
3. Alan Guttmacher Institute. *Sex and America's Teenagers.* Washington, DC: The Alan Guttmacher Institute; 1994.
4. Bell TA, Holmes KK. Age-specific risks of syphilis gonorrhea and hospitalized pelvic inflammatory disease in sexually experienced US women. *Sex Transm Dis* 1984; 7:291–295.
5. Centers for Disease Control and Prevention. *Sexually transmitted disease surveillance 1996.* Atlanta: Centers of Disease Control and Prevention Division of STD Prevention; 1997.
6. Eng TR, Butler WT, eds. *The Hidden Epidemic: Confronting Sexually Transmitted Disease.* Washington, DC: National Academy Press; 1997.
7. Cates W, Stone KM. Family planning sexually transmitted diseases and contraceptive choice: A literature update—Part I. *Fam Plann Perspect* 1992; 24:75–84.
8. Centers for Disease Control and Prevention. Condoms for the prevention of sexually transmitted diseases. *Morb Mortal Wkly Rep* 1988; 37:133–137.
9. Centers for Disease Control and Prevention. Update: Barrier protection against HIV infection and other sexually transmitted diseases. *JAMA* 1993; 270(8):933–934.
10. Sonenstein FL, Pleck JH, Ku LC. Sexual activity condom use and AIDS awareness among adolescent males. *Fam Plann Perspect* 1989; 21:152–158.
11. Anderson JE, Kann L, Holtzman D, et al. HIV/AIDS knowledge and sexual behavior among high school students. *Fam Plann Perspect* 1990; 22:252–255.
12. Hingson RW, Strunin L, Berlin B, Heeren T. Beliefs about AIDS use of alcohol and drugs and unprotected sex among Massachusetts adolescents. *Am J Public Health* 1990; 80:295–299.
13. Jemmott LS, Jemmott JB III. Sexual knowledge attitudes and risky sexual behavior among inner-city black male adolescents. *J Adolesc Res* 1990; 5:346–369.
14. Centers for Disease Control and Prevention. Youth risk behavior surveillance—United States 1997. *Morb Mortal Wkly Rep* 1998; 47(No. SS-3):1–89.
15. Pratt W, Mosher W, Bachrach C, Horn M. Understanding US fertility: Findings from the National Survey of Family Growth Cycle III. *Population Bull* 1984; 39:1–42.
16. Taylor H, Kagay M, Leichenko S. *American Teens Speak: Sex Myths TV and Birth Control.* New York: Planned Parenthood Federation of America Inc; 1986.
17. Zelnik M, Kantner JF, Ford K. *Sex and Pregnancy in Adolescence.* Beverly Hills, CA: Sage; 1981.
18. Hatcher RA, Trussell J, Stewart F, et al. *Contraceptive Technology,* 16th ed., rev. New York: Irvington Publishers Inc; 1994.
19. Becker MH, ed. The health belief model and personal health behavior. *Health Educ Monogr* 1974; 2:324–473.
20. Fishbein M, Ajzen I. *Belief, Attitude, Intention and Behavior.* Boston: Addison-Wesley; 1975.
21. Ajzen I, Fishbein M. *Understanding Attitudes and Predicting Social Behavior.* Englewood Cliffs, NJ: Prentice-Hall; 1980.
22. Ajzen I. From intentions to actions: A theory of planned behavior. In: Kuhl J, Beckmann J, eds. *Action–Control: From Cognition to Behavior.* Heidelberg: Springer; 1985:11–39.
23. Ajzen I. The theory of planned behavior. *Organizational Behavior Human Decision Processes* 1991; 50:179–211.
24. Madden TJ, Ellen PS, Ajzen I. A comparison of the theory of planned behavior and the theory of reasoned action. *Pers Soc Psychol Bull* 1992; 18:3–9.
25. Bandura A. *Social Foundations of Thought and Action: A Social Cognitive Theory.* Englewood Cliffs, NJ: Prentice-Hall; 1986.
26. Bandura A. Self-efficacy mechanism in human agency. *Am Psychol* 1982; 37:122–147.
27. Bandura A. Social cognitive theory and exercise of control over HIV infection. In: DiClemente R, Peterson J, eds. *Preventing AIDS: Theories and Methods of Behavioral Interventions.* New York: Plenum Press; 1994: 25–60.

28. Prentice-Dunn S, Rogers RW. Protection motivation theory and preventive health: Beyond the health belief model. *Health Educ Res* 1986; 1:153–161.

29. Fisher JD, Fisher WA. Changing AIDS risk behavior. *Psychol Bull* 1992; 111:455–474.

30. Adler NE, Kegeles SM, Irwin CE, Wibbelsman C. Adolescent contraceptive behavior: An assessment of decision processes. *J Pediatrics* 1990; 116:463–471.

31. Fisher WA, Fisher JD, Rye BJ. Understanding and promoting AIDS-preventive behaviors: Insights from the theory of reasoned action. *Health Psychol* 1995; 14:255–264.

32. Stanton BF, Li X, Black MM, et al. Longitudinal stability and predictability of sexual perceptions intentions and behaviors among early adolescent African Americans. *J Adolesc Health* 1996; 18(1):10–19.

33. Basen-Engquist K, Parcel GS. Attitudes norms and self-efficacy: A model of adolescents' HIV-related sexual risk behavior. *Health Educ Q* 1992; 19(2):263–277.

34. Bryan AD, Aiken LS, West SG. Increasing condom use: Evaluation of a theory-based intervention to prevent sexually transmitted diseases in young women. *Health Psychol* 1996; 15(5):371–382.

35. Sheppard BH, Hartwick J, Warshaw PR. The theory of reasoned action: A meta-analysis of past research with recommendations for modifications and future research. *J Consumer Res* 1988; 15:325–343.

36. O'Leary A, Goodhart F, Jemmott LS, Boccher-Lattimore D. Predictors of safer sex on the college campus: A social cognitive theory analysis. *J Am College Health* 1992; 40:254–264.

37. Pendergrast RA Jr, DuRant RH, Gaillard GL. Attitudinal and behavioral correlates of condom use in urban adolescent males. *J Adolesc Health* 1992; 13(2):133–139.

38. Jemmott JB III, Jemmott LS, Hacker CI. Predicting intentions to use condoms among African-American adolescents: The theory of planned behavior as a model of HIV risk associated behavior. *J Ethn Dis* 1992; 2:371–380.

39. DiClemente RJ, Lodico M, Grinstead OA, et al. African-American adolescents residing in high-risk urban environments do use condoms: Correlates and predictors of condom use among adolescents in public housing developments. *Pediatrics* 1996; 98(2 Pt 1):269–278.

40. Catania JA, Dolcini MM, Coates TJ, et al. Predictors of condom use and multiple partnered sex among sexually active adolescent women: Implications for AIDS-related health interventions. *J Sex Res* 1989; 26:514–524.

41. DiClemente RJ, Durbin M, Siegel D, et al. Consistent condom use among middle adolescents in a predominantly minority inner-city school district. *Pediatrics* 1992; 89:197–202.

42. Pleck JH, Sonenstein FL, Ku LC. Adolescent males' condom use: Relationships between perceived costs-benefits and consistency. *J Marriage Fam* 1991; 53:733–745.

43. Jemmott III JB, Jemmott LS, Spears H, et al. Self-efficacy, hedonistic expectancies, and condom-use intentions among inner-city black adolescent women: A social cognitive approach to AIDS risk behavior. *J Adolesc Health* 1992; 13:512–519.

44. Jemmott LS, Jemmott III JB. Increasing condom use intentions among sexually active inner-city black adolescent women: Effects of an AIDS prevention program. *Nurs Res* 1992; 41:273–279.

45. Pleck JH, Sonenstein FL, Ku LC. Changes in adolescent males' condom use and attitudes 1988-1991. *Fam Plann Perspect* 1993; 25(3):106–110,117.

46. Valdiserri RO, Arena VC, Proctor D, Bonati FA. The relationship between women's attitudes about condoms and their use: Implications for condom promotion programs. *Am J Public Health* 1989; 79:499–503.

47. DiClemente RJ. Predictors of HIV-preventive sexual behavior in a high-risk adolescent population: The influence of perceived peer norms and sexual communication on incarcerated adolescents' consistent use of condoms. *Am J Adolesc Health* 1991; 12:385–390.

48. Plichta SB, Weisman CS, Nathanson CA, et al. Partner-specific condom use among adolescent women clients of a family planning clinic. *J Adolesc Health* 1992; 13:506–513.

49. Morrison DM. Adolescent contraceptive behavior: A review. *Psychol Bull* 1985; 98:538–568.

50. Milan RJ, Kilmann PR. Interpersonal factors in premarital contraception. *J Sex Res* 1987; 23:289–321.

51. Fox GL, Inazu JK. Patterns and outcomes of mother–daughter communication about sexuality. *J Soc Issues* 1980; 36:7–29.

52. Jemmott JB III, Jones JM. Social psychology and AIDS among ethnic minority individuals: Risk behaviors and strategies for changing them. In: Pryor JB, Reeder GD, eds. *The Social Psychology of HIV Infection*. Hillsdale, NJ: Lawrence Erlbaum Associates; 1993: 183–224.

53. Centers for Disease Control and Prevention. State-specific pregnancy rates among adolescents—United States 1992–1995. *Morb Mortal Wkly Rep* 1998; 47(24):497–504.

54. Ku LC, Sonenstein FL, Pleck JH. Young men's risk behaviors for HIV infection and STDs 1988 through 1991. *Am J Public Health* 1993; 83:1609–1615.

55. Weisman CS, Nathanson CA, Ensminger M, et al. AIDS knowledge perceived risk and prevention among adolescent clients of a family planning clinic. *Fam Plann Perspect* 1989; 21:213–217.

56. Centers for Disease Control and Prevention. Premarital sexual experience among adolescent women—United States 1970–1988. *Morb Mortal Wkly Rep* 1991; 39:929–932.

57. Leigh BC, Morrison DM, Trocki K, Temple MT. Sexual behavior of American adolescents: Results from a US national survey. *J Adolesc Health* 1994; 15:117–125.

58. Soskolne V, Aral SO, Magder LS, et al. Condom use with regular and casual partners among women attending family planning clinics. *Fam Plann Perspect* 1991; 23:222–225.

59. Jemmott JB III, Jemmott LS. Alcohol and drug use during sex and HIV risk-associated sexual behavior among inner-city black male adolescents. *J Adolesc Res* 1993; 8:41–57.

60. Lowry R, Holtzman D, Truman B, et al. Substance use and HIV-related sexual behaviors among US high school students: Are they related? *Am J Public Health* 1994; 84:1116–1120.

61. MacDonald TK, Zanna MP, Fong GT. Why common sense goes out the window: Effects of alcohol on intentions to use condoms. *Pers Soc Psychol Bull* 1996; 22:763–775.

62. Gerrard M, Gibbons FX, Bushman BJ. Relation between perceived vulnerability to HIV and precautionary sexual behavior. *Psychol Bull* 1996; 119(3):390–409.

63. Gillmore MR, Morrison DM, Richey CA, et al. Effects of a skill-based intervention to encourage condom use among high-risk heterosexually active adolescents. *AIDS Educ Prev* 1997; 9(1 Suppl):22–43.

64. Festinger L. *A Theory of Cognitive Dissonance*. Stanford, CA: Stanford University Press; 1957.

65. Stone J, Aronson E, Crain AL, et al. Inducing hypocrisy as a means of encouraging young adults to use condoms. *Pers Soc Psychol Bull* 1994; 20(1):116–128.

66. Rosenthal R. *Meta-analytic Procedures for Research*. Beverly Hills, CA: Sage; 1984.

67. Hedges LV, Olkin I. *Statistical Methods for Meta-analysis*. New York: Academic Press; 1985.

68. Cohen J. *Statistical Power Analysis for the Behavioral Sciences*. Hillsdale, NJ: Erlbaum Associates; 1988.

69. Jemmott JB III, Jemmott LS, Fong GT. Abstinence and safer sex HIV risk-reduction interventions for African American adolescents: A randomized controlled trial. *JAMA* 1998; 279:1529–1536.

70. Jemmott III JB, Jemmott LS, Fong GT, McCaffree K. Reducing HIV risk-associated sexual behavior among African-American adolescents: Testing the generality of intervention effects. *Am J Community Psychol* 1999; 27:161–187.

71. Rotheram-Borus MJ, Koopman C, Haignere C, Davies M. Reducing HIV sexual risk behaviors among runaway adolescents. *JAMA* 1991; 266:1237–1241.

72. St. Lawrence J, Brasfield T, Jefferson K, et al. Cognitive behavioral intervention to reduce African-American adolescent's risk for HIV infection. *J Consult Clin Psychol* 1995; 63:221–237.

73. Sellers DE, McGraw SA, McKinlay JB. Does the promotion and distribution of condoms increase teen sexual activity? Evidence from an HIV prevention program for Latino youth. *Am J Public Health* 1994; 84(12):1952–1959.

74. St. Pierre TL, Mark MM, Kaltreider DL, Aikin KJ. A 27-month evaluation of a sexual activity prevention program in Boys and Girls Clubs across the nation. *Fam Relations* 1995; 44:69–77.

75. Kirby D, Korpi M, Barth RP, Cagampang HH. The impact of the Postponing Sexual Involvement curriculum among youth in California. *Fam Plann Perspect* 1997; 29:100–108.

76. Stanton B, Li X, Ricardo I, et al. A randomized, controlled effectiveness trial of an AIDS prevention program for low-income African-American youths. *Arch Pediatr Adolesc Med* 1996; 150:363–372.

77. Stanton B, Fang X, Li X, et al. Evolution of risk behaviors over two years among a cohort of urban African-American adolescents. *Arch Pediatr Adolesc Med* 1997; 151(4):398–406.

78. Baron RM, Kenny DA. The moderator–mediator variable distinction in social psychological research: Conceptual, strategic, and statistical considerations. *J Pers Soc Psychol* 1986; 51:1173–1182.

79. Sanderson CA, Jemmott JB III. Moderation and mediation of HIV prevention interventions: Relationship status intentions and condom use among college students. *J Appl Soc Psychol* 1996; 26:2076–2099.

80. Jemmott III JB, Jemmott LS, Fong GT. Reductions in HIV risk-associated sexual behaviors among black male adolescents: Effects of an AIDS prevention intervention. *Am J Public Health* 1992; 82:372–377.

81. Eagly AH, Chaiken S. *The Psychology of Attitudes*. Fort Worth, TX: Harcourt Brace Jovanovich; 1993.

82. O'Leary A, Jemmott LS, Goodhart F, Gebelt J. Effects of an institutional AIDS prevention intervention: Moderation by gender. *AIDS Educ Prev* 1996; 8(6):516–528.

83. Sikkema KJ, Winett RA, Lombard DN. Development and evaluation of an HIV-risk reduction program for female college students. *AIDS Educ Prev* 1995; 7(2):145–159.

84. Kalichman SC, Carey MP, Johnson BT. Prevention of sexually transmitted HIV infection: A meta-analytic review of the behavioral outcome literature. *Ann Behav Med* 1996; 18:6–15.

85. Kim N, Stanton B, Li X, et al. Effectiveness of the 40 adolescent AIDS risk-reduction interventions: A quantitative review. *J Adolesc Health* 1997; 20:204–215.

86. Rotheram-Borus MJ, Gwadz M, Fernandez MI, Srinivasan S. Timing of HIV interventions on reductions in sexual risk among adolescents. *Am J Community Psychol* 1998; 26:73–96.

87. Cook TD, Campbell DT. *Quasi-experimentation: Design and Analysis Issues for Field Settings*. Chicago: Rand McNally; 1979.

88. Kauth MR, St. Lawrence JS, Kelly JA. Reliability of retrospective assessments of sexual HIV risk behavior: A comparison of biweekly, three-month, and twelve-month self-reports. *AIDS Educ Prev* 1991; 3:207–214.

89. Ford CA, Millstein SG, Halpern-Felsher BL, Irwin CE Jr. Influence of physician confidentiality assurances on adolescents' willingness to disclose information and seek future health care: a randomized controlled trial. *JAMA* 1997; 278(12):1029–1034.

90. Fisher JD, Fisher WA, Misovich SJ, et al. Changing AIDS risk behavior: Effects of an intervention emphasizing AIDS risk reduction information, motivation, and behavioral skills in a college student population. *Health Psychol* 1996; 15:114–123.

91. Rickert VI, Gottlieb A, Jay MS. A comparison of three clinic-based AIDS education programs on female adolescents' knowledge attitudes and behavior. *J Adolesc Health* 1990; 11:298–303.

92. Crowne D, Marlowe D. *The Approval Motive*. New York: Wiley; 1964.

93. Orr DP, Fortenberry JD, Blythe MJ. Validity of self-reported sexual behaviors in adolescent women using biomarker outcomes. *Sex Transm Dis* 1997; 24(5):261–266.

94. Shew ML, Remafedi GJ, Bearinger LH, et al. The validity of self-reported condom use among adolescents. *Sex Transm Dis* 1997; 24(9):503–510.

95. Kelly JA, Murphy DA, Sikkema KJ, et al. Randomised controlled community-level HIV-prevention intervention for sexual risk behaviour among homosexual men in US cities. *Lancet* 1997; 350:1500–1505.

96. Orr DP, Langefeld CD, Katz BP, Caine VA. Behavioral intervention to increase condom use among high-risk female adolescents. *J Pediatrics* 1996; 128(2):288–295.

97. Smith PB, Weinman ML, Parrilli J. The role of condom motivation education in the reduction of new and reinfection rates of sexually transmitted diseases among inner-city female adolescents. *Patient Educ Couns* 1997; 31(1):77–81.

98. Buimer M, van Doorum GJ, Ching S, et al. Detection of *Chlamydia trachomatis* and *Neisseria gonorrhoeae* by ligase chain reaction-based assays with clinical specimens from various sites: Implications for diagnostic testing and screening. *J Clin Microbiol* 1996; 34:2395–2400.

99. Cohen DA, Nsuami M, Etame RB, et al. A school-based chlamydia control program using DNA amplification technology. *Pediatrics* 1998; 101(1):E1.

100. Oh MK, Smith KR, O'Cain M, et al. Urine-based screening of adolescents in detention to guide treatment for gonococcal and chlamydial infections. Translating research into intervention. *Arch Pediatr Adolesc Med* 1998; 152(1):52–56.

101. Magura S, Kang SY, Shapiro JL. Outcomes of intensive AIDS education for male adolescent drug users in jail. *J Adolesc Health* 1994; 15(6):457–463.

102. Jemmott LS, Jemmott III JB, McCaffree K. *Be Proud! Be Responsible! Strategies to Empower Youth to Reduce Their Risk for AIDS*. New York: Select Media Publications; 1995.

6

Interventions for High-Risk Youth

MARGUERITA LIGHTFOOT
and MARY JANE ROTHERAM-BORUS

INTRODUCTION

Currently, almost 3,000 adolescents have been diagnosed with AIDS and more than 16,000 youth have been identified as seropositive for human immunodeficiency virus (HIV).[1] This represents an almost fourfold increase in the last 5 years in the number of adolescent AIDS cases. However, the latter number reflects seropositive youth in only 26 states; most states do not have HIV reporting laws. Given the long incubation period of the HIV virus, the World Health Organization (WHO) estimates that 50% of infections worldwide and 25% of HIV infections in the United States are acquired during adolescence.[2] Therefore, the actual number of seropositive youth is likely to be substantially higher.

Nationally, we have recognized the need for primary HIV prevention programs designed specifically for adolescents.[3] School districts, community agencies, and agencies that serve adolescents at high risk for acquiring HIV have initiated prevention programs,[4] and there have been substantial positive changes in response to these prevention programs: condom use has increased substantially, and youth are informed regarding HIV and recognize the consequences of HIV infection.[5] While there has been a substantial number of primary prevention interventions, there has been far less attention on recognizing the importance of the continuum of care for adolescents. In particular, it is critical to develop interventions for: (1) the early detection of infected youth, and (2) the prevention of transmission of HIV and increased health-related behaviors among youth living with HIV (YLH). The recent advances in antiretroviral medications make implementation of a continuum of services for adolescents imperative.

Consequently, prevention strategies must address not only uninfected individuals, but those who are already infected. Primary versus secondary prevention services for adolescents differ in their targeted outcomes, motivations addressed by the intervention, and delivery format. The implementation of a continuum of services for adolescents will require substantial changes in public policies regarding adolescents. This chapter will review the epidemiology and the existing interventions that address points in the continuum of care for seronegative and seropositive youth, providing a theoretical framework for designing HIV prevention interventions for these youth and pointing to new challenges facing prevention researchers: mounting early detection programs, developing coordinated, comprehensive, and continuous HIV systems of care, and broadly disseminating programs.

MARGUERITA LIGHTFOOT and MARY JANE ROTHERAM-BORUS • Department of Social and Community Psychiatry, University of California, Los Angeles, California 90024.

Handbook of HIV Prevention, edited by Peterson and DiClemente.
Kluwer Academic/Plenum Publishers, New York, 2000.

EPIDEMIOLOGY

Estimates of the number of YLH are based on studies of adolescents considered at high risk for HIV: gay and bisexual youth[6,7] and runaway and homeless youth.[8] The HIV seroprevalence rates for these high-risk subgroups are 6 to 10 times higher than the seropositivity rates reported for the general population of adolescents.[9,10] The factors responsible for HIV among adolescents in high-risk subpopulations has been clear; these youth engage in sexual and substance use behaviors associated with the transmission of HIV.[11] We will review the epidemiology of each of these adolescent subgroups (see Tables 1 and 2).

Gay and Bisexual Youth

Sexual activity between males is the primary HIV risk factor for one third of adolescent males with acquired immunodeficiency syndrome (AIDS) and two thirds of the 20- to 24-year-old males with AIDS.[12] Unfortunately, like many other young people at risk, young gay and bisexual men do not consider their peers to be at risk for infection and often do not have peer or other social support networks to encourage and reinforce safer sex practices.[12]

The existing data on sexual behavior among male gay and bisexual youth, typically available from convenience samples, indicate that these youth initiate sex at early ages (around 12.5 years) and have many sexual partners (median = 8 at age 15 years[13,14]). Survey data indicate that gay and lesbian youth[14–18] engage in a substantial number of sexual risk acts. For example, Remafedi[17] found that 63% of gay male youth report unprotected anal intercourse. The sexual behaviors among gay and bisexual youth are particularly problematic because of the high seroprevalence rate of HIV among partners of young gay youth. Many gay male youth have sexual relationships with older adult gay men,[19] who are more likely to be infected.[1]

The substance use patterns of gay youth further increase their HIV risk. The relationship between sex and alcohol–drug use is important because substance use is common among gay youth. For example, in one study[20] substance use was higher among homosexual and bisexual male youth than adolescents in general in a 1991 national household survey.[21] Although alcohol and noninjection drug use are not directly linked to HIV infection, use of drugs and alcohol can greatly increase adolescents' sexual risk behaviors. For example, frequent use of alcohol and drugs is associated with unprotected sex, and those gay youth with the largest number of partners are more likely to barter sex for money or drugs.[19] In addition, substance use often disinhibits sexual restraints,[22] further increasing the HIV risk of gay youth.

Among AIDS cases for young gay men, aged 13–25, the racial demographics have changed markedly over time. For example, in 1984, whites accounted for 49% of the AIDS cases, while 27% were among African Americans and 12% Latino. Of the 1501 AIDS cases in 1995, African Americans accounted for 40%, whites 37%, and Latinos 22%. In general, the largest increases in AIDS cases were reported by metropolitan areas,[12] and seroprevalence studies in New York and San Francisco suggest much higher seroprevalence rates among young African-American and Latino gay men than among their white counterparts.[6,7]

Runaway and Homeless Youth

Among the adolescent runaway and homeless subpopulation, HIV seropositivity ranges from 2 to 17%,[23–25] and considerable evidence demonstrates that a sizable proportion of runaway and homeless adolescents engage in behaviors associated with transmission of HIV.[26–31]

Having multiple sex partners is characteristic of this adolescent subgroup. A far greater

Table 1. A Summary of Sexual Behavior Patterns of High-Risk Youth

Study	Time period	N	Mean age	Age of initiation	No. sexual encounters (mean)	No. partners median (mean)	Never/inconsistent condom use (%)	Always/consistent condom use (%)
Nationally								
Youth Risk Behavior Study[99]	3 mo		9–12 grade	9% before age 13				54% at last intercourse
Runaways								
Midwestern[31]	6 mo	108	15		18.7/7	1 (3.4)	8	46
Los Angeles[28]	3 mo	446	19.8	11		2	34	37
New York City[27]	3 mo	145	15.5		20	1 (3.0)	22	24
Los Angeles[100]	30 days	409	13–23			11.7	Anal: 80 / Vaginal: 64.5	
New York City, San Francisco, Los Angeles[101]	3 mo	478	18.8		Males anal: 16.3 / Males vaginal: 12.1 / Females anal: .8 / Females vaginal: 14.5	Males: 5.1 / Females: 1.5		Males: 77% / Females: 79.5%
Los Angeles[30]	Lifetime	620	10–24 yrs	57% by age 15				
Gay, lesbian, and bisexual youth								
New York City, Los Angeles, San Francisco[20]	3 mo	131	16.8	12.4	Males: 23.9/8.0 / Females: 6.7/1.7	Males: 2.0 (10.3) / Females: 1.0 (1.7)	Receptive anal: 44 / Active anal: 60	
New York[102]	Lifetime	156	18.3	Males: 12.9 / Females: 13.3				
Minnesota[12]	6 mo	239	19.9			1	Vaginal: 10 / Anal: 53	
San Francisco[103]	6 mo	99	22.57			3	57	
Seropositives								
New York City, Los Angeles, Miami, San Francisco[44]	3 mo	350	21.3	14		1	30.6	30.6
New York City[47]	Lifetime	72	15–24				Vaginal: 48 / Anal: 63	Vaginal: 13 / Anal: 11

Table 2. A Summary of Substance Use Behavior Patterns of High-Risk Youth

Study	Time period	N	Mean age	Abstinent alcohol and drugs (%)	Alcohol use (%)	Marijuana use (%)	Hard drug use (%)	Injection drug use (%)
Nationally								
NIDA Drug Survey[104]	Lifetime	16,300	12th grade		87.0	35.3	26.7	
	30 days				51.0	15.5	7.9	
Youth Risk Behavior Study[99]	Lifetime				80.4	42.4	16	2.0
	30 days				51.6	25.3		
Runaways								
Midwestern[31]	6 mo	108	15	32	30	9		
New York City[105]	Lifetime	150	18.5		41% drug and alcohol abuse		27	
Hollywood[106]	Lifetime	90	16.1		30% biweekly	70% at least 5 times	43% more than 5 times	
Los Angeles[28]	Lifetime	446	19.8	2.9				30.6
Gay								
New York City[20]	3 mo	131	16.8	29	69	33	14	0
New York City[102]	Lifetime	154	18.3	9	83	56	26	
Minnesota[17]	6 mo	239	19.9		55 ≥ 5 drinks in 2 weeks	67	23	
Seropositive youth								
New York City, Los Angeles, Miami, San Francisco[44]	3 mo	102	21.1		63	41	36	12
New York City[47]	Lifetime	72	15–24	8	87	61	18–42	

proportion of runaways have had more than 10 sexual partners during their lifetime[32] compared to national samples.[33,34] Runaway and homeless adolescents are also more likely to engage in survival sex. Studies have found that 22% of runaways in Los Angeles[35] and 26% in New York City[14] are involved in survival sex, as compared with 1% in a national sample.[36] Among young men reporting male-to-male sex, HIV prevalence ranged from 13 to 17% in two homeless and runaway youth centers and two sexually transmitted disease (STD) clinics located in four metropolitan areas.[25]

One of the most alarming risk factors among runaway and homeless youth is their inconsistent use of condoms. Consistent condom use among runaways is low, about 20%,[27] and STDs are common among homeless youth.[37] Only 24% of male street youth in Los Angeles always used condoms with opposite-sex partners, and 40% never used condoms with opposite sex partners.[28] Sugerman et al.[38] found that among a sample of runaway and homeless adolescents in Houston, 20% reported consistent condom use and 33% reported rarely or never using condoms. These data are particularly worrisome considering the high levels of survival sex and multiple partners among these adolescents.

Also alarming is the high level of alcohol and drug use among runaway youth. Yates et al.[35] found that 84% of homeless and runaway youth use alcohol and drugs. Although alcohol and noninjection drug use are not directly linked to HIV infection, use of drugs and alcohol can greatly influence adolescents' sexual risk behaviors. For example, two thirds of the runaway and homeless youth in Los Angeles were high on drugs more than half the time during survival sex, and one fourth were high on drugs more than half the time during recreational sex.[28] In addition, runaway and homeless youth in New York City[11] were far more likely to report substance use than national samples of teenagers,[39] increasing the likelihood of unprotected sex.

HIV-Seropositive Youth

Many adults living with HIV do not change their sexual and substance use risk behaviors after being informed of their serostatus,[40,41] and findings are similar for YLH.[42–44] Youth who continue to engage in HIV risk-related behaviors may spread the disease and reduce their chances of maintaining a healthy lifestyle. About one third of young gay–bisexual men who are seropositive report that they had recently engaged in unprotected anal intercourse with sexual partners,[7] similar to the 29% reported by Kelly et al.[45] About 35% of gay men living with HIV from the Multisite AIDS Cohort Study cohort engaged in unprotected insertive anal intercourse in the prior 6 months.[46]

Even when considerable time has lapsed since a seropositive diagnosis, youth continue to engage in a substantial number of HIV-related risk acts, both sexual and substance use, and these behaviors are common and stable across time.[44] Compared to a national study of adolescent males,[36] YLH had approximately five times the number of sexual partners than those in the national sample; the median number of lifetime sexual partners for YLH in the Rotheram-Borus et al.[44] study was 57 for males (who were all under the age of 23 years), and the median number of partners for females was 8. Furthermore, YLH are at increased risk of reinfection and transmission of HIV to others due to their inconsistent use of condoms. Only about 10 to 30% of YLH consistently use condoms.[44,47]

Although few YLH continue to share needles after their infection, many have used alcohol or drugs in the previous 3 months.[44] Over 60% of YLH have used alcohol, 41% have used marijuana, and almost 40% have used drugs such as cocaine and heroin. Again, given that the use of drugs and alcohol can greatly influence adolescents' sexual risk behaviors, the danger of reinfection or transmission of the virus is increased when YLH engage in alcohol or drug use.

In summary, early and frequent unprotected sexual behavior increasingly has placed adolescents at risk for HIV,[1] other STDs,[48] and teen pregnancy.[49] Youth considered at risk for these outcomes are more likely to be sexually active at early ages, to have unprotected intercourse, to be sexually abused, to be emotionally distressed, and to be abusing alcohol or drugs. Although within-group differences exist, HIV risk and other risk-related behavioral patterns overlap for gay, runaway, and seropositive youth. For example, gay youth are overrepresented in runaway and homeless populations.[50] Thus, it is difficult to determine how specific subgroups of youth at high risk differ from each other.

However, based on seroprevalence data and reported AIDS cases, adolescents at risk for contracting HIV are likely to be young gay or bisexual males (61% of nonhemophiliac adolescent male AIDS cases)[1] and runaway or homeless youth.[23,24] Further, given the continued risk behavior of seropositive youth, these data indicate the necessity to intervene in the continuum of care for adolescents by: (1) implementing broad scale interventions for early detection; (2) identifying alternative prevention messages for increased and sustained condom use; and (3) intervening with providers to enhance broad scale dissemination of prevention programs for adolescents.

THEORETICAL BASIS FOR BEHAVIOR CHANGE

There is substantial evidence that adolescents, even those at very high risk, reduce their HIV risk acts and increase condom use in response to attending HIV prevention programs.[51-55] The National Institutes of Health,[3] based on a review by Jemmott and Jemmott,[5] concluded that interventions conducted with heterosexual adolescents can significantly affect HIV risk-related sexual behavior, including condom acquisition, condom use, unprotected sexual intercourse, frequency of sexual intercourse, and the number of sexual partners. Intervention services in the reviewed studies were administered in a number of service settings: schools, medical clinics, weekend programs, homeless shelters, and community-based organizations. Effective interventions were: (1) tailored to the subgroup at risk (e.g., African-American adolescents) based on research with members of the study's population, and (2) explicit in their theoretical basis.

Social cognitive theories have been used most commonly to guide interventions delivered to adolescents: the theory of reasoned action,[56,57] the health belief model,[58] the theory of self-efficacy,[59] and social action theory.[60] These theories highlight, as determinants of HIV risk-related behavior change, the importance of beliefs, outcome expectancies, perceived norms, skills, self-efficacy, self-regulation skills, and behavioral intentions. When the desired behavior change is identified, the resources, skills, attitudes, and knowledge necessary for survival in the youth's living situation are analyzed. Youth's outcome expectancies, perceptions of peer norms, social skills, feelings of self-efficacy, and behavioral intentions to act safely have been linked to behavior change.[5] Yet, when one considers the activities and exercises that constitute effective programs, the assumptions about changing behavior are much more complex than the specific social cognitive components outlined by traditional theory. Each of the social cognitive theories only addresses the targeted outcomes of increasing condom use and decreasing the number of sexual acts and sexual partners. However, in changing the behavior of these youth, the interventionists have used more complex behavior change programs. Although the principles of behavior change are used effectively in interventions (i.e., successive approximation, rehearsal, modeling, setting realistic goals, establishing cognitive dissonance as a means of motivating behavior, providing social and tangential rewards, and rewarding goal achievement), often the multiple levels of an individual's motivation and behaviors also are addressed.

Within the context of the intervention, youth begin to distinguish their social identities and roles and rules for interpersonal interactions and behaviors. This process is integral in identifying motivations and agents for behavior change. Efficacious interventions reframe and redevelop youth's views of themselves and how they relate to those around them. Personal integration theory[61] suggests that the success of an intervention is dependent on the degree to which youth are able to reexamine and reshape their social identity, roles, interpersonal rules, and behaviors. When examining these constructs within the context of the youth's physical, social, and emotional environment, youth will be able to identify their personal view and shift toward accomplishing safe outcomes. For example, the desirable rules for living as a homeless youth might include willingness to enroll in a job training program, stop bartering sex for drugs and money, and reduce substance use that would inhibit the youth's ability to maintain a job and housing.

Personal integration theory[61] suggests that in order for these programs to effect long-term change they must successfully change not only the target behaviors but the social routines, interpersonal rules, social roles, and social identities of youth that surround the target behaviors. It is critical that program developers explicitly articulate the components of their programs that involve changing behaviors. By not recognizing the complexity of the programs that are implemented, service providers are often unable to replicate the interventions mounted by researchers. As an example of the intensiveness of the programs that have been found to successfully change behavior, we will briefly describe HIV intervention programs delivered to the high-risk groups that are the focus of this chapter.

Gay and Bisexual Youth

Rotheram-Borus et al.[62] designed, conducted, and evaluated an intensive HIV prevention intervention at a community-based agency that provided recreational and social services to gay youth. The specific goals of the intervention were to help gay youth (1) abstain from unsafe behavior, (2) use a condom when engaging in sexual activities, (3) avoid sex with partners who are at risk for being HIV-positive, and (4) resist getting high before engaging in sexual activities. The intervention targeted sexual risk acts because there was little injecting drug use among gay youth in New York City. Based on social learning theory,[63,64] the intervention addressed general and personalized knowledge of HIV, coping skills (including problem-solving and self-efficacy), acquiring condoms and health care resources, and an analysis of barriers to implementing safer sex acts (e.g., contextual factors, outcome expectancies, dysfunctional attitudes). The intervention was delivered by skilled trainers in small-group sessions that lasted from 90 to 120 minutes each.

It is important to note that for each of the targeted behaviors, activities were developed to (1) enhance positive actions, (2) change interpersonal rules, (3) redefine social roles, and (4) help youth examine the meaning and social identity attached to each risk act. For example, in order to resist getting high before engaging in sexual activities, youth identified the contexts in which sex was likely to occur after alcohol or drug use. Persons, places, and activities that were linked to alcohol and sex also were identified. These contexts and triggers were examined over the course of the intervention so that the interpersonal relationships that typically unfolded in these settings were identified, and the importance of these settings to maintaining youth's social identities were articulated and listed. Examining the social meaning of the behaviors almost always involved recognizing youth's comfort and ability to disclose their sexual orientation. Settings that were most likely to link substances and sexuality were often gay-identified settings. Being in gay-identified settings, therefore, meant that youth had to negotiate, without alcohol, their romantic relationship prior to the initiation of the sexual contact. Rehearsal of new repertoires of sexual routines involved not only the target behaviors of using condoms but also modification of the meaning of going to gay-identified sites, the social routines within casual interpersonal relationships, and the social roles that youth and their partners adopted.

After receiving this intervention, the patterns of sexual risk acts in the cohort of 136 gay youth were examined over 2 years.[65] Retention in the intervention was high: 88% of the youth completed at least three of the four assessments. Over 1 year, significant reductions occurred in the number of unprotected same-gender anal and oral sex acts. Also, the youth significantly reduced their number of sexual partners following the intervention and maintained this reduction in partners over 1 year. When individual patterns of HIV-related risk from receptive and insertive anal sexual behavior were examined over 1 year, it was found that 45% of youth were abstinent or used condoms for each sexual encounter.

Runaway and Homeless Youth

Similar positive behavior changes were observed in a study conducted to investigate the efficacy of an HIV prevention program delivered in shelters for homeless and runaway youth (M. J. Rotheram-Borus, R. Van Rossem, M. Gwadz, C. Koopman, and M. Lee, unpublished data, 1999). This study examined HIV-related sexual and substance use risk acts among 312 runaway and homeless youth, about half male, aged 11 to 17 years over 2 years in New York City. Recruitment sites were randomized for either the intervention or as a control. The sample consisted of 167 youth in the intervention condition and 145 adolescents in the nonintervention control condition. Runaways participated in small groups that offered an opportunity for behavior change.

Again, similar to the interventions for gay youth, the social identities of youth, and their social roles, routines, and behaviors were each targeted in order to change substance use and sexual behavior patterns over time. An example of the changes that were identified can be demonstrated by examining the difference between the social identity of "druggie" and "junkie," two subgroups of youth who participated in the intervention. Being able to define oneself as a druggie meant having a certain degree of social responsibility, self-esteem, and altruism. Youth who were druggies used clean syringes when they injected drugs, often picked up their discarded needles, and encouraged others to use clean needles. The interpersonal social routines in which drugs were used did not include sharing drugs. The social role of druggies within their peer network was that of caretakers. Youth who were druggies were more likely to provide "works" for their friends. In contrast, a junkie had a lower social status in their peer network, did not consistently keep clean needles on their person, did not have clean needles to share with others, and discarded needles in a casual manner. The intervention delineated the social roles that were different for these two subgroups and also encouraged the adoption of a social identity as a druggie and discouraged the adoption of the role of a junkie. Unfortunately, youth with either social identity did not use condoms during sex. The social role was limited to their substance use pattern. Therefore, the intervention not only attempted to enhance the positive aspects of the druggies' social identity, it also attempted to insert the social routines and definitions of sexual responsibility into the social role of a junkie or druggie. Youth acquired these social routines by practicing how to negotiate safer sex with others through role-playing, mobilizing support for beliefs and attitudes that reinforce safer sex acts and abstinence from substance use, and maintaining positive social support networks for sustained behavior change. Similar differences, including the need for shifting social definitions (social identities, roles, routines, and behavior patterns), were found for social identities that were based primarily on youth's sexual behaviors.

The benefits of the HIV prevention program were observed for both sexual risk acts and substance use. Significant reductions in the number of unprotected sexual acts, and in a weighted index of substance use (taking into account the seriousness of the drug used as well as frequency of use) were found based on intervention condition. The number of sexual acts unprotected by condoms decreased significantly more in the intervention compared to the control group. Overall, females in the intervention group demonstrated greater reductions in sexual risk and substance use compared to males, and African Americans reported greater reductions in substance use than other ethnic groups.

HIV-Seropositive Youth

As noted earlier, it is crucial for interventions to address the continuum of care for adolescents. Secondary prevention of HIV involves stopping the spread of the virus by infected persons. In addition, continued high-risk behavior by YLH is a concern because it increases the youth's risk of exposure to STDs and the possibility of reinfection with a new strain of the virus, which in turn may accelerate disease progression.[66,67] A study conducted by Rotheram-Borus et al.[44] examined the efficacy of a secondary prevention intervention to reduce sexual and substance use risk acts among YLH, and thereby reduce the transmission of HIV to uninfected individuals. YLH who were linked to adolescent clinical care sites in New York City, Los Angeles, and San Francisco were recruited. Youth recruited at each site were randomly assigned within site by cohort (i.e., a group of 15–20 youth) to receive the intervention immediately or 12 months later. Unprotected sex, substance use, and social cognitive mediators of transmission acts (i.e., outcome expectancies for sexual and substance use behavior, social norms, and self-efficacy in the negotiation of safer sex acts and ability to negotiate lower or no substance use) were examined among 187 YLH aged 13 through 23 years (27% African American, 35% Latino) who were randomly assigned to an intervention or a lagged control group (76% follow-up at 3 months). About half the youth (53%) were asymptomatic, most youth were out of school, and about two thirds considered their economic and living conditions to be adequate or comfortable.

Again, this intervention influenced the social roles, interpersonal rules, social identities, and actions or behavior of the YLH. A salient social identity YLH were asked to confront was that of being an unlovable and isolated person, a person others would not want to have sex with or be in a relationship with due to the risk of contracting HIV. Often youth engaged in unprotected sex because they anticipated a lack of companionship due to their serostatus; they were willing to risk transmission for intimacy. Youth were asked to reconstruct their conceptualization of what it means to be a caring, lovable person who protects their sexual partners. The intervention encouraged youth to form a self-identity as a lovable person hwho cares enough about others not to infect them with HIV through unprotected sex, and being a lovable person translates into finding sexual partners who care for who they are, not what they carry in their bodies.

At the 15-month follow-up, youth who attended the intervention reported significantly fewer sexual partners, fewer HIV-negative sexual partners, a lower proportion of sexual acts unprotected by condoms, and less substance use (as reflected in a weighted index of use) than those in the lagged group. Those who attended the intervention were also significantly higher in safer sex and substance use self-efficacy, and behavioral intentions for safer sex were significantly higher at the follow-up interview compared to the lagged group. The authors concluded that delivering systematic behavioral interventions to YLH already linked to intensive medical care further reduced the risk of HIV transmission to others, and interventions for YLH need broad scale implementation. The number of youth who were hesitant to participate in a group format and the difficulty of recruiting a sufficient number of youth to form groups also suggest that other formats need to be examined in the future.

The limited data on gay, runaway, and seropositive youth suggest that HIV prevention programs are likely to be successful with these youth. Each of the successful programs was intensive (at least 12 sessions), included social skills training, had multiple goals (e.g., reducing drug/alcohol use, increasing condom use), was delivered in small groups or institutional settings where learning could be reinforced by peers and adults, and was designed to be engaging and fun. These results are similar to the results of prevention programs for smoking,[68] heart disease,[69] and for adolescents at risk for drug abuse.[70] While researchers have demonstrated that these programs can be successful, there are new challenges confronting HIV prevention researchers, challenges that demand dramatic revisions of the types of programs currently being mounted and evaluated.

Other Considerations

It is important to note that to maintain safe behaviors among gay, runaway, and seropositive youth, it is critical to anticipate relapse and design programs to prevent it.[71,72] In the previously reviewed HIV intervention study of runaways and gay male adolescents, the authors found relapse to unsafe sexual practices.[62] There is evidence among adult gay men[73-76] that relapse of high-risk sexual behavior is common. Among gay men, relapse was especially likely among the younger males,[74] suggesting it may be an even greater problem among adolescents. Adolescent relapse after substance abuse treatment is also high.[77] Therefore, relapse prevention would address identifying ongoing barriers to safe acts and recognizing that day-to-day change is difficult, using peers for motivational support, focusing on consistently implementing safe acts and health maintenance practices, and strengthening and building self-rewards to maintain safe behaviors.

In addition, most successful intervention programs have been delivered in small groups.[78] Small-group interventions offer the opportunity for social support and for learning to be reinforced by peers. Youth have the opportunity to share successful strategies with each other, which can be highly reinforcing and effective for many youth. However, some youth may be concerned with further stigmatization and therefore may not want to attend group meetings. Anonymity and confidentiality are central issues for some youth, similar to gay men.[79] For others, issues related to scheduling reduce attendance; it is often difficult to find one time each week that youth who are working, participating in other recreational activities, and so on, could attend. Overall, small groups, especially those designed for YLH, may not be feasible in small cities, where sufficient numbers of youth are available. Additionally, delivering tailored interventions in a group setting can be problematic. Youth may form unhealthy bonds with other groups members (e.g., drug exchanging), and managing or facilitating adolescents in a group setting is difficult. Therefore, other methods of delivery also should be considered.

Two possible modes for intervention delivery are anonymous telephone groups and individual sessions. Each of these strategies has been demonstrated to be efficacious with adults. Roffman et al.[80] have demonstrated that gay men will participate over time in telephone intervention groups with ongoing significant reductions in risk acts over time. Kelly et al.[45] also established that individual counseling for gay men will result in reductions of HIV-related risk acts. Rotheram-Borus[32] found that delivering an intensive, 10- to 15-session HIV prevention program that incorporated individual sessions in homeless shelters was successful at modifying youth's condom use and high-risk sexual patterns, behaviors typically difficult to change among adolescents. More than 70% participated over time in their interventions. Therefore, evidence suggests that HIV intervention programs can be successfully delivered individually or over the telephone, although this has not been evaluated with adolescents.

Finally, although interventions focus on establishing healthy routines, stable routines require that basic survival needs are met first. At-risk youth whose basic needs are not met will understandably focus their attention not on the desired behavior change but on finding food and shelter, and they are less likely to attend an intervention meeting. Therefore, HIV prevention programs in community settings for youth also must recognize and provide for these basic needs.

FUTURE DIRECTIONS

From the first identification of HIV as a life-threatening virus in 1981, the challenges presented by the HIV pandemic have shifted constantly for policy makers, researchers, and the infected. Early detection of HIV is increasingly needed as one component of prevention programs. A number of recent scientific advances have stimulated major practical and ethical challenges to current HIV testing practices and heightened the importance of systematically examining issues of early detection of HIV as well as the need for coordinated and comprehensive treatment interventions.[81,82] First, those identified as HIV seropositive can potentially be helped to prolong the duration and quality of their life by early intervention with combination antiretroviral therapies.[83–87] Second, the period of new infection has been identified as a time when there are high levels of viral load[88]; this period is likely to be associated with an increased likelihood of transmitting the HIV virus to others.[89] It is critical to reduce the likelihood of transmission during this period by identifying those who are newly infected and teaching both those at high risk and the service provider community to recognize the physical signs of early infection.[90] Third, those who have developed stratified models on the impact of viral transmission have demonstrated the importance of stopping risk behaviors among the infected, particularly considering the extended life expectancies of those infected and of the increasing number of young people becoming infected with HIV. There are substantial fears that decreases in viral load associated with antiretrovirals may lead to increased risk acts among the HIV infected, even among those who have changed their HIV risk acts previously (G.F. Lemp, personal conversation, February 1997). Finally, given that viral load appears to be related to transmission, projections of the epidemic that consider variations in viral load and transmission of the virus across different stages of illness among the infected must be generated.

Unless early detection is realized, most infected adolescents will remain unaware of their serostatus. Among adults, it is estimated that one third of those who are infected in the United States are unaware of their serostatus.[91] Because the time from infection until the development of AIDS has been estimated as 11.5 years,[92–94] many adults may have been infected during adolescence, and youth will have many sexual and substance use partners from the time they are infected until becoming symptomatic and aware of their serostatus. Nationally, the possibility exists to identify the 10,000–20,000 newly infected adolescents per year,[2] but this goal remains unrealized. Wortley et al.[95] found that more than half (51%) of those infected with HIV find out that they are infected within 1 year of their diagnosis with AIDS (about 10 years after infection); this figure is even higher among women (60%). More than a third (36%) of persons discover that they are infected with HIV at the time they are diagnosed with AIDS.[95] About 70% of HIV-positive gay men (ages 17–22) in San Francisco and Berkeley, California, are unaware of their serostatus,[7] and 36% of infected heterosexuals at clinics for those with STDs are unaware.[96] Thus, for the infected to take advantage of the new therapeutic advances, there must be an increased emphasis on early detection and a reconsideration of the role of HIV testing within existing prevention programs.

HIV testing needs to be part of a comprehensive prevention program for adolescents. A majority of prevention programs, particularly programs for adolescents, rely exclusively on condom use as a means of prevention. In countries where there are higher seroprevalence rates, the impact of increased condom use will be far less than the potential preventive impact of early HIV detection on a routine basis.[81] The Swiss national HIV prevention program[97] has demonstrated substantial improvements in knowledge, condom use, and nonstigmatization of disease over 7 years. In particular, this program led to decreased sexual activity among adolescents and increased condom use among young people. However, HIV testing was not initially included in this campaign. HIV testing is one additional component of the prevention arsenal and a vehicle for the infected to enter into the HIV system of care. For example, testing can be part of a multistage practice of personal protection: use condoms until committed to a single partner, both people test for HIV, use condoms another 6 months, get retested for HIV, and then stop using condoms if both people are uninfected.[98] This strategy recognizes that lifetime condom use is an unrealistic expectation and offers an additional prevention strategy for the 95% of adolescents who eventually will want to have children. These data suggest that a new era in prevention must unfold, one that includes testing for HIV as a basic tool within our prevention strategies for adolescents.

Finally, primary prevention must be broadly disseminated among adolescent service providers. Almost all existing prevention programs for adolescents focus on encouraging youth to recognize their HIV risk and seek services. However, in order for broad scale dissemination of prevention programs to occur, service providers must proactively contact youth in order to detect HIV, screen for risk, and implement intensive prevention programs. Among service providers for adolescents, the majority of HIV-identified providers are focused on providing medical care to the infected (M. J. Rotheram-Borus, O. Grusky, T. M. Mann, and M. Lightfoot, unpublished data, 1998); about 25% provide HIV testing services and 12% provide prevention services. The most typical type of service delivered is distributing brochures and single guest lectures about HIV (i.e., AIDS 101). Fewer than 10% of providers are delivering HIV prevention programs in a small-group setting that involves multiple sessions. Thus, even though almost all research with adolescents at high risk has focused on small-group intensive interventions, almost all practice in the field has focused on one-time, informational presentations on HIV. These data suggest the importance of implementing programs with service providers similar to those that have been evaluated for youth.

Youth at high risk for HIV are likely to be at risk for a cluster of negative behavioral outcomes: mental health problems, substance use, school and unemployment problems, and early parenthood. If HIV is addressed in an isolated fashion without recognizing the interaction of problem behaviors related to HIV, it is unlikely that long-term behavior change can be sustained. While a range of HIV services (detection, prevention, care, and aftercare) may be available for some adolescents in AIDS epicenters, there is little research or planning that involves the sectors most likely to care for adolescents at high risk (i.e., substance abuse treatment, juvenile justice, special education classes at school, clinics for STDs, child welfare services, gay-identified youth agencies, and mental health). Future prevention programs with adolescents must begin to focus on the needs for cross-sector coordination and the organization of a comprehensive set of services. Only when such networks are established can adolescents at high risk be expected to maintain their behaviors as their paths take them through different service providers and life situations.

SUMMARY

Accumulating evidence demonstrates the urgent need for HIV prevention services tailored for runaway, homeless, gay, and HIV-infected youth. Similarly, there is substantial research evidence that intensive, cognitive behavioral programs delivered with integrity can reduce HIV-related sexual and substance use behaviors over sustained periods of time. Although general knowledge of HIV and recognition of HIV as a personal threat are prerequisites to behavior change by youth, additional skills are necessary to translate this knowledge into behavior change. As suggested by the personal integration theory, the reconstruction of social roles, social identities, and interpersonal rules are important in implementing safe behaviors. Prevention programs that fail to address the adolescent in a holistic manner are more likely to fail, particularly among at-risk populations of gay, runaway, and seropositive youth. Interventions that build skills coupled with the motivation for change, while paying particular attention to the differences in the sources of motivation as a result of HIV serostatus, allow gay, runaway, and seropositive youth to make positive changes and engage in healthy lifestyles.

However, a new set of challenges has emerged recently for prevention researchers. Advances in HIV therapeutics have significantly increased the benefits of knowing one's serostatus. Knowledge of one's seropositivity benefits both the individual (by the implementation of combination therapies) and society (because most of those who know they are infected reduce their transmission behaviors). However, interventions have not kept pace with the advances in HIV therapeutics and have neglected the continuum of care for youth. For the infected to take advantage of the new therapeutic advances, there must be an increased emphasis on early detection and a reconsideration of the role of HIV testing within existing prevention programs.

Rather than attempting to demonstrate that it is possible to change adolescents' behaviors, it is time to broadly implement prevention programs with providers in real-world settings. There is substantial evidence that providers will require as much information, training, and skills as was invested in implementing effective programs for youth. Interventions for providers must recognize the need for examining intra- and interorganizational relationships in service sectors serving youth, help providers acquire new knowledge, attitudes, and skills in order to implement programs for youth, and directly address structural features in the organization of service settings. HIV systems of care must be implemented that are comprehensive, coordinated, and continuous. These are new challenges that have not previously been addressed by researchers, demonstrating that the challenges in working with runaway, gay, and seropositive youth are ongoing.

REFERENCES

1. Centers for Disease Control and Prevention. HIV/AIDS among young gay and bisexual men. Atlanta, GA: Centers for Disease Control and Prevention; 1995 September.
2. Office of National AIDS Policy. Youth & HIV/AIDS. An American agenda: A report to the president. Washington, DC: Office of National AIDS Policy; 1996.
3. National Institutes of Health. Interventions to prevent HIV risk behaviors. Bethesda, MD: National Institutes of Health; 1997.
4. Kirby D, Collins J, Rugg D, et al. School based programs to reduce sexual risk behaviors: A review of effectiveness. *Public Health Rep* 1994; 109:339–360.
5. Jemmott JB, Jemmott LS. Behavioral interventions with heterosexual adolescents. In: *NIH Consensus Development Conference: Interventions to Prevent HIV Risk Behaviors*. Bethesda, MD: National Institutes of Health; 1997:75–80.
6. Dean L, Meyer I. HIV prevalence and sexual behavior in a cohort of New York City gay men (aged 18–24). *J AIDS Human Retrovirol* 1995; 8:208–211.
7. Lemp GF, Hirozawa AM, Givertz D, et al. Seroprevalence of HIV and risk behaviors among young homosexual and bisexual men. The San Francisco/Berkeley Young Men's Survey. *JAMA* 1994; 272:449–454.
8. Stricof RL, Kennedy JT, Nattell TC, et al. HIV seroprevalence in a facility for runaway and homeless adolescents. *Am J Public Health* 1991; 81:50–53.
9. DiClemente RJ. Epidemiology of AIDS, HIV seroprevalence and HIV incidence among adolescents. *J School Health* 1992; 62:325–330.
10. St. Louis M, Hayman C, Miller C, et al. HIV infection in disadvantaged adolescents in the US: Findings from the Job Corps screening program. Abstracts from the 5th International Conference on AIDS; Montreal, Quebec, Canada; 1989. Abstract no. MDPI. Unpublished.
11. Koopman C, Rosario M, Rotheram-Borus MJ. Alcohol and drug use and sexual behaviors placing runaways at risk for HIV infection. *Addict Behav* 1994; 19:95–103.
12. Centers for Disease Control and Prevention. US HIV and AIDS cases reported through December 1995. *HIV/AIDS Surveillance Report* 1995; 7(Pt 2):6–23.
13. Rotheram-Borus MJ, Rosario M, Meyer-Bahlburg HFL, et al. Sexual and substance use acts of gay and bisexual male adolescents in New York City. *J Sex Res* 1994; 31:47–57.
14. Rotheram-Borus MJ, Meyer-Bahlburg H, Rosario M, et al. Lifetime sexual behaviors among predominantly minority male runaways and gay/bisexual adolescents in New York City. *AIDS Educ Prev* 1992; Fall(suppl): 34–42.
15. Meyer HI, Dean L. Patterns of sexual behavior and risk taking among young New York City gay men. *AIDS Educ Prev* 1995; 7:13–23.
16. Peplau LA, Cochran SD, Mays VM. A national survey of the intimate relationships of African-American lesbians and gay men: A look at commitment, satisfaction, sexual behavior, and HIV disease. In: Greene B, ed. *Ethnic and Cultural Diversity among Lesbians and Gay Men. Psychological Perspectives on Lesbian and Gay Issues*, 3. Newbury Park, CA: Sage; 1997:11–38.
17. Remafedi G. Cognitive and behavioral adaptations to HIV/AIDS among gay and bisexual adolescents. *J Adolesc Health* 1994; 15:142–148.
18. Silvestre AJ, Kingsley LA, Wehman P, et al. Changes in HIV rates and sexual behavior among homosexual men, 1984 to 1988/92. *Am J Public Health* 1993; 83:578–580.
19. Harry J, DeVall W. Age and sexual culture among homosexually oriented males. *Arch Sex Behav* 1978; 7:199–209.
20. Rotheram-Borus MJ, Rosario M, Meyer-Bahlburg HFL, et al. Sexual and substance use acts of gay and bisexual male adolescents in New York City. *J Sex Res* 1994; 31:47–57.
21. National Institute on Drug Abuse. *National Household Survey on Drug Abuse: Population Estimates 1991*. Revised November 20, 1992. Washington, DC: US Government Printing Office; 1992. Publication No.: (ADM) 92-1887.
22. Fullilove RE, Fullilove MT, Bowser BP, Gross SA. Risk of sexually transmitted disease among black adolescent crack users in Oakland and San Francisco, California. *JAMA* 1990; 263:851–855.
23. Stricof R, Novick LF, Kennedy J. HIV-1 seroprevalence in facilities for runaway and homeless adolescents in four states: Florida, Texas, Louisiana, and New York. Presented at 7th International Conference on AIDS; San Francisco, CA; 1990.
24. Shalwitz JC, Goulart M, Dunnigan K, Flannery D. Prevalence of sexually transmitted diseases (STD) and HIV in a homeless youth medical clinic in San Francisco. Paper presented at the Sixth Annual International Conference on AIDS; San Francisco, CA; Abstract No.: SC571, 1990.

25. Sweeney P, Lindegren ML, Buehler JW, et al. Teenagers at risk of human immunodeficiency virus type 1 infection. Results from seroprevalence surveys in the United States. *Arch Pediatr Adolesc Med* 1995; 149: 521–528.

26. Goodman E, Berecochea JE. Predictors of HIV testing among runaway and homeless adolescents. *J Adolesc Health* 1994; 15:566–572.

27. Rotheram-Borus MJ, Koopman C. Sexual risk behavior, AIDS knowledge, and beliefs about AIDS among runaways. *Am J Public Health* 1991; 81:208–210.

28. Pennbridge J, Freese T, MacKenzie R. High-risk behaviors among male street youth in Hollywood, California. *AIDS Educ Prev* 1992; Fall(suppl):24–33.

29. Athey JL. HIV infection and homeless adolescents. *Child Welfare* 1991; 70:517–528.

30. Yates GL, Mackenzi RG, Pennbridge J, Swofford A. A risk profile comparison of homeless youth involved in prostitution and homeless youth not involved. *J Adolesc Health* 1991; 12:545–548.

31. Zimet GD, Sobo EJ, Zimmerman T, et al. Sexual behavior, drug use, and AIDS knowledge among Midwestern runaways. *Youth Soc* 1995; 26:450–462.

32. Rotheram-Borus MJ. Reducing sexual behaviors among runaways at risk for AIDS. Presented at National Institute of Mental Health Conference on Interventions; Washington, DC; 1989.

33. Turner CF , Miller HG, Moses LE, eds. *AIDS: Sexual Behavior and Intravenous Drug Use*. National Research Counsel: Secondary analysis of Kantner and Zelnik's 1979 National Survey of Metropolitan Youths. Washington, DC: National Academy Press; 1989.

34. Miller HG, Turner CF, Moses LE. *AIDS: The Second Decade*. Washington, DC: National Academy Press; 1990.

35. Yates G, MacKenzie R, Pennbridge J, Cohen E. A risk profile comparison of runaway and non-runaway youth. *J Public Health* 1988; 78:820–821.

36. Sonenstein FF, Pleck JH, Ku LC. Sexual activity, condom use and AIDS awareness among adolescent males. *Fam Plann Perspect* 1989; 21:152–158.

37. General Accounting Office. Homelessness and runaway youth receiving services at federally funded shelters. Washington, DC: General Accounting Office; 1989.

38. Sugerman ST, Hergenroeder A, Chacko M, Parcel G. Acquired immunodeficiency syndrome and adolescents: Knowledge, attitudes, and behaviors of runaway and homeless youths. *Am J Dis Child* 1991; 145:431–436.

39. National Institute on Drug Abuse. *National Household Survey on Drug Abuse: Population Estimates 1990*. Washington, DC: Government Printing Office; 1991. DHHS Publication No. (ADM) 91-1732.

40. Fox R, Odaka NJ, Brookmeyer R, Polk BF. Effect of HIV antibody disclosure on subsequent sexual activity in homosexual men. *AIDS* 1987; 1:241–246.

41. Ostrow DG, Monjan A, Joseph J, et al. HIV-related symptoms and psychological functioning in a cohort of homosexual. *Am J Psychiatry* 1989; 146:737–742.

42. Futterman D, Hein K, Kipke M, et al. HIV+ adolescents: HIV testing experiences and changes in risk related sexual and drug use behavior. In: *Abstracts of the Sixth International Conference on AIDS*, 3. Abstract No.: SC 663. 1990:254. San Francisco: University of California, San Francisco.

43. Hein K. AIDS in adolescence: Exploring the challenge. *J Adolesc Health* Care 1989; 10:10–35.

44. Rotheram-Borus MJ, Murphy DA, Coleman CL, et al. Risk acts, health care, and medical adherence among HIV+ youths in care over time. *AIDS Behav* 1997; 1:43–52.

45. Kelly JA, Murphy DA, Sikkema KJ, Kalichman SC. Psychological interventions to prevent HIV infection are urgently needed. New priorities for behavioral research in the second decade of AIDS. *Am Psychol* 1993; 48:1023–1034.

46. Robins AG, Dew MA, Davidson S, et al. Psychosocial factors associated with risk sexual behavior among HIV-seropositive gay men. *AIDS Educ Prev* 1994; 6:483–492.

47. Hein K, Dell R, Futterman D, et al. Comparison of HIV+ and HIV− adolescents: Risk factors and psychosocial determinants. *Pediatrics* 1995; 95:96–104.

48. Cates W. Teenagers and sexual risk taking: The best of times and the worst of times. *J Adolesc Health* 1991; 12: 84–94.

49. Dryfoos JG. A review of interventions to prevent pregnancy. In: Stiffman AR, Feldman RA, eds. *Contraception, Pregnancy, and Parenting. Advances in Adolescent Mental Health*, vol 4. London, England: Jessica Kingsley Publishers; 1990:121–135.

50. Remafedi G. Adolescent homosexuality: Psychosocial and medical implications. *Pediatrics* 1987; 79:331–337.

51. Kelly JA, Murphy DA, Washington CD, et al. The effects of HIV/AIDS intervention groups for high-risk women in urban clinics. *Am J Public Health* 1994; 84:1918–1922.

52. DiClemente RJ, Wingood GM. A randomized controlled trial of an HIV sexual risk-reduction intervention for young African-American women. *JAMA* 1995; 274:1271–1276.

53. Kelly JA, St. Lawrence JS, Stevenson LY, et al. Community AIDS/HIV risk reduction: The effects of endorsements by popular people in three cities. *Am J Public Health* 1992; 82:1483–1489.
54. Jemmott JB, Jemmott LS. Interventions for adolescents in community settings. In: DiClemente RJ, Peterson JL, eds. *Preventing AIDS: Theories and Methods of Behavioral Interventions.* New York: Plenum Press; 1994:141–174.
55. Rotheram-Borus MJ, Koopman C, Haignere C, Davies M. Reducing HIV sexual risk behaviors among runaway adolescents. *JAMA* 1991; 266:1237–1241.
56. Ajzen I, Fishbein M. The prediction of behavior from attitudinal and normative variables. *J Exp Soc Psychol* 1970; 6:466–487.
57. Ajzen I, Fishbein M. A Bayesian analysis of attribution processes. *Psychol Bull* 1975; 82:261–277.
58. Janz NK, Becker MH. The health belief model: A decade later. *Health Educ Q* 1984; 11:1–47.
59. Bandura A. *Social Foundations of Thought and Action: A Social Cognitive Theory.* Englewood Cliffs, NJ: Prentice-Hall; 1986.
60. Ewart CK. Social action theory for a public health psychology. *Am Psychol* 1991; 46:931–946.
61. Rotheram-Borus MJ. Putting research into practice: A case study of the sexual health of homeless youth. The Seventh Biennial Meeting of the Society for Research on Adolescence. San Diego, CA; March 1998.
62. Rotheram-Borus MJ, Rosario M, Reid H, Koopman C. Predicting patterns of sexual acts among homosexual and bisexual youths. *Am J Psychiatry* 1995; 152:588–595.
63. Bandura A. *Self-Efficacy: The Exercise of Control.* New York: WH Freeman & Co; 1997.
64. Bandura A. Perceived self-efficacy in the exercise of control over AIDS infection. In: Mays VM, Albee GW, Schneider SF, eds. *Primary Prevention of AIDS: Psychological Approaches,* vol 13. Newbury Park, CA: Sage; 1989:128–141.
65. Rotheram-Borus MJ, Reid H, Rosario M. Factors mediating changes in sexual HIV risk behaviors among gay and bisexual adolescents. *Am J Public Health* 1994; 84:1938–1946.
66. Augenbraun MH, McCormack WM. Sexually transmitted diseases in HIV-infected persons. *Infect Dis Clin North Am* 1994; 8:439–448.
67. Irwin KL, Pau CP, Lupo D, et al. Presence of human immunodeficiency virus (HIV) type 1 subtype A infection in a New York community with high HIV prevalence: A sentinel site for monitoring HIV genetic diversity in North America. *J Infect Dis* 1997; 176:1629–1633.
68. Walter HJ, Vaughan RD, Wynder EL. Primary prevention of cancer among children: Changes in cigarette smoking and diet after six years of intervention. In: Steptoe A, Wardle J, eds. *Psychosocial Processes and Health: A Reader.* Cambridge, England: Cambridge University Press; 1994:325–335.
69. Perry S, Fishman B, Jacobsberg L, et al. Effectiveness of psychoeducational interventions in reducing emotional distress after human immunodeficiency virus antibody testing. *Arch Gen Psychiatry* 1991; 48:143–147.
70. Botvin GJ. Defining "success" in drug abuse prevention. 50th Annual Scientific Meeting of the Committee on Problems of Drug Dependence. *NIDA Res Monogr* 1988; 90:203–212.
71. Becker MH. Theoretical models of adherence and strategies for improving adherence. In: Shumaker SA, Schron EB, Ockene JK, et al., eds. *The Handbook of Health Behavior Change.* New York: Springer; 1990:5–43.
72. Ekstrand ML, Stall RD, Coates TJ, McKusick L. Risky sex relapse, the next challenge for AIDS prevention programs: The AIDS Behavioral Research Project. In: *Abstracts of the VI International Conference on AIDS.* 1989:699. Unpublished.
73. Roffman R. AIDS prevention with gay men. Paper presented at a meeting of the National Institute of Mental Health. Bethesda, MD; 1991.
74. Kelly J, St. Lawrence J, Brasfield T, et al. Psychological factors that predict AIDS high-risk versus AIDS precautionary behavior. *J Consult Clin Psychol* 1990; 58:117–120.
75. Ostrow DG, Whitaker RE, Frasier K, et al. Racial differences in social support and mental health in men with HIV infection: A pilot study. *AIDS Care* 1991; 3:55–62.
76. Stall R, Ekstrand M. The quantitative/qualitative debate over "relapse" behavior: Comment. *AIDS Care* 1994; 6:619–624.
77. Schinke SP, Botvin GJ, Orlandi MA. *Substance Abuse in Children and Adolescents: Evaluation and Intervention.* Newbury Park, CA: Sage; 1991.
78. Dryfoos JG. Medical clinics in junior high school: Changing the model to meet demands. *J Adolesc Health* 1994; 15:549–557.
79. Roffman RA, Stephens RS, Simpson EE. Relapse prevention with adult chronic marijuana smokers. Special issue: Relapse: Conceptual, research and clinical perspectives. *J Chem Depend Treat* 1989; 2:241–257.
80. Roffman RA, Beadnell B, Ryan R, Downey L. Telephone group counseling in reducing AIDS risk in gay and bisexual males. In: Lloyd GA, Kuszelewicz MA, eds. *HIV Disease: Lesbians, Gays and the Social Services.* New York: Harrington Park Press/Haworth Press; 1995:145–157.

81. Frerichs RR. Personal screening for HIV in developing countries. *Lancet* 1994; 343:960–962.

82. Bayer R, Stryker J, Smith MD. Testing for HIV infection at home. *N Engl J Med* 1995; 332:1296–1299.

83. Eron JJ, Benoit SL, Jemsek J, et al. Treatment with lamivudine, zidovudine, or both in HIV-positive patients with 200 to 500 CD4+ cells per cubic millimeter. *N Engl J Med* 1995; 333:1662–1669.

84. Kaplan JE, Masur H, Jaffe HW, Holmes KK. Reducing the impact of opportunistic infections in patients with HIV infection. New guidelines. *JAMA* 1995; 275:347–348.

85. Kinloch-de Loes S, Perrin L. Therapeutic interventions in primary HIV infection. *J AIDS Human Retrovirol* 1995; 10(suppl 1):S69–76.

86. Sharp D. Vancouver AIDS meeting highlights combination attack on HIV. *Lancet* 1996; 348:115.

87. Stephenson J. New anti-HIV drugs and treatment strategies buoy AIDS researchers. *JAMA* 1996; 275:579–580.

88. Ho DD. Therapy of HIV infections: Problems and prospects. *Bull NY Acad Med* 1996; 73:37–45.

89. Fang G, Burger H, Grimson R, et al. Maternal plasma human immunodeficiency virus type 1 RNA level: A determinant and projected threshold for mother-to-child transmission. *Proc Natl Acad Sci USA* 1995; 92:12100–12104.

90. Clark SJ, Saag MS, Decker WD, et al. High titers of cytopathic virus in plasmas of patients with symptomatic primary HIV-1 infection. *N Engl J Med* 1991; 324:954–960.

91. UNAIDS/WHO Working Group on Global HIV/AIDS and STD Surveillance, compilers. *UNAIDS: Report on the Global HIV/AIDS Epidemic—December 1997*. World AIDS Day; 1997 Nov 26; Geneva, Switzerland.

92. Alcabes P, Munoz A, Vlahov D, Friedland G. Maturity of human immunodeficiency virus infection and incubation period of acquired immunodeficiency syndrome in injecting drug users. *Ann Epidemiol* 1994; 4:17–26.

93. Ghirardini A, Puopolo M, Rossetti G, et al. Survival after AIDS among Italian hemophiliacs with HIV infection. *AIDS* 1995; 9:1351–1356.

94. Nageswaran A, Kinghorn GR, Shen RN, et al. Hospital service utilization by HIV/AIDS patients and their management cost in a provincial genitourinary medicine department. *Int J STD AIDS* 1995; 6:336–344.

95. Wortley PM, Chu SY, Diaz T, et al. HIV testing patterns: Where, why and when were persons with AIDS tested for HIV? *AIDS* 1995; 9:487–492.

96. Simon PA, Weber M, Ford WL, et al. Reasons for HIV antibody test refusal in a heterosexual sexually transmitted disease clinic population. *AIDS* 1996; 10:1549–1553.

97. Dubois-Arber F, Jeannin A, Konings E, Paccaud F. Increased condom use without other major changes in sexual behavior among the general population in Switzerland. *Am J Public Health* 1997; 87:558–566.

98. Kutchinsky B. *The Role of HIV Testing in AIDS Prevention*. Copenhagen, Denmark: University of Copenhagen; 1988.

99. Trends in sexual risk behavior among high school students—United States, 1990, 1991, and 1993. *Morb Mort Wkly Rep* 1995; 44(7):124–125,131–132.

100. Kipke M, O'Connor S, Palmer R, MacKenzie R. Street youth in Los Angeles: Profile of a group at high risk for human immunodeficiency virus infection. *Arch Pediatr Adolesc Med* 1995; 149:513–519.

101. Rotheram-Borus MJ, Marelich W, Srinivasan S. HIV risk among homosexual, bisexual, and heterosexual male and female youths. *Arch Sex Behav* 1999; 28:159–177.

102. Rosario M, Hunter J, Gwadz M. Exploration of substance use among lesbian, gay, and bisexual youth: Prevalence and correlates. *J Adolesc Res* 1997; 12:454–476.

103. Hays R, Kegeles S, Coates T. High HIV risk-taking among young gay men. *AIDS* 1990; 4:901–907.

104. National Institute on Drug Abuse (1992). National household survey on drug abuse: Population estimates 1991, revised Nov. 20, 1992. (Publication No. (ADM)92-1887). Washington, DC: US Government Printing Office.

105. Feitel B, Margetson N, Chamas J, Lipman C. Psychosocial background and behavioral and emotional disorders of homeless and runaway youth. *Hosp Comm Psychiatry* 1992; 43:155–159.

106. Mundy P, Robertson M, Robertson J, Greenblatt M. The prevalence of psychotic symptoms in homeless adolescents. *J Am Acad Child Adolesc Psychiatry* 1990; 29:724–731.

7

The Role of Drug Abuse Treatment in the Prevention of HIV Infection

DAVID S. METZGER, HELEN NAVALINE, and GEORGE E. WOODY

INTRODUCTION

The acquired immunodeficiency syndrome (AIDS) epidemic has had a profound impact on the community of injection drug users (IDUs) in the United States. The human immunodeficiency virus (HIV) is believed to have been introduced into this risk group in the mid-1970s,[1,2] and within two decades estimates suggest that over 300,000 IDUs had become infected. During this time over 100,000 IDUs are believed to have died of AIDS-related causes. Injection drug use has become the leading cause of infection among newly diagnosed AIDS cases.[3]

The AIDS epidemic among IDUs has brought with it numerous attempts to reduce HIV transmission through implementation of a range of interventions including education of drug users about the way the virus is transmitted and methods for reducing risk of infection; increased access to HIV testing and counseling; condom, bleach, and needle distribution; and expanded outreach to drug users who are not in treatment. No intervention, however, has been as widely applied or as carefully evaluated as substance abuse treatment. From the earliest days of the epidemic, drug treatment has been advocated as a cornerstone of the AIDS prevention effort in the United States.[4]

TREATMENT AS PREVENTION

Typically, treatment programs are not considered prevention programs; treatment is usually applied when prevention has failed. In the case of substance abuse treatment, however, there is real potential for treatment to achieve primary prevention goals. Drug treatment has played two important yet distinct roles in the prevention of HIV infection. First, by reducing the frequency of injection, substance abuse treatments have been shown to aid in the direct prevention of HIV transmission. Second, by gaining access to IDUs, treatment programs have served as a primary contact point for public health interventions and information dissemination.

DAVID S. METZGER, HELEN NAVALINE, and GEORGE E. WOODY • Center for Studies of Addiction, Opiate/AIDS Research Division, University of Pennsylvania/VA Medical Center, Philadelphia, Pennsylvania 19104.

Handbook of HIV Prevention, edited by Peterson and DiClemente.
Kluwer Academic / Plenum Publishers, New York, 2000.

Reducing Injection Frequency

To understand the potential of drug treatment as primary prevention, it is necessary to consider the way in which the virus is transmitted among IDUs. Drug use is implicated in the transmission of HIV via direct and indirect transmission routes. Needle sharing, a direct method of transmission, involves the reuse of a contaminated syringe. Infection occurs when residual blood containing virus from an infected individual remains in a needle or syringe and is injected along with the drug solution into an uninfected user. Although the reuse of syringes was rarely studied prior the AIDS epidemic, data from retrospective surveys suggest that the practice was extremely common prior to the initiation of educational initiatives targeting the IDU community.[5,6]

Drug-related transmission of HIV also may occur when injection paraphernalia other than needles and syringes are reused. These "indirect" methods include the transmission of virus via the use of contaminated water to rinse a syringe or mix a drug solution. Also, virus can be transferred via the "cooker" used to heat and dissolve the drug or the "cotton" used to strain the drug solution as it is drawn into the syringe. Virus also can be transmitted when injectors, who often pool money to buy drugs, divide the drug solution by using one syringe to fill others. Since the drug can be more accurately divided in its liquid form, the use of a syringe facilitates fair division and distribution. This practice, known as "frontloading" or "backloading," depending on which end of the syringe is removed, can result in the transfer of infected blood from the syringe used to distribute the solution.[7,8]

Both direct and indirect methods of viral transmission occur at the time of injection. Thus, by assisting drug users to effectively eliminate or reduce the frequency of injection, substance abuse treatment can have a primary prevention impact on both direct and indirect risks of HIV infection. There is a substantial body of literature pointing to the efficacy of drug treatment in reducing substance use.[9,10] In addition, data from the past 15 years have clearly established an association between treatment participation and lower risk of HIV infection.

Access to a Hidden Population

Substance abuse treatment programs also have played an important role in the prevention of HIV transmission by serving as a location within which interventions could reach IDUs. As one of the very few organizations with an interest in maintaining involvement with drug users, drug treatment programs have provided a structure for the delivery of prevention messages and supplies. Many of the early efforts directed at understanding the scope of the epidemic and monitoring its spread were based in treatment programs.[11-13] Also, drug treatment programs were the location of many of the first prevention interventions targeted at IDUs. In many ways, the treatment program served as an outpost in the struggle to slow the spread of HIV infection among the drug-using community.

A major limitation to using treatment programs as HIV prevention delivery vehicles is that only a minority of drug users are in treatment. It is estimated that 10 to 20% of IDUs are in treatment at any given time. However, treated drug users often remain enmeshed in the social networks of those who continue to use drugs, and as such represent a link to those in the community who are not in treatment. Also, given the typically brief treatment experiences of IDUs, most individuals who received interventions while in treatment will leave and carry the prevention messages with them back to the community. Thus, by working with IDUs who are in treatment, it is possible to impact the injection practices of those drug users who are out of treatment.

Treatment Variability

It is important to note that there is great variability among substance abuse treatment programs. The treatment modalities most often used by drug injectors include methadone maintenance, outpatient drug-free residential programs, therapeutic communities, and detoxification services. These program types vary not only across modalities but within modalities as well. Treatment programs use a variety of methods to achieve a variety of objectives. They vary with respect to duration, philosophy, and use of pharmacological adjuncts. They also vary with respect to effectiveness.[9]

In a similar vein, it is common for policy makers and researchers to simply refer to drug users as being "in treatment" or "out of treatment." This conceptualization does not reflect changes that typically occur in drug users' treatment status over time. When patterns of treatment participation are examined, only a minority of users remain in what might be termed stable patterns of treatment. Most individuals who enter treatment do not remain in treatment longer than 6 months. Thus, long-term stable treatment is relatively rare.

DRUG TREATMENT PARTICIPATION AND HIV RISK REDUCTION

Keeping in mind the diversity of substance abuse treatments and the complex manner in which they are implemented and used, the underlying mechanism of HIV protection supported by available data is rather simple: Individuals who enter effective treatments reduce their drug use. Lower rates of use lead to fewer instances of drug-related risk behavior. In turn, lower rates of drug-related risk behaviors result in fewer exposures, and thus infections with HIV. In this model, the individual's use of substances is the causal factor in a chain of events that culminates in exposure to and infection with HIV. Effective treatments break this chain by reducing the frequency of drug use.

The remainder of this chapter will summarize research findings that have examined the relationship between treatment participation and HIV risk reduction, as well as methodological challenges to such research. The data are derived from two broad research approaches: (1) studies that have examined frequency of drug use and related risk behaviors of drug users in and out of treatment, and (2) studies that have used serological data from cohorts of drug users to evaluate the role of treatment in the prevalence and incidence of HIV infection.

Most of the published research has evaluated the impact of methadone treatment. This modality serves opiate-dependent drug users, many of whom were at high risk of HIV infection from injection drug use during the first 15 years of the epidemic. A few studies are beginning to emerge that have evaluated the sexual risk reduction impacts of treatments for noninjection drug use, behaviors that may well define the future of the epidemic among drug users.

Frequency of Injection Drug Use following Treatment Entry

The association between treatment participation and reductions in drug use frequency has been repeatedly reported in the literature.[14–16] Perhaps the most consistent finding has been the association between participation in methadone treatment and lower rates of injection frequency.

Nowhere is this association more clearly articulated than in the data from a 3-year study that examined the drug use patterns of 633 male IDUs participating in methadone maintenance.[17,18] The study participants were drawn from the active caseloads and intake rosters of six methadone maintenance treatment programs in New York City, Philadelphia, and Baltimore. All subjects completed a baseline interview and 506 completed a follow-up interview 1 year later. The results of these interviews allowed investigators to identify a clear pattern of drug use in which nearly all subjects reported daily injection prior to treatment entry. Following treatment entry, rapid reductions in injection frequency were observed and continued for those who remained in treatment. Thirty-seven percent of these subjects reported their last injection occurred just prior to, or during, their time of entry into the program. It is important to note that, for most subjects, the cessation of injection was not immediate on treatment entry. Similarly, some subjects never ceased injection while in treatment. Of those interviewed at follow-up, 29% reported injecting an average of 11 days during the month prior to the interview. While drug was not completely eliminated, when compared to the pretreatment levels of use, the impact of treatment was dramatic: 71% of the subjects had no injections during the prior month and 60% had no injections during the prior year.

A similar pattern of reduction in drug use following treatment entry has been reported more recently in analyses of data from drug users recruited in 15 cities as part of the National Institute on Drug Abuse's Cooperative Agreement studies.[19] These analyses included 2973 drug users who had been recruited while they were out of treatment and followed 6 months later. Once enrolled, all subjects were randomly assigned to either a standard intervention that consisted of comprehensive risk reduction counseling and HIV testing delivered in two sessions or an enhanced intervention that provided additional risk reduction counseling and referral. During the 6-month follow-up interval, 250 (8.4%) had entered and remained in treatment for at least 90 days. Of these, 60% received methadone treatment, 28% outpatient drug-free treatment, and 29% residential treatment (approximately 20% had been in multiple treatment programs). When the drug use patterns of these treated subjects were compared to those who had not entered treatment, significantly lower rates of use were found. Compared to the untreated subjects, those who had entered treatment had injected heroin, cocaine, and speedball (mixture of cocaine and heroin) at significantly lower rates. Significantly lower rates of crack smoking were also found. Additionally, those who had been in treatment for 90 days or more were three times more likely to report no drug use at all and nearly four times more likely to provide a urine specimen with no detectable drugs. Analyses further revealed that participation in enhanced interventions did not account for significant reductions in drug use, and thus, their treatment participation is the most plausible explanation for the reduction in drug use.

Together, the data from these studies highlight the reductions in injection drug use that occur following treatment entry. While such finding are very encouraging, they are by no means definitive and raise many questions about the causal forces that account for these changes.

Drug Use after Treatment

Drug dependence is a chronic disorder and many studies have now documented high rates of relapse following cessation of treatment. Because of the close association between injection drug use and HIV risk behaviors, relapse to drug use often reflects relapse to HIV risk behaviors as well. In fact, drug use following a period of abstinence may involve a higher likelihood of risk behavior since such events are more likely to be unplanned and precipitated by involvement with active users. Also, those with long periods of abstinence may not have ready access to sterile injection equipment.

As mentioned earlier, Ball et al.[18] noted dramatic reductions in drug use following entry into methadone treatment. Equally dramatic was the rapid return to injection by those in the study who left treatment. Using data collected from subjects who left treatment, an 82% annualized relapse rate, defined as return to injection drug use, was derived.

Despite the high relapse rates that occur following treatment, no study has documented a complete return to pretreatment levels of drug use, particularly when the frequency of drug use is measured and the duration of treatment controlled.

Several large, multisite studies have examined the impact of substance abuse treatment by comparing the frequency of drug use during the year prior to treatment with drug use during the year after leaving treatment. Analyses of data from 9989 drug users from 37 treatment programs participating in the Treatment Outcome Prospective Study (TOPS) provide insight on treatment impact during the earliest days of the epidemic.[15] These analyses revealed a rate of weekly or daily heroin use during the year following treatment (16.7%) one fourth that of the pretreatment rate (63.5%). It is important to note that these findings were from methadone patients who had remained in treatment for longer than 3 months. Length of time in treatment was an important predictor of effect size.

More recently, the Center for Substance Abuse Treatment (CSAT) reported the results of the National Treatment Improvement Evaluation Study (NTIES).[20] This 5-year study interviewed 4411 individuals at entry into treatment and again 1 year after leaving treatment. The study included participants entering methadone maintenance, methadone detoxification, outpatient drug-free, short-term residential, long-term residential, and correctional treatment facilities. As in the TOPS data, analyses of changes in drug use patterns revealed dramatically lower rates of heroin use during the year following treatment. This was true for all modalities and all drug types. Heroin use decline 47%, cocaine use dropped 55%, and crack smoking was reduced by 51%.

Importantly, the NTIES data also documented significant reductions in sexual risk behaviors during the year following treatment. Exchange of money or drugs for sex declined 56% from its pretreatment rate of 16.7%, and heterosexual sex with multiple partners and not always using condoms decreased from 43.5% to 28.5%, a 34% decline.

Together, these data suggest that while relapse to drug use is very common among substance abusers who leave treatment, the posttreatment rates of use do not return to pretreatment levels. Thus, there is an overall decline in the rate of drug use and related risk behaviors.

Risk Reduction and Treatment Participation

Do the reductions in drug use observed among those who enter treatment lead to reductions in HIV risk behavior? The available data would suggest that is often the case. Participation in treatment has been found to be associated not only with reductions in injection drug use, but with reductions in needle sharing as well. These data highlight the ability of treatment to interrupt high-risk practices associated with drug use.

In a large community-based survey conducted by Capplehorn and Ross,[21] 1200 IDUs from Sydney, Australia, were interviewed regarding their injection practices and treatment participation. Analyses of these data revealed two important findings. First, those IDUs who were in methadone treatment were 50% less likely to report sharing a syringe. Second, and perhaps more importantly, the protective effects of treatment disappeared when those who had stopped injecting were removed from the analyses. Those who were in treatment and continuing to inject were as likely to report needle sharing as those not in treatment. These data not only document the lower rates of risk behavior among IDUs in treatment, they also suggest that it is the reduction in drug use, not safer injection practices, that accounts for the protective effects of treatment.

These authors also summarized the results of eight other studies in which needle sharing among IDUs in methadone treatment was compared to their untreated counterparts from the same communities. These studies were conducted in Australia, Europe, and the United States between 1985 and 1995. With one exception, these studies each observed significantly lower rates of sharing among those in methadone treatment. Rates were from one third to one half of those found among the out-of-treatment subjects.

Lower rates of risk behaviors have been reported by others and the consistency of their results is notable. Abdul-Quader et al.[22] found that both frequency of drug injection and the practice of injecting in shooting galleries were significantly reduced proportionate to the amount of time spent in methadone maintenance treatment. In another study, conducted in New Haven, Connecticut, 107 methadone-maintained IDUs and 314 IDUs who were not in treatment were surveyed regarding their risk behaviors. Frequency of injections were found to be 50–65% ($P < .001$) higher among the out-of-treatment subjects.[23]

Treatment of Noninjection Drug Use and Risk Reduction

Although our discussion in this chapter is focused primarily on injection drug use, there are data emerging from the treatment of noninjection drug use (e.g., crack smoking and alcohol) that suggest an association between treatment and reductions in risky sexual behaviors. Data from these interventions are important for several reasons. First, they provide further opportunity to examine the protective effects of substance abuse treatment participation. Despite the fact that noninjection drug use involves the sexual transmission of HIV, there is a close association between unprotected sexual activity and substance use, particularly cocaine and alcohol. Second, most injection drug users also use noninjection drugs. Thus, in many cases, the treatments are serving similar, if not the same, populations.

A study of HIV risk behavior change among individuals receiving alcohol treatment was reported by Avins et al.[24] In this study, 700 alcohol-dependent subjects completed a baseline assessment and follow-up an average 13 months later. In comparing baseline and follow-up data, significant reductions in both sexual and drug-related risks were found. These included a 15% reduction in reports of multiple sex partners, a 58% reduction in injection drug use, a 26% reduction in the number of partners who were IDUs, and a 77% increase in consistent condom use.

In a similarly designed study, Shoptaw and colleagues[25] in Los Angeles found significant reductions in risk behaviors among 232 cocaine-abusing or -dependent individuals who received up to 6 month of weekly drug counseling. Despite the fact that no formal HIV prevention interventions were delivered, those who completed treatment showed significant decreases in sexual risk behavior, primarily the result of a reduction in the number of sexual partners. Among those who demonstrated a treatment effect, the sexual risk reductions accompanied reductions in cocaine use as monitored by urinalysis.

The findings of these studies are consistent with the data from evaluations of treatment of injection drug use: Effective substance abuse treatments lead to reductions in drug use, which in turn lead to reductions in drug-related risk behaviors.

Prevention Interventions within Treatment Settings

As mentioned earlier, one of the important prevention roles played by drug treatment has been to provide a location for the delivery of prevention interventions to drug users at risk of

HIV infection. Many of the early educational initiatives targeted at drug users were based in treatment programs, as were the first large-scale efforts to provide HIV counseling and testing to IDUs. While these efforts are generally considered to have achieved a rapid increase in the awareness of AIDS and basic prevention messages among IDUs, the ability to assess their impact has been limited by the absence of adequate evaluation data.[16,26]

Many of the initial treatment-based prevention initiatives were begun early in the epidemic when implementation was more urgent than research and evaluation. Thus, many interventions were implemented without adequate research designs that could provide valid and reliable data regarding impact. Second, HIV risk reduction interventions are now provided as components within the drug treatment setting. The coexisting effects of drug treatment make it extremely difficult to monitor and control the impact of risk reduction interventions. It has been difficult to separate the effects of these interventions from the impact of drug treatment itself.[27]

In this regard, it is important to note that the AIDS epidemic has had an impact on the way in which treatment programs operate. Prevention messages have been incorporated into routine drug counseling. Program goals and structures in many cases have been adjusted to give priority to HIV-infected participants.[28] Medical services within treatment programs have received more attention in an effort to directly provide or arrange for the delivery of clinical care to HIV-infected program participants.[29] Thus, many treatment programs have attempted to incorporate prevention messages and medical service provision into their service delivery, rather than delivering distinct HIV and AIDS prevention interventions.

BIOLOGICAL OUTCOMES: HIV PREVALENCE AND INCIDENCE AND TREATMENT PARTICIPATION

A variety of observational and "nonrandomized" experimental strategies have been used to examine prevalence and incidence of HIV infection among IDUs and its relationship to participation in substance abuse treatment. These approaches have produced findings consistent with the self-report behavioral data from drug users in and out of treatment.

Perhaps the first report linking treatment participation to lower rates of HIV infection appeared in 1984, shortly after the virus had been isolated and antibody testing became available.[30] In describing prevalence rates among individuals from known risk groups, antibody test results from 86 "heavy IV drug users" in New York City found 75 (87%) to be infected. In contrast, less than 10% of 35 methadone-maintained drug users were found to be infected. All of the methadone patients had been in treatment for greater than 3 years and had "greatly reduced" their IV drug use.

In 1985, Novick et al.[2] reported on the findings of HIV testing from stored samples of blood that had been collect between 1978 and 1983 from IDUs participating in a study of chronic liver disease. Of the 48 subjects who were in methadone treatment at the time they were studied, 23% tested positive for HIV. This rate dropped to 17% among those who had been in treatment for 5 years or longer. Of those not in treatment at the time of study, 47% tested positive for antibody to HIV.

In 1988, Brown et al.[31] noted that rates of HIV varied with length of time in treatment. Among the 360 injectors studied, those who had been in treatment for longer periods of time had significantly lower rates of infection. In fact, the patients who had been in treatment for less than 1 year were 1.5 times more likely to test positive for HIV. While overall, the rate of infection was highest among African-American subjects, the relationship between prevalence and duration of treatment was consistent across racial groups.

Together, data from these early prevalence studies suggested that methadone treatment was a valuable intervention in reducing HIV infection among IDUs. Beyond this, for the first time evidence of the public health significance of substance abuse treatment was beginning to emerge. It was also becoming clear that treatment duration was a critical factor in understanding the protective effects of treatment.

By the end of the 1980s, several studies had reported on low rates of HIV infection among individuals who had continually been in methadone treatment during the period of rapid spread of HIV infection. In 1988, in New York City, 58 individuals who had been in methadone treatment for an average of 17 years were tested and found to be uninfected with HIV. During the time they had been treated, the prevalence of HIV infection among IDUs in New York had risen to over 50%.[32] Similarly, Blix and Gronbladh[33] examined HIV testing data collected in 1984 from methadone patients in Uppsala, Sweden. Only two infections (3%) were found among 67 patients who had been admitted prior to 1979. During this time HIV infection rates had risen to 38% among IDUs. Importantly, both infected individuals were women in relationships with IDU men. The 65 HIV-negative patients, all of whom remained in treatment, remained uninfected as of 1990.

In an observational study of HIV seroincidence among 681 IDUs, Moss et al.[34] examined the characteristics that best distinguished those who seroconverted from those who remained uninfected. Subjects in this study were methadone patients who had been tested at least twice while in treatment in San Francisco between 1985 and 1990. The study identified 22 seroconverters for an average annual seroconversion rate of 1.9% per person year of study. It is important to note that the incidence rate was 4% per person year among African-American subjects.

The risk factors that were found to be significantly associated with seroconversion included having more than five sexual partners per year, ever using a shooting gallery, and having less than 1 year of methadone maintenance treatment. In fact, over three times the rate of infection was found among those with less than 1 year of treatment when they were compared with those with a year or more of methadone maintenance treatment.

In a case–control study, nested within a prospective evaluation of 952 seronegative IDUs, 40 incident cases were matched to 40 subjects who remained seronegative.[35] In analyses directed at identifying differences between cases and controls, duration of methadone treatment and methadone dosage were found to have dramatic protective effects. For every 3 months spent out of treatment, the risk of getting infected with HIV increased by 70%. Further, the higher the methadone dosage, the lower the risk of infection. In multivariate analyses, these variables remained the most salient characteristics in explaining differences between cases and controls.

In Philadelphia, a prospective longitudinal study of HIV infection and risk behaviors among in- and out-of-treatment drug users was initiated in 1989.[36] In this study, 152 IDUs were randomly selected from a methadone treatment program and 103 out-of-treatment IDUs were recruited using a chain referral technique. Consistent with prior work, this study found significantly lower rates of needle sharing, injection frequency, shooting gallery use, and visits to crack houses among the methadone maintained IDUs.

At entry into this study, 18% of the out-of-treatment subjects and 11% of the methadone-maintained clients tested positive for antibodies to HIV. After 18 months of study, 33% of the out-of-treatment cohort were infected, while 15% of the methadone clients tested positive ($P < .01$). The incidence of new infection was strongly associated with participation in methadone treatment. When incidence rates were examined in relation to whether or not the subjects remained in treatment, changed their treatment status, or remained out of treatment, dramatically different rates of incident HIV cases were observed. Those who remained out of treatment were nearly six times more likely to have become infected than were those who remained in treatment during the first 18 months of the study. Among those who remained in methadone treatment for the entire 18-month study period, 3.5% became infected. Among those who remained out of treatment, 22% became infected with HIV.

Recently, Friedman et al.[37] reported the results of analyses directed at examining the factors associated with seroconversion among 6882 IDUs who had at least two HIV tests. Subjects were participants in the National AIDS Demonstration Research Projects and the AIDS Targeted Outreach Models projects and were drawn from 15 cities characterized as either high prevalence (> 20%) or low prevalence (< 8%) based on the baseline infection rates. Having been in any drug treatment program during the follow-up interval was the only variable significantly "protective" and it was the only variable that reached significance in both high- and low-prevalence cities.

CONCLUSION

Numerous studies now have documented that significantly lower rates of risk behaviors are practiced by drug users who are in treatment. This has been the finding when in-treatment IDUs were compared to untreated IDUs, when drug use patterns during treatment were compared to pretreatment patterns, and when drug use patterns during treatment were compared to posttreatment drug use practices. Importantly, these self-report behavioral differences are consistent with seroprevalence and seroincidence data.

Despite the consistency of these findings, one cannot escape the dilemma that without randomized controlled clinical trials, the differences cannot be attributed unequivocally to the treatment process. The most serious threat to the conclusion that drug treatment reduces the risk of HIV infection, comes from the possibility of selection bias. It could be argued that those individuals who seek and enter drug treatment are "by nature" more likely to practice safer behaviors than those who do not enter treatment.

The available data, however, do not provide strong support for such an interpretation. The findings presented here indicate that both pre- and posttreatment drug use behaviors are dramatically elevated when compared to drug use and related risk behaviors during treatment. Investigators also have identified a "dose–response" relationship between treatment duration, intensity, and methadone dosage and participation in risk behavior.[38,39] Thus, while methodological challenges may serve a useful purpose in encouraging more rigorous research, they should not prevent us from forming well-reasoned conclusions based on the preponderance of evidence.

A final note on the prevention potential of substance abuse treatment programs. In addition to the direct delivery of drug treatment, these programs have had an important role in the implementation of many other prevention initiatives. As one of the few organized social institutions with access to drug users at risk of HIV infection, treatment programs have in many ways become community-based staging areas for risk reduction interventions directed at IDUs. There is growing awareness that individuals who are in treatment provide access to a much larger community of out-of-treatment drug users. Similar to the disproportionate impact that is achieved when even a partially effective vaccine is given to many individuals, significant preventive impact is possible through the effective treatment of those drug users engaged in a treatment program. Despite their small numbers, drug users in treatment provide a bridge to the larger community of drug users.

Unfortunately, funding for the support of substance abuse treatment programs has eroded during the course of the AIDS epidemic; there are now fewer treatment programs available and within programs fewer services.[40] Residential services have been particularly affected and detoxification program regimens now typically extend only a few days. Thus, to maximize the preventive potential of drug and alcohol treatment, it will be necessary to first establish funding mechanisms that allow for an expansion of the treatment system and provide a stable base for program operations.

The strength of the data presented here derives its power from the consistency of findings among behavioral studies and studies that have used HIV infection as a biological marker. While these findings are impressive, they do not address some of the fundamental issues involved in understanding treatment. At the same time we must continue to investigate the "active ingredients" of substance abuse treatment and to increase research attention on those factors associated with treatment entry and retention. Research needs to address the issue of access to treatment. If treatment programs are to maximize their impact, access is critical. However, little is known about the forces that attract users into treatment and the barriers that impede treatment entry. Beyond cost and space constraints, there is a need to better understand drug users' perceptions regarding drug treatment.

In reviewing the literature on the role of treatment in the prevention of HIV infection, it is important to note that emphasis on HIV prevention initiatives have forced the treatment community to adopt a broader perspective of its work. Although it has become more common to hear reference to the role of drug treatment in slowing the spread of this epidemic, this is a new phenomenon. Prior to the AIDS epidemic, drug treatment had little recognition or support outside a small community of physicians, health care workers, counselors, recovering people, and active users. One legacy of the AIDS epidemic may be the increased awareness of the link between the health of marginalized communities, such as IDUs, and the health of the nation.

REFERENCES

1. Des Jarlais DC, Friedman SR, Hopkins W. Risk reduction for the acquired immunodeficiency syndrome among intravenous drug users. *Ann Intern Med* 1985; 103:755–759.
2. Novick DM, Kreek MJ, Des Jarlais DC, et al. Abstract of clinical research findings: Therapeutic and historical aspects. *NIDA Res Monogr* 1985; 67:318–320.
3. Holmberg SD. Estimated prevalence and incidence of HIV in 96 large US metropolitan areas. *Am J Public Health* 1996; 86:642–654.
4. Cooper JR. Methadone treatment and acquired immunodeficiency syndrome. *JAMA* 1989; 262:1664–1668.
5. Vlahov D, Anthony JC, Celentano D, et al. Trends of HIV-1 risk reduction among initiates into intravenous drug use 1982–1987. *Am J Drug Alcohol Abuse* 1991; 17:39–48.
6. McCusker J, Stoddard A, Koblin B, et al. Time trends in high-risk injection practices in a multi-site study in Massachusetts: Effects of enrollment site and residence. *AIDS Educ Prev* 1992; 4:108–119.
7. Marmor M, Des Jarlais DC, Cohen H, et al. Risk factors for infection with human immunodeficiency virus among intravenous drug abusers in New York City. *AIDS* 1987; 1:39–44.
8. Koester S, Hoffer L. "Indirect sharing" additional risks associated with drug injection. *AIDS Public Policy* 1994; 2:100–105.
9. Institute of Medicine. *Treating Drug Problems*, vol. 1. Washington, DC: National Academy Press; 1990.
10. McLellan AT, Woody G, Metzger D, et al. Evaluating the effectiveness of addiction treatments: reasonable expectations, appropriate comparisons. *Milbank Q* 1996; 74:51–85.
11. Kozel NJ, Adams EH. Epidemiology of drug abuse: An overview. *Science* 1986; 234:970–974.
12. Hahn RA, Onorato I, Jones TS, Dougherty J. Prevalence of HIV infection among intravenous drug users in the United States. *JAMA* 1989; 261:2677–2684.
13. Battjes RJ, Pickens RW, Amsel Z. HIV infection and AIDS risk behaviors among intravenous drug users entering methadone treatment in selected US cities. *J Acquir Immune Defic Syndr* 1991; 4:1148–1154.

14. Orr MF, Glebatis D, Friedmann P, et al. Incidence of HIV infection in a New York City methadone maintenance treatment program. *JAMA* 1996; 276:99.
15. Hubbard RL, Marsden ME, Cavanaugh E, et al. Role of drug-abuse treatment in limiting the spread of AIDS. *Rev Infect Dis* 1988; 10:377–384.
16. McCusker J, Stoddard AM, Hindin RN, et al. Changes in HIV risk behavior following alternative residential programs of drug abuse treatment and AIDS education. *Ann Epidemiol* 1996; 6:119–125.
17. Ball JC, Lange RL, Myers CP, Friedman SR. Reducing the risk of AIDS through methadone maintenance treatment. *J Health Soc Behav* 1988; 29:214–226.
18. Ball JC, Ross A. *The Effectiveness of Methadone Maintenance Treatment.* New York: Springer-Verlag; 1991.
19. Booth RE, Crowley T, Zhang Y. Substance abuse treatment entry, retention and effectiveness: Out-of-treatment opiate injection drug users. *Drug Alcohol Depend* 1996; 42:11–20.
20. Center for Substance Abuse Treatment. *NTIES: National Treatment Improvement Evaluation Study Preliminary Report: The Persistent Effects of Substance Abuse Treatment—One Year Later.* Washington, DC: US Dept Health and Human Services; 1996.
21. Caplehorn JRM, Ross MW. Methadone maintenance and the likelihood of risky needle sharing. *Int J Addic* 1995; 30:685–698.
22. Abdul-Quader AS, Friedman SR, Des Jarlais DC, et al. Methadone maintenance and behaviors by intravenous drug users that can transmit HIV. *Contemp Drug Prob* 1987; 14:425–433.
23. Meandzija B, O'Connor P, Fitzgerald B, et al. HIV infection and cocaine use in methadone maintained and untreated injection drug users. *Drug Alcohol Depend* 1994; 36:109–113.
24. Avins AL, Woods WJ, Lindan CP, et al. HIV infection and risk behaviors among heterosexuals in alcohol treatment programs. *JAMA* 1994; 271:515–518.
25. Shoptaw S, Frosch DL, Rawson RA, Ling W. Cocaine abuse counseling as HIV prevention. *AIDS Educ Prev* 1997; 9:509–518.
26. Calsyn DA, Sazon J, Freeman G, Whittaker S. Ineffectiveness of AIDS education and HIV antibody testing in reducing high-risk behaviors among injection drug users. *Am J Public Health* 1992; 82:573–575.
27. Booth RE, Watters JK. How effective are risk-reduction interventions targeting injecting drug users? *AIDS* 1994; 8:1515–1524.
28. Sorenson JL, Miller MS. Impact of HIV risk and infection on delivery of psychosocial treatment services in outpatient programs. *J Subst Abuse Treat* 1996; 13:387–395.
29. Selwyn PA. Impact of HIV infection on medical services in drug abuse treatment programs. *J Subst Abuse Treat* 1996; 13:397–410.
30. Centers for Disease Control and Prevention. Antibodies to a retrovirus etiologically associated with acquired immunodeficiency syndrome (AIDS) in populations with increased incidences of the syndrome. *Morb Mortal Wkly Rep* 1984; 33:377–379.
31. Brown LS, Burkette W, Primm BJ. Drug treatment and HIV seropositivity. *NY State J Med* 1988; 88:156.
32. Novick DM, Joseph H, Croxon TS, et al. Absence of antibody to human immunodeficiency virus in long-term, socially rehabilitated methadone maintenance patients. *Arch Intern Med* 1990; 150:97–99.
33. Blix O, Gronbladh L. Impact of methadone maintenance treatment on the spread of HIV among IV heroin addicts in Sweden. In: Loimer N, Schmid R, Springer A, eds. *Drug Addiction and AIDS.* New York: Springer-Verlag Wien; 1991:200–205.
34. Moss AR, Vranizan K, Gorter R, et al. HIV seroconversion in intravenous drug users in San Francisco, 1985–1990. *AIDS* 1994; 8:223–231.
35. Serpelloni G, Carriere MP, Rezza G, et al. Methadone treatment as a determinant of HIV risk reduction among injecting drug users: A nested case-controlled study. *AIDS Care* 1994; 6:215–220.
36. Metzger DS, Woody GE, McLellan AT, et al. Human immunodeficiency virus seroconversion among in- and out-of-treatment intravenous drug users: An 18-month prospective follow-up. *J Acquir Immune Defic Syndr* 1993; 6:1049–1056.
37. Friedman SR, Jose B, Deren S, et al. Risk factors for HIV seroconversion among out-of-treatment drug injectors in high and low seroprevalence cities. *Am J Epidemiol* 1995; 142:864–874.
38. McLellan AT, Arndt IO, Metzger DS, et al. Effects of psychological services in substance abuse treatment. *JAMA* 1993; 269:1953–1959.
39. Yancovitz SR, Des Jarlais DC, Peskoe-Peyser N, et al. Randomized trial of an interim methadone maintenance clinic. *Am J Public Health* 1991; 81:1185–1191.
40. Etheridge RM, Craddock SG, Dunteman GH, Hubbard RL. Treatment services in two national studies of community-based drug abuse treatment programs. *J Subst Abuse* 1995; 7:9–26.

8

HIV/AIDS Prevention for Drug Users in Natural Settings

DON C. DES JARLAIS, JOSEPH GUYDISH, SAMUEL R. FRIEDMAN, and HOLLY HAGAN

INTRODUCTION

Now, in the second decade of the human immunodeficiency virus (HIV) epidemic, injection drug use and related risk behaviors continue to spread HIV to drug users, their sexual partners, and their children. In this chapter we briefly describe the epidemiology of HIV infection among injection drug users (IDUs), including the health impacts of infection in this population, and the factors that facilitate or impede transmission. Second, we describe key strategies for HIV prevention among IDUs, beginning with consideration of stereotypes about IDUs and social desirability as they affect research among IDUs. We then describe research concerning three broad preventive strategies (methadone maintenance, street outreach, and syringe exchange), with examples of how these strategies have been tailored to the needs of special populations and of how they have been integrated to achieve greater potential impact. Third, we discuss limitations of research on HIV prevention among IDUs, including standards for assessing prevention programs and problematic issues in preventing HIV infection in this population. Finally, we comment on the philosophy of harm reduction as an important conceptual development that grew out of HIV prevention efforts and at the same time provides a common denominator for HIV prevention strategies among IDUs.

EPIDEMIOLOGY OF HIV INFECTION AMONG IDUs

HIV has been reported among injecting drug users in 80 countries.[1] This is a substantial increase over the 59 countries with HIV infection among IDUs in 1989.[2] In some European countries, such as Spain and Italy, injecting drug use has long been the most common risk factor for HIV infection and acquired immunodeficiency syndrome (AIDS).[3] In the United States, injecting drug use has been associated with approximately one third of the cumulative cases of AIDS.[4] Over half of the US heterosexual transmission cases have involved transmission from an injecting drug user, and over half of the perinatal transmission cases have

DON C. DES JARLAIS • Chemical Dependency Institute, Beth Israel Medical Center, New York, New York 10003. *JOSEPH GUYDISH* • Institute for Health Policy Studies, University of California, San Francisco, California 94109. *SAMUEL R. FRIEDMAN* • National Development and Research Institutes, New York, New York 10048. *HOLLY HAGAN* • Seattle/King County Department of Health, Seattle, Washington 98104.

Handbook of HIV Prevention, edited by Peterson and DiClemente. Kluwer Academic / Plenum Publishers, New York, 2000.

occurred in women who injected drugs themselves or were the sexual partners of injecting drug users. In the most recent estimate of new HIV infections in the United States, approximately half of all new infections in the country are occurring among injecting drug users.[5]

Health Impacts of HIV Infection among IDUs

In sharp contrast to HIV infection among homosexual–bisexual men, HIV infection among IDUs leads to a wider variety of illnesses than the original opportunistic infections that were used to define AIDS. HIV infection has been associated with increased morbidity and/or increased mortality for tuberculosis, bacterial pneumonia, endocarditis,[6] and cervical cancer (through a possible interaction with human papilloma virus).[7] The 1987 and 1993 revisions of the Centers for Disease Control (CDC) surveillance definition for AIDS were based in part on the studies of the wider spectrum of HIV-related illnesses among IDUs. Prior to these revisions, many IDUs were dying from HIV-related illnesses without ever being classified as having AIDS.[6]

The mechanisms through which HIV infection leads to this wider spectrum of illnesses have not yet been identified. Tuberculosis (TB) infection is controlled primarily through cell-mediated immunity, so that one would expect HIV infection to lead to increased reactivation of latent TB infection and increased susceptibility to TB infection. HIV infection also can affect humoral immune functioning,[8] so that resistance to many infectious agents may be compromised. The lifestyle of many IDUs also may put them at greater risk for exposure to a wide variety of pathogens and reduce immune functioning through mechanisms such as poor nutrition.

Whether continued use of psychoactive drugs influences the course of HIV infection among IDUs has been an important question since AIDS was first noticed among IDUs. A wide variety of psychoactive substances have at least some *in vitro* effects on components of the immune system. Studies comparing progression of HIV infection among IDUs and among men infected through male-with-male sex, however, generally have shown no differences in the rate of CD4 cell count loss or development of AIDS.[9] At present, it does not appear that continued use of psychoactive drugs per se has any strong effect on the course of HIV infection among IDUs. Immune system activation, however, may increase replication of HIV,[10] so that very high frequencies of nonsterile injections or the development of other infections such as bacterial pneumonia may increase progression of HIV infection.

Transmission of HIV among IDUs

In many areas, HIV has spread extremely rapidly among IDUs, with the HIV seroprevalence rate (the percentage of IDUs infected with HIV) increasing from less than 10% to 40% or greater within a period of 1 to 2 years.[11] Several factors have been associated with extremely rapid transmission of HIV among IDUs: (1) lack of awareness of HIV/AIDS as a local threat; (2) restrictions on the availability and use of new injection equipment; and (3) mechanisms for rapid, efficient mixing within the local IDU population. Without an awareness of AIDS as a local threat, injecting drug users are likely to use each other's equipment very frequently. Indeed, prior to an awareness of HIV/AIDS, providing previously used equipment to another IDU is likely to be seen as an act of solidarity among IDUs or as a service for which one may legitimately charge a small fee.

There are various types of legal restrictions that can reduce the availability of sterile injection equipment, and thus lead to increased multiperson use ("sharing") of drug injection equipment. In some jurisdictions, medical prescriptions are required for the purchase of needles and syringes. Possession of needles and syringes also can be criminalized as "drug paraphernalia," putting users at risk of arrest if needles and syringes are found in their possession. Even if laws permit sales of needles and syringes without prescriptions, pharmacists may choose not to sell without prescriptions or not to sell to anyone who "looks like a drug user." Similarly, police may harass drug users found carrying injection equipment even if there are no laws criminalizing the possession of narcotics paraphernalia.

"Shooting galleries" (places where IDUs can rent injection equipment, which is then returned to the gallery owner for rental to other IDUs) and "dealer's works" (injection equipment kept by a drug seller, which can be lent to successive drug purchasers) are examples of situations that provide rapid, efficient mixing within an IDU population. The mixing is rapid in that many IDUs may use the gallery or the dealer's injection equipment within very short periods of time. Several studies have indicated that the infectiousness of HIV is many times greater in the 2- to 3-month period between initial infection and the development of severe immunosuppression.[12] Thus, the concentration of new infections in these settings may synergistically interact with continued mixing and lead to highly infectious IDUs transmitting HIV to large numbers of other drug injectors. Efficient mixing refers to the sharing of drug injection equipment with few restrictions on who shares with whom. Thus efficient mixing serves to spread HIV across potential social boundaries, such as friendship groups, which otherwise might have served to limit transmission. Based on retrospective interviews we conducted with IDUs in New York City, approximately one quarter of all injections occurred in shooting galleries during the period of rapid HIV transmission (1978 to 1984).[13]

HIV/AIDS PREVENTION FOR IDUs

Stereotypes and Social Desirability in IDU Research

The common stereotype that IDUs are not at all concerned about health led to initial expectations that they would not change their behavior because of AIDS. In sharp contrast to these expectations, reductions in risk behavior were observed among IDU participants in a wide variety of early prevention programs, including outreach/bleach distribution,[14,15] "education only,"[16,17] drug abuse treatment,[18] syringe exchange,[19] increased over-the-counter sales of injection equipment,[20,21] and HIV counseling and testing.[22,23]

It also is important to note that there is evidence that IDUs will reduce HIV risk behavior in the absence of any specific prevention program. IDUs in New York City reported risk reduction prior to the implementation of any formal HIV prevention programs.[24,25] IDUs had learned about AIDS through the mass media and the oral communication networks within the drug-injecting population, and the illicit market in sterile injection equipment had expanded to provide additional equipment.[26]

Rather than having to overcome indifference to AIDS among IDUs, the scientific problem became one of understanding and quantifying the change processes. The differences in research design and measurement instruments in these early studies generally have precluded any comparisons regarding the differential effectiveness of the different HIV prevention programs. It also was difficult to determine how a specific prevention program might be contributing to behavior change processes and the effects of the behavior change on the rate of new HIV infections among IDUs and their sexual partners.

Possible "social desirability" effects also were an important potential problem in interpreting the early behavior change studies. It was clear that subjects were reporting reduced risk behavior, but this might have been that the subjects simply learned what the researchers wanted to hear and were providing the socially desirable responses without any meaningful changes in risk behavior. Research conducted as part of the World Health Organization (WHO) Multi-Centre study show significantly lower HIV infection rates among IDUs who reported changing their behavior in response to AIDS than the rates among IDUs who did not report changing their behavior in response to AIDS.[27,28] While there was important variation across sites, the overall protective effect adjusted odds ratio of self-reported behavior change against infection with HIV was 0.50. Social desirability effects still must be considered in any research on highly stigmatized behaviors such as injecting drug use and the "sharing" of drug injection equipment, but there is evidence for the construct validity of self-reported AIDS risk reduction among IDUs.

Strategies for Preventing HIV among IDUs

Over the last few years, sufficient data have been accumulated to provide estimates of the likely HIV incidence after implementation of three types of prevention programs: methadone maintenance treatment, street outreach, and syringe exchange.

Methadone Maintenance Treatment

Many different types of drug abuse treatment, including residential therapeutic communities, outpatient drug-free counseling, and methadone maintenance, have been shown to reduce the use of illicit drugs, including the injection of illicit drugs.[29,30] Thus, it is quite reasonable to expect that participation in drug treatment would lead to reductions in unsafe drug injection and then to reductions in HIV incidence. While this expectation should hold for all types of drug treatment that have been shown to be effective in reducing drug injection, there are sufficient data to assess only methadone maintenance treatment with respect to rates of new HIV infection.

A variety of studies have shown that participation in methadone maintenance treatment is associated with lower rates of HIV risk behavior and with lower HIV seroprevalence compared to persons not in drug abuse treatment. Table 1 shows HIV incidence data among methadone patients in selected cities. The rate among methadone maintenance patients in the Swedish study[18] is particularly striking, given that HIV seroprevalence increased from 0 to approximately 50% over the same time period among a group of heroin injectors who applied to the methadone program but could not be accepted because the program was already at capacity. The incidence rate among the Philadelphia methadone patients is not low, but in the

Table 1.   HIV Incidence among Methadone
Maintenance Patients

Location	Rate per 100 person-years at risk	Reference
Sweden	0.00	18
Los Angeles	0.07	32
New York	0.88	33
Philadelphia	2.30	31
Amsterdam	4.00	34

same study HIV incidence among a comparison group of drug injectors who were not in methadone maintenance was six times as high.[31]

The very low rate seen in Los Angeles is undoubtedly a function of the low HIV seroprevalence among drug injectors in the Los Angeles area.[32] The incidence rate in the New York City program[33] also must be considered low given the high HIV seroprevalence in the city (between 40 and 50% at the time of data collection).

Amsterdam clearly has a relatively high HIV incidence rate among its methadone patients, and this rate is not different from the rate among IDUs in Amsterdam who did not participate in methadone maintenance programs.[34] This may be due to several factors, including low methadone doses prescribed for the patients (below where cross-tolerance to heroin and protection from heroin use occurs) and cocaine injection among the patients (methadone provides no pharmacological protection against cocaine use). Since these data were collected, the Amsterdam program has increased the dosages of methadone that are prescribed.

Street Outreach

Street outreach HIV prevention strategies were initially developed to address the prevention needs of out-of-treatment IDUs, and early programs began in the United States in the mid-1980s.[35] Early street outreach efforts focused on HIV prevention and education messages, and were soon supplemented with distribution of bleach (to decontaminate syringes) and condoms. Outreach programs were designed and implemented quickly and used to interrupt the spread of HIV while other interventions could be developed.[36] The main objective for many of the early outreach programs was to provide information and prevention materials in a nonjudgmental context that would educate and support IDUs in lowering their HIV risk behavior. Outreach workers were trained to enter high-risk communities, develop relationships with members of social groupings of IDUs, and begin the process of education. Outreach programs originally conducted in San Francisco, Chicago, New York City, and Baltimore were expanded and the technology was disseminated across the United States through the National AIDS Demonstration Research/AIDS Targeted Outreach Model (NADR/ATOM) program.

The NADR/ATOM project was begun in 1987, and eventually included 41 projects in nearly 50 different cities.[37] In all of the cities, the project involved street outreach to IDUs not in treatment programs. The eligibility requirements for subjects to be enrolled in the research component of the NADR/ATOM projects required that the person must have injected illicit drugs in the previous 6 months and must not have been in drug abuse treatment in the preceding 1 month. Approximately 40% of the more that 30,000 subjects enrolled in the NADR/ATOM projects reported that they had never been in drug abuse treatment.

Many of the NADR/ATOM projects used experimental designs to test psychological theories of health behavior change. All subjects were provided with a "standard" intervention to reduce HIV risk behavior, which included information about HIV and AIDS, a baseline risk assessment, and the option of HIV counseling and testing. Some of these subjects were then randomly assigned to an "enhanced" condition, which typically involved several additional hours of counseling–education–skill training, that incorporated components of the psychological theories of health behavior. Subjects were followed at 6-month intervals to assess changes in HIV risk behaviors and the incidence of new HIV infections.

With respect to changes in HIV risk behaviors, there were two strong and consistent findings. First, almost all the NADR/ATOM projects showed substantial reductions in injection risk behavior from the baseline assessment to the follow-up interviews, with the percentage of IDUs reporting that they did not "always use a sterile needle" declining from 64 to 41%, while those reporting ever sharing needles declined from 54 to 23% (in the month prior to interview).[38]

The second general finding was that few of the different projects showed significant differences in risk reduction between the standard intervention and the enhanced intervention. The general lack of differences between the standard and the enhanced interventions should not be interpreted as meaning that the psychological theories of health behavior are not relevant to HIV risk reduction among IDUs. Rather, these results suggest two other possible explanations. First, after the provision of basic information about AIDS (as in the standard intervention), 2 to 6 hours of additional education and counseling does little to further "strengthen" anti-AIDS attitudes, perceptions, and intentions.

A second explanation is that risk reduction among IDUs—again, after basic HIV/AIDS education—is primarily a function of social processes rather than the characteristics of individual IDUs. Thus, information about HIV/AIDS, new attitudes toward risk behaviors, and skills in practicing new behaviors would have been transmitted among active IDUs influencing persons who had not participated in the enhanced conditions.

The NADR/ATOM studies included follow-up of the participants with repeated HIV counseling and testing to detect new HIV infections. Table 2 presents data on new HIV infections among participants in NADR/ATOM projects for which these outcome data are available.[39] (The cities are not identified individually, because researchers in those cities are preparing individual research reports.)

There are two clear findings from the NADR/ATOM HIV incidence (new infection) studies. First, the new infection rates are substantially lower in the cities where the initial

Table 2. HIV Seroprevalence and HIV Seroconversions per 100 Person-Years at Risk among Injecting Drug User in 14 Localities,[a] by Legal Status of Over-the-Counter Syringe Sales

Number HIV−	Number HIV+	% HIV+	Seroconversions	Person-years at risk[b]	Seroconversions per 100 person-years at risk
\multicolumn{6}{l}{Localities where over-the-counter sales are illegal}
288	311	51.9	4	49.3	8.11
1088	908	45.5	6	146.1	4.10
855	589	40.8	3	81.9	3.66
669	194	22.5	17	262.8	6.47
1222	76	5.9	2	956.1	0.21
787	14	1.7	0	109.0	0.00
\multicolumn{6}{l}{Localities where over-the-counter sales are legal}
1760	138	7.3	7	184.0	3.80
652	43	6.2	5	187.0	2.67
1968	61	3.0	8	732.5	1.09
651	17	2.5	0	225.3	0.00
2099	31	1.5	2	765.1	0.26
891	13	1.4	3	983.4	0.31
372	4	1.1	0	18.0	0.00
514	5	1.0	0	53.7	0.00

[a]The principal investigators of specific sites are preparing detailed analyses of their data on seroconversion rates. Data are publicly available (with locality identifiers removed) through Nova Research Company, Bethesda, Maryland.
[b]Numbers presented are person-years at risk by locality do not add up to those for the summary table due to rounding error.

(background) HIV seroprevalence rates were low. Second, both background HIV seroprevalence and the new infection rates are generally much lower in areas that permit over-the-counter sales of sterile injection equipment (i.e., do not have prescription requirements for the sale of injection equipment).

The higher new infection rates in areas with higher HIV seroprevalence are easily understood in epidemiological terms. An uninfected person who engages in risk behavior ("sharing" of drug injection equipment or unprotected sexual intercourse) is more likely to encounter an HIV-infected risk partner. Indeed, even within the low-seroprevalence cities, in the NADR/ATOM seroincidence data, there was a direct relationship between higher background seroprevalence and higher incidence.[39]

The overall incidence rate also was much lower in areas with legal over-the-counter sales of injection equipment (0.79 per 100 person-years at risk) than in areas that had prescription requirements for sale of injection equipment (1.99 per 100 person-years at risk) (Friedman et al., unpublished data). Current HIV seroprevalence is the product of past seroincidence (plus changes in the composition of the IDU population) and the presence of over-the-counter sales was also strongly linked with current seroprevalence (so strongly that multivariate analyses were not possible).

One must be cautious in drawing conclusions about causal relationships between over-the-counter sales of injection equipment and lower rates of HIV incidence. The data in Table 2, however, strongly suggest that over-the-counter sales may be one factor in facilitating safer injection among IDUs. Studies from France,[20,40] Glasgow, Scotland,[21] and Connecticut[41] show HIV risk reduction associated with over-the-counter sales, supporting the interpretation of a causal role for over-the-counter sales in reducing HIV transmission among IDUs.

One NADR/ATOM program deserves additional consideration. The NADR program in Chicago not only had one of the strongest theoretical bases, but the Chicago research group was able to collect 4 years of HIV incidence data in the cohort of IDUs who participated in the program.[42] There was a dramatic drop in injection risk behavior over the 4-year period, from 95% of the subjects reporting recent injection risk behavior in the start of the project to only 15% reporting recent injection risk behavior by the fourth year. HIV incidence in the cohort fell from approximately 9 per 100 person-years at risk during the first year of the cohort follow-up to approximately 2 per 100 person-years at risk for the rest of the follow-up period. Most importantly, there was a strong relationship between self-reported injection risk behavior and actual HIV seroconversion: All the subjects who become infected with HIV were from among those who reported current injection risk behavior. All subjects who reported that they had stopped injection risk behavior avoided HIV infection. The study did not include a comparison group, so that caution is needed in making causal inferences. Nevertheless, the dramatic drop in reported injection risk behavior and the strong association between HIV incidence and reported injection risk behavior suggest that this project did lead to a substantial reduction in HIV transmission among IDUs in the study.

Many of the NADR/ATOM programs distributed small bottles of bleach to IDUs for disinfection of used injection equipment. Bleach is a relatively strong viricide, but there is some doubt as to whether the bleach disinfection as practiced by IDUs in the field actually protects against HIV infection. Studies from Baltimore[43] and New York City[44] failed to show any relationship between self-reported use of bleach to disinfect injection equipment and protection from infection with HIV. There are, of course, numerous difficulties in attempting to find such a relationship. Reporting on the frequency and circumstances of using bleach may not be very accurate. Drug users may not know how to "properly" use bleach to disinfect injection equipment (the current recommendation is for 30 seconds of contact time of full-strength bleach in the needle and syringe). Even if the drug injectors know how to properly use bleach, they may not be using it properly under "field conditions."[45]

Thus, the effectiveness of the outreach–bleach distribution programs in lowering rates of new HIV infections among IDUs may be a result of participants obtaining more sterile injection equipment (from pharmacies or on the illicit market) rather than resulting from the actual use of bleach to disinfect used injection equipment.

Syringe Exchange

Syringe exchange programs play a unique role in HIV prevention. The exchange transaction converts a relatively worthless object (used syringes) into a valued object (clean syringes). With this incentive, exchange programs can attract a large proportions of IDUs in a community and attract out-of-treatment IDUs who may not be exposed to HIV prevention strategies based in treatment programs.[46] Syringe exchange programs are relatively inexpensive,[47] and they have potential to be highly effective and cost-effective. Once syringe exchange is developed in a community, it not only provides clean injection equipment to individual IDUs, but also can reinforce social norms that proscribe needle sharing. When IDUs attend such programs on a regular basis, the program becomes a community-based platform for the delivery of other health and prevention services. As with other street outreach prevention efforts, the relationship between IDUs and exchange staff is often ongoing and nonjudgmental. In the context of this relationship and by providing treatment referrals on request, syringe exchange programs facilitate entry into drug treatment.[48]

The first syringe exchange program was established in Amsterdam, the Netherlands, in 1984, to slow the spread of hepatitis B among IDUs.[49] With growing recognition of the HIV epidemic, at least 23 countries implemented exchange programs as an HIV prevention strategy.[50] Also like street outreach interventions, syringe exchange programs were the subject of extensive evaluation shortly after they emerged in, for example, England and Scotland.[51]

The first US syringe exchange program was initiated in Tacoma, Washington, in 1988,[52] yet the development of research efforts in the United States initially lagged behind that in many countries. Until 1992, it was not possible to use federal funds to even conduct research on syringe exchange programs, and the ban on federal support for syringe exchange programs is still in place.[50]

Table 3 presents recent studies of HIV incidence among syringe exchange participants. First, as with the outreach–bleach distribution programs, HIV incidence is quite low in areas with low background HIV prevalence. Among other factors, HIV incidence is related to the probability of a seronegative IDU sharing equipment with a seropositive IDU. Because of this, it may be that almost any HIV prevention program will appear to be effective in a low-seroprevalence area. Conversely, the presence of syringe exchange programs (or other good access to sterile injection equipment) may itself be an important reason why HIV seroprevalence and HIV incidence has remained low in many populations of IDUs.

IDUs from the Montreal and Vancouver exchange have an HIV incidence rate notably above that of the other cites in Table 3. The Montreal and Vancouver programs appear to attract a subgroup of IDUs with extremely high initial risk levels,[53–55] including high rates of cocaine injection, high levels of unprotected commercial sex work, and unstable housing (which may make it difficult to have clean needles available at the time of drug injection). Still, additional data are needed to fully explain the Montreal and Vancouver incidence rates, and new studies are presently being initiated in these cities.

Table 3. Recent Studies of HIV Incidence among Syringe Exchange Participants

City	HIV prevalence[a]	Measured HIV seroconversion[b]	Estimated HIV seroconversion[c]	Reference
Lund	Low	0		92
Glasgow	Low		0–1 (2)	93
Sydney	Low		0–1 (2)	93
Toronto	Low		102 (1)	93
England and Wales (except London)	Low		0–1 (1)	94
Kathmandu	Low	0		95
Tacoma, WA	Low	<1		96
Portland, OR	Low	<1		97
Montreal	Moderate	5–13		54
London	Moderate		1–2 (3)	94
Vancouver, BC	Moderate	18		55
Amsterdam	High	4		Van den Hoek, personal communication
Chicago, IL	High	3		Wiebel, personal communication
New York, NY	Very high	1.5		57
New Haven, CT	Very high		3 (4)	98

[a]Low = 0–5%; moderate = 6% to 20%; high = 21% to 40%; very high = 41+%.
[b]Cohort study and/or repeated testing of participants in per 100 person-years at risk.
[c]Estimated from: (1) stable, very low <2% seroprevalence in area; (2) self-reports of previous seronegative test and a current HIV blood/saliva test; (3) stable or declining rate of seroprevalence; (4) from HIV testing of syringes collected at exchange per 100 person-years at risk.

At the same time, HIV incidence data from the three US high-HIV seroprevalence cities (New Haven, Chicago, and New York) with syringe exchange programs must be considered extremely encouraging with respect to reducing HIV transmission in high-seroprevalence areas. The data from New Haven are generally consistent with the previously developed mathematical model to assess the effectiveness of the New Haven syringe exchange program.[56]

A major difficulty in interpreting the HIV incidence studies of syringe exchange participants is the lack of meaningful comparison groups. In almost all the areas, IDUs who do not use the syringe exchanges purchase sterile injection equipment from pharmacies, for example, in the United Kingdom, Sydney, Montreal, and Amsterdam. In the New York City study, however, only the IDUs who used the syringe exchanges had legal access to sterile injection equipment, as New York has a prescription law requirement. The New York City study did show a significantly higher HIV incidence rate among IDUs who did not use the syringe exchanges: 5.3/100 person-years at risk.[57] The New York City study is the first to show a difference in HIV incidence between IDUs who had full legal access to sterile injection equipment for injecting illicit drugs versus IDUs who used illegal sources for obtaining their injection equipment.

A study of incident hepatitis B and hepatitis C infection among IDUs in Tacoma, Washington, also provides support for the effectiveness of syringe exchange programs on reducing transmission of blood-borne viruses.[58] Tacoma/Pierce County is one of the four counties in the US CDC Hepatitis Surveillance System, and thus has among the best data on hepatitis incidence in the United States. A case–control design was used. Cases of hepatitis B and C among IDUs were identified through the surveillance reporting system. Controls were identified among IDUs attending the drug treatment and HIV counseling clinics in the county. Demographic data, drug injection history data, and whether the subject had ever used the local syringe exchange program were abstracted from the clinics' records.

Multiple logistic regression analyses were used to identify statistically independent factors differentiating the incident IDU hepatitis cases from the controls. Failure to use the local syringe exchange was strongly associated with both incident hepatitis B and C. After statistical control for age, gender, race–ethnicity, and duration of injection, the odds ratio for acute infection with hepatitis B among IDUs who had never used the exchange compared with any use of the exchange was over 5 for hepatitis C; the adjusted odds ratio also was over 5 for "never" versus "ever" using the exchange.

Of course, the HIV seroincidence data in Table 3 and the hepatitis data from the Tacoma study are far from constituting "experimental proof" of the effectiveness of syringe exchange programs in reducing transmission of blood-borne viruses. Nevertheless, these data clearly indicate that IDUs will use syringe exchange programs to successfully protect themselves against infection with blood-borne viruses.

Tailoring Programs to Special Populations

To this point, we have described HIV prevention and risk reduction programs in general categories of methadone maintenance, street outreach, and syringe exchange. Each of these general types of programs, however, have been modified in some cases to meet the needs of special populations. Drug abuse treatment programs in general and methadone maintenance programs in particular have been modified extensively in the past 10 years to incorporate a variety of HIV prevention strategies into the treatment process. These include, for example, HIV counseling and testing,[59] individual counseling concerning HIV risk,[60] and HIV education–counseling using group therapy models[61]; provision of prevention information to family, friends, or IDUs not enrolled in treatment, and interventions targeting female sexual partners of IDUs in treatment.[62] Similarly, street outreach projects have been designed to intervene with special populations, such as high-risk youth,[63] and to target social networks of IDUs rather than individuals.[64] Syringe exchange programs have been adapted to increase penetration into local IDU communities and volume of syringes distributed,[65] and to use surrogate or "secondary" exchange strategies to reach IDUs who may not attend traditional street-based exchanges.[66] Below we discuss in more detail a single example of adapting syringe exchange strategies to the needs of a special at-risk population: young IDUs.

Nearly 20% of cumulative US AIDS cases are reported among persons between the ages of 13 and 29.[67] The lag time between HIV infection and AIDS diagnosis indicates that most of these cases were infected as adolescents or young adults. One estimate is that 25% of new HIV infections occur in youth under the age of 22.[68] While many adolescents engage in some risk taking behaviors, those who use drugs and homeless and runaway youth have increased risk of HIV infection. Adolescents who use drugs may also report increased sexual risk behavior.[69] Among homeless and runaway youth, HIV risk factors include sexual risk behavior,[70] and higher rates of drug use[71] and injection drug use.[72] Many high-risk youth have life histories including sexual abuse and intergenerational drug use. The daily life of street youth is often chaotic and characterized by survival sex, violent relationships, and other traumatic events.[73] The HIV prevention needs of youth are often ignored or nullified by controversy related to HIV education for youth, condom distribution among youth, and providing clean needles to young injectors.

To date, relatively few youth have participated in syringe exchange programs in the

United States. Indeed, this lack of participation by youth in syringe exchange program is an important part of the evidence that syringe exchange programs do not lead to an increase in illicit drug injection. (If the availability of sterile syringes led youth to begin injecting, then one would expect the new injectors to be participating in the exchange programs.) In order to reach youth who are injecting drugs, many programs are now developing special outreach programs to young injectors. Youth-specific syringe exchange services have been reported in Boulder, Los Angeles, New York, San Francisco, Santa Cruz, Seattle, Toronto, and Vancouver.[74]

Integrating Multiple Prevention Programs

While assisting drug injectors to practice safer injection and providing drug abuse treatment to reduce drug injection per se are often perceived as contradictory strategies, in practice they have been complementary strategies. One of the most important lessons of the early outreach programs was that the process of teaching drug injectors how to practice safer injection uncovered previously hidden demand for entry into drug abuse treatment. This unexpected demand for drug abuse treatment led to a program in which New Jersey outreach workers distributed vouchers that could be redeemed for no-cost detoxification treatment.[16] Over 95% of the vouchers were redeemed by drug users entering treatment, many of whom had never before been in drug abuse treatment.

There also are examples of syringe exchange programs that have become important sources of referral to abuse treatment programs. For example, the New Haven program reports 33% of the first 569 participants were referred to drug treatment.[56] The Tacoma syringe exchange program has become the leading source of referrals to the local drug treatment program.[75] The capacity of outreach–bleach distribution programs and syringe exchange programs to make effective referrals to drug treatment programs primarily may depend on the availability of treatment in the local area and whether the programs can afford the appropriate staff to make and follow through on referrals.

While much progress has been made in providing referrals from outreach–bleach distribution programs to drug abuse treatment programs, HIV prevention efforts in many countries, including the United States, are still hampered by a lack of "referrals" from drug abuse treatment programs to bleach distribution and syringe exchange programs. While drug abuse treatment programs lead to substantial and well-documented reductions in illicit drug use,[30] it would be unrealistic to expect that all IDUs who enter treatment programs will abstain from further illicit drug injection. Indeed, the majority are likely to fail to complete treatment and/or to use illicit drugs while in treatment. Some US drug treatment programs currently include information about the locations and hours of operation of local bleach distribution and syringe exchange programs as part of the AIDS education provided to all entrants into treatment. In general, however, drug abuse treatment programs in the United States and in many developing countries have not yet developed strategies for reducing HIV risk among persons who relapse back to drug injection.

LIMITATIONS OF PREVENTION RESEARCH

Standards for Assessing HIV Prevention Programs for IDUs

Evaluation of HIV prevention programs is critical to reducing HIV transmission. The resources available for HIV prevention are limited; in many developing countries, these resources are severely limited. Thus, expending resources on ineffective programs will involve great opportunity-lost costs. Randomized clinical trials are the current gold standard for evaluating public health and medical interventions. There are many good reasons, however, not to use randomized clinical trials for HIV prevention efforts. First, effective HIV prevention often occurs at a community level rather than at an individual level. This means that the community (or local population of IDUs) is the appropriate unit of analysis for evaluating prevention programs. While community-level randomized clinical trials are possible, they are usually very difficult and expensive to conduct. Second, HIV prevention may be highly dependent on the local context. As noted above, both street outreach programs and syringe exchange programs are very likely to be associated with low HIV incidence if they are implemented in populations with low seroprevalence. Thus, a very large sample of communities may be needed to assess a particular type of HIV prevention program in different community contexts. Third, for many aspects of HIV prevention, present knowledge would make a randomized clinical trial unethical, for example, providing access to condoms versus denying access to condoms, providing access to sterile injection equipment versus denying access to sterile injection equipment. Randomized clinical trials thus should be used when there is great uncertainty whether a specific type of prevention program will be effective and, if the program is effective, it is likely to have a large public health impact. Given the multiple difficulties in conducting randomized clinical trials for HIV prevention, we would suggest the following criteria for evaluating the public health effectiveness of HIV prevention programs:

1. There is sound biological, psychological, or sociological theory underlying the intervention. For example, at the biological level, syringes obtained from pharmacies or exchanges will not contain HIV, and HIV does not penetrate latex condoms. At a psychological level, persons with accurate information about how HIV is and is not transmitted will be more likely to be able to reduce their risk behavior; persons who have options in selecting methods for reducing risk are more likely to change their risk behavior. At a social level, drug injectors do influence each other's behavior, and thus can act as influence agents to reduce the risk behavior of their peers.
2. The prevention program is popular with the target audience. It attracts and retains large numbers of persons at risk for HIV transmission.
3. Participants in the program achieve a low HIV transmission rate. A low incidence rate must be determined with respect to HIV seroprevalence in the local population of IDUs. We would suggest that in areas where the seroprevalence is under 10%, a low incidence rate would be 1% per year or less. In areas with higher seroprevalence rates, we would suggest that a low incidence rate would be 2% per year or less.

Problematic Issues in Preventing HIV Infection among IDUs

Much has been learned in the last decade of research on prevention of HIV infection among IDUs. Most importantly, all studies to date have shown that the large majority of IDUs will modify their behavior to reduce the chances of becoming infected with HIV. The theoretical bases for HIV prevention efforts have expanded from "factual education" to psychological and social change theories. Prevention programs are increasingly providing the means for behavior change (for safer injection and for reducing drug injection).

Despite the progress in terms of research findings, increasing sophistication of prevention programs, and actual reduction in HIV transmission, there still are a number of problem areas with respect to prevention of new HIV infections among IDUs in some industrialized countries—the United States in particular—and in many developing countries.

HIV Prevention in High Seroprevalence Areas

Current prevention programs for IDUs in low seroprevalence areas appear capable of achieving control over HIV transmission.[76] These programs cannot prevent all new HIV infections, but it does appear that they can maintain low seroprevalence indefinitely. In these low HIV seroprevalence areas, almost all the remaining risk behavior among IDUs occurs among persons who are HIV seronegative and therefore without transmission of the virus. In high HIV seroprevalence areas, however, even moderate levels of injection risk behavior are likely to involve persons of different HIV serostatus, and thus lead to transmission of the virus. Recent analyses conducted by Holmberg[5] of the CDC suggest that transmission of HIV among IDUs in high seroprevalence areas may account for the plurality of new HIV infections in the United States.

A new generation of HIV prevention programs thus may be needed for IDUs in high HIV seroprevalence areas. In addition to more intensive programs focusing on safer injection, there is a need for programs to reduce the numbers of persons injecting illicit drugs in high seroprevalence areas. Massive expansion of drug abuse treatment could lead to large reductions in the numbers of persons who are injecting illicit drugs. Programs to reduce initiation into drug injection also would be useful for high seroprevalence areas, as these would also lead to a reduction over time in the numbers of injecting drug users.[77]

Sexual Transmission of HIV

While there is highly consistent evidence that IDUs will make large changes in their injection risk behavior in response to concerns about AIDS, changes in sexual behavior appear to be much more modest. All studies that have compared changes in injection risk behavior with changes in sexual risk behavior found greater changes in injection risk behavior.[78] In general, IDUs appear more likely to make risk reduction efforts (reduced numbers of partners, increased use of condoms) for casual sexual relationships rather than in primary sexual relationships.[78]

One factor that appears to be important in increasing condom use among IDUs is an altruistic desire to avoid transmitting HIV to a noninjecting sexual partner. In both Bangkok[79] and New York City,[80] IDUs who know (or have reason to suspect) that they are HIV-positive are particularly likely to use condoms in relationships with sexual partners who do not inject illicit drugs. Most programs that have urged IDUs to use condoms thus far have focused on the self-protective effects of condom usage. Appealing to altruistic feelings of protecting others from HIV infection may be an untapped source of motivation for increasing condom use.

Heterosexual transmission from IDUs to their sexual partners who do not inject drugs has occurred in the United States since the first heterosexual IDUs were infected with HIV. The use of crack cocaine is often associated with high frequencies of unsafe sexual behaviors. In cities like New York and Miami, where there are large numbers of HIV-infected IDUs who also use crack cocaine, the use of crack without injection drug use itself has become an important risk factor for infection with HIV.[81] While intervening in the nexus of injection drug use–crack use–unsafe sex will be quite difficult, one strategy that might be used is to provide prompt treatment for genital ulcerative sexually transmitted diseases such as syphilis. The presence of these ulcerative sexually transmitted diseases appears to greatly increase the likelihood of HIV transmission.[82]

It is also worth noting that additional strategies are needed for increasing safer sex among IDUs who engage in male-with-male sexual activities. IDUs who also engage in male-with-male sex can act as a bridge population between non-drug-injecting men who engage in male-with-male sex and the larger IDU population. In many industrialized countries, HIV seroprevalence among men who engage in male-with-male sex is substantially higher than among exclusively heterosexual IDUs. There are indications of "slippage" back to high-risk sexual behavior among men-who-have-sex-with-men in San Francisco[83,84] and Amsterdam.[85] If slippage back to unsafe sex should occur among men who have sex with men in the United States as a whole, this could lead to more HIV infections among IDU men who engage in male-with-male sex, followed by more transmission from these men to other IDUs.

Provision of Prevention Services

While there are important questions still to be answered with respect to how to do HIV prevention among IDUs, the biggest single problem may simply be the scarcity of HIV prevention services for IDUs in the world. For example, in the United States, the Presidential Commission on the HIV Epidemic recommended in 1988 that drug abuse treatment be provided to all persons who desire it. The US National Commission on AIDS made the same recommendation in 1991.[86] The National Commission on AIDS also recommended the removal of legal barriers to the purchase and possession of sterile injection equipment. Although there has been some expansion of syringe exchange services in the United States in the last several years, the commissions' recommendations would appear as valid today as when they were initially made.

HARM REDUCTION

The worldwide epidemic of HIV infection among IDUs has led to important conceptual developments on injecting drug use as a health problem. HIV and AIDS have dramatically increased the adverse health consequences of injecting drug use, and thus have led to seeing psychoactive drug use as more of a health problem and not just a criminal justice problem. At the same time, HIV infection can be prevented without requiring the cessation of injecting drug use. The potential separation of a severe adverse consequence of drug use from the drug use itself has encouraged analysis of other areas in which adverse consequences of drug use might be reduced without requiring cessation of drug use.

The ability of many IDUs to modify their behavior to reduce the chances of HIV infection also has led to consideration of drug addicts as both concerned about their health and as capable of acting on that concern (without denying the compulsive nature of drug dependence).

These ideas have formed much of the basis for what has been termed the "harm reduction" perspective on psychoactive drug use.[87-90] Harm reduction is an evolving set of ideas, without firm definitional boundaries. It is important to recognize, however, that harm reduction does not include unrestricted legalization of currently illegal drugs. To permit the commercial exploitation of drugs like heroin and cocaine in a manner similar to the current commercial exploitation of nicotine would undoubtedly lead to increased social and individual harms.

The Harm Reduction Coalition,[91] a nonprofit organization, defines harm reduction as:

> a set of strategies and tactics that encourage users to reduce the harm done to themselves and communities by their licit and illicit substance abuse. In allowing users access to the tools with which to become healthier, we recognize the competency of their efforts to protect themselves, their loved ones and their communities.

Consequently, harm reduction is concerned with both licit and illicit drug use and with the impact of drug use on individual users and on the larger community. It recognizes that users often will act to reduce drug-related harm if given the means to do so, and it advocates the development of innovative strategies to support this goal. It is not inconsistent with drug abuse treatment. By encouraging users to carefully consider harms associated with their behavior, harm reduction strategies may accelerate entry into treatment for some users. Conversely, it recognizes the possibility of reducing drug-related harm even for users who choose not to enter drug treatment.

Harm reduction, as an articulated philosophy, has largely followed rather than preceded the implementation of interventions described in this chapter. In the wake of the HIV epidemic and as programs were put in place with the goal of interrupting HIV transmission among active drug users (rather than treating drug use itself), harm reduction developed as a philosophy underlying these interventions.

ACKNOWLEDGMENTS.   Sections of this chapter were originally prepared as reports to the United Kingdom Department of Health and for the United States Congress Office of Technology Assessment. Additional support was provided by grant DA R01 03574 from the National Institute on Drug Abuse, and by grant U95 TI00669 from the Center for Substance Abuse Treatment.

REFERENCES

1. Des Jarlais DC, Stimson GV, Hagan H, et al. Emerging infectious diseases and the injection of illicit psychoactive drugs. *Curr Issues Public Health* 1996; 2:102–137.
2. Des Jarlais DC, Friedman SR. AIDS and IV drug use. *Science* 1989; 245:578–579.
3. European Centre for Epidemiological Monitoring of AIDS. *Third Quarterly Report.* World Health Organization, Geneva, Switzerland; 1996.
4. Centers for Disease Control and Prevention. *HIV/AIDS Surveillance Report.* Surveillance Branch of the HIV/ AIDS Prevention–Surveillance and Epidemiology, National Center for HIV, STD, and TB Prevention, Atlanta, GA; 1995.
5. Holmberg S. The estimated prevalence and incidence of HIV in 96 large US metropolitan areas. *Am J Public Health* 1996; 86:642–654.
6. Stoneburner R, Des Jarlais DC, Benezra D, et al. A larger spectrum of severe HIV-1-related disease in intravenous drug users in New York City. *Science* 1988; 242:916–919.
7. Vermund SH, Kelley KF, Klein RS, et al. High risk of human papillomavirus infection and cervical squamous intraepithelial lesions among women with symptomatic human immunodeficiency virus infection. *Am J Obstet Gynecol* 1991; 165:392–400.
8. Zolla-Pazner S, Des Jarlais DC, Friedman SR, et al. Nonrandom development of immunologic abnormalities after infection with human immunodeficiency virus: Implications for immunologic classification of the disease. *Proc Natl Acad Sci* 1987; 84:5404–5408.
9. Margolick JB, Munoz A, Vlahov D, et al. Direct comparison of the relationship between clinical outcome and change in CD4+ lymphocytes in human immunodeficiency virus-positive homosexual men and injecting drug users. *Arch Intern Med* 1994; 154:868–875.
10. Zagury D, Bernard J, Leonard R, et al. Long-term cultures of HTLV-III-infected T cells: A model of cytopathology of T-cell depletion in AIDS. *Science* 1986; 231:850–853.
11. Des Jarlais DC, Friedman SR, Choopanya K, et al. International epidemiology of HIV and AIDS among injecting drug users. *AIDS* 1992; 6:1053–1068.
12. Jacquez J, Koopman J, Simon C, et al. Role of the primary infection in epidemic HIV infection of gay cohorts. *J Acquir Immunodefic Syndr* 1994; 7:1169–1184.
13. Des Jarlais DC, Friedman SR, Sotheran JL, et al. Continuity and change within an HIV epidemic: Injecting drug users in New York City, 1984 through 1992. *JAMA* 1994; 271:121–127.

14. Thompson PI, Jones TS, Cahill K, et al. Promoting HIV prevention outreach activities via community-based organizations. Sixth International Conference on AIDS, June 1990; San Francisco, CA.
15. Wiebel W, Chene D, Johnson W. Adoption of bleach use in a cohort of street intravenous drug users in Chicago. Sixth International Conference on AIDS, June 1990; San Francisco, CA.
16. Jackson J, Rotkiewicz L. A coupon program: AIDS education and drug treatment. Third International Conference on AIDS, 1987; Washington, DC.
17. Ostrow DG. AIDS prevention through effective education. *Daedalus* 1989; 118:229–254.
18. Blix O, Gronbladh L. AIDS and IV heroin addicts: The preventive effect of methadone maintenance in Sweden. Fourth International Conference on AIDS, 1988; Stockholm, Sweden.
19. Buning EC, Hartgers C, Verster AD, et al. The evaluation of the needle/syringe exchange in Amsterdam. Fourth International Conference on AIDS, 1988; Stockholm, Sweden.
20. Espinoza P, Bouchard I, Ballian P, et al. Has the open sale of syringes modified the syringe exchanging habits of drug addicts? Fourth International Conference on AIDS, 1988; Stockholm, Sweden.
21. Goldberg D, Watson H, Stuart F, et al. Pharmacy supply of needles and syringes—The effect on spread of HIV in intravenous drug misusers. Fourth International Conference on AIDS, 1988; Stockholm, Sweden.
22. Cartter ML, Petersen LR, Savage RB, et al. Providing HIV counseling and testing services in methadone maintenance programs. *AIDS* 1990; 4:463–465.
23. Higgins DL, Galavotti C, O'Reilly KR, et al. Evidence for the effects of HIV antibody counseling and testing on risk behaviors. *JAMA* 1991; 266:2419–2429.
24. Friedman SR, Des Jarlais DC, Sotheran JL, et al. AIDS and self-organization among intravenous drug users. *Int J Addict* 1987; 22:201–219.
25. Selwyn P, Feiner C, Cox C, et al. Knowledge about AIDS and high-risk behavior among intravenous drug abusers in New York City. *AIDS* 1987; 1:247–254.
26. Des Jarlais DC, Friedman SR, Hopkins W. Risk reduction for the acquired immunodeficiency syndrome among intravenous drug users. *Ann Intern Med* 1985; 103:755–759.
27. Des Jarlais DC, Choopanya K, Vanichseni S, et al. AIDS risk reduction and reduced HIV seroconversion among injection drug users in Bangkok. *Am J Public Health* 1994; 84:452–455.
28. Des Jarlais DC, Friedman P, Hagan H, et al. The protective effect of AIDS-related behavioral change among injection drug users: A cross-national study. *Am J Public Health* 1996; 86:1780–1785.
29. Gerstein D, Harwood H, eds. *Treating Drug Problems.* Washington, DC: National Academy Press; 1990.
30. Hubbard RL, Marsden ME, Rachal JV, et al. *Drug Abuse Treatment: A National Study of Effectiveness.* Chapel Hill: The University of North Carolina Press; 1989.
31. Metzger D, Woody G, McLellan AT, et al. Human immunodeficiency virus seroconversion among in- and out-of-treatment intravenous drug users: An 18 month prospective follow-up. *J Acquir Immune Defic Syndr* 1993; 6:1049–1056.
32. Kerndt P, Weber M, Ford W. HIV incidence among injection drug users enrolled in a Los Angeles methadone program. *JAMA* 1995; 278:1831–1832.
33. Orr M, Friedmann P, Glebatis D, et al. Incidence of HIV infection among clients of a methadone maintenance program in New York City. *JAMA* 1996; 276:99.
34. van Ameijden EJC, van den Hoek A, Coutinho RA. Risk factors for HIV seroconversion in injecting drug users in Amsterdam, the Netherlands. Seventh International Conference on AIDS, 1991; Florence, Italy.
35. Watters JK, Feldman HW, Biernacki P, et al. Street-based AIDS prevention for intravenous drug users in San Francisco: Prospects, obstacles and options. In: *Community Epidemiology Working Group Proceedings.* Rockville, MD; Department of Health and Human Services, National Institute on Drug Abuse; 1986:46–55.
36. Watters JK, Guydish JG. HIV/AIDS prevention for drug users in natural settings. In: DiClemente RL, Peterson JL, eds. *Preventing AIDS: Theories and Methods of Behavioral Interventions.* New York: Plenum Press; 1994: 209–225.
37. Brown BS, Beschner GM, eds. *Handbook on Risk of AIDS: Injection Drug Users and Sexual Partners.* Westport, CT: Greenwood Press; 1993.
38. Stephens RC, Simpson DD, Coyle SL, et al. Comparative effectiveness of NADR interventions. In: Brown BS, Beschner GM, eds. *Handbook on Risk of AIDS: Injection Drug Users and Sexual Partners.* Wesport, CT: Greenwood Press; 1993:519–556.
39. Friedman SR, Jose B, Deren S, et al. Risk factors for human immunodeficiency virus seroconversion among out-of-treatment drug injectors in high and low seroprevalence cities. *Am J Epidemiol* 1995; 142:864–874.
40. Ingold FR, Ingold S. The effects of the liberalization of syringe sales on the behavior of intravenous drug users in France. *Bull Narc* 1989; 41:67–81.
41. Groseclose SL, Weinstein B, Jones TS, et al. Impact of increased legal access to needles and syringes on practices

of injecting-drug users and police officers—Connecticut, 1992–1993. *J Acquir Immune Defic Syndr* 1995; 10: 2–89.

42. Wiebel W, Jimenez A, Johnson W, et al. Positive effect on HIV seroconversion of street outreach intervention with IDU in Chicago, 1988–1992. Ninth International Conference on AIDS, 1993; Berlin, Germany.

43. Vlahov D, Astemborski J, Solomon L, et al. Field effectiveness of needle disinfection among injecting drug users. *J Acquir Immune Defic Syndr* 1994; 7:760–766.

44. Titus S, Marmor M, Des Jarlais DC, et al. Bleach use and HIV seroconversion among New York City injection drug users. *J Acquir Immune Defic Syndr* 1994; 7:700–704.

45. Gleghorn AA, Jones TS, Doherty MC, et al. Acquisition and use of needles and syringes by injecting drug users in Baltimore, Maryland. *J Acquir Immune Defic Syndr Hum Retrovirol* 1995; 10:97–103.

46. Guydish J, Lurie P. Chapter 9. Who are the IDUs who use NEPs? In: Lurie P, Reingold A, eds. *The Public Health Impact of Needle Exchange Programs in the United States and Abroad*, vol. I. Berkeley: School of Public Health, University of California; San Francisco: Institute for Health Policy Studies, University of California. Final report prepared for the Centers for Disease Control and Prevention; September 1993:263–289.

47. Kahn JG. How much does it cost to operate NEPs? In: Lurie P, Reingold A eds. *The Public Health Impact of Needle Exchange Programs in the United States and Abroad*, vol. I. Berkeley: School of Public Health, University of California; San Francisco: Institute for Health Policy Studies, University of California. Final report prepared for the Centers for Disease Control and Prevention; September 1993:247–261.

48. Sorensen J, Lurie P. Do NEPs act as bridges to public health services? In: Lurie P, Reingold A, eds. *The Public Health Impact of Needle Exchange Programs in the United States and Abroad*, vol. I. Berkeley: School of Public Health, University of California; San Francisco: Institute for Health Policy Studies, University of California. Final report prepared for the Centers for Disease Control and Prevention; September 1993:225–243.

49. Buning EC. Effects of Amsterdam needle and syringe exchange. *Int J Addict* 1991; 26:1303–1311.

50. Lane S. How and why did NEPs develop? In: Lurie P, Reingold A eds. *The Public Health Impact of Needle Exchange Programs in the United States and Abroad*, vol. I. Berkeley: School of Public Health, University of California; San Francisco: Institute for Health Policy Studies, University of California. Final report prepared for the Centers for Disease Control and Prevention; September 1993:141–171.

51. Stimson GV, Alldritt LJ, Dolan KA, et al. *Injecting Equipment Exchange Schemes: Final Report*. London, UK: The Centre for Research on Drugs and Health Behaviour; 1998.

52. Hagan H, Reid T, Des Jarlais DC, et al . The incidence of HBV infections and syringe exchange programs. *JAMA* 1991; 266:1646–1647.

53. Lamothe F, Bruneau J, Soto J, et al. Risk factors for HIV seroconversion among injecting drug users in Montreal: The Saint-Luc cohort experience. Tenth International Conference on AIDS, 1994; Yokohama, Japan.

54. Hankins C, Gendron S, Tran T. Montreal needle exchange attenders versus non-attenders: What's the difference? Tenth International Conference on AIDS, 1994; Yokohama, Japan.

55. Strathdee SA, Patrick DM, Currie SL, et al. Needle exchange is not enough: lessons from the Vancouver injecting drug use study. *AIDS* 1997; 11:F59–F65.

56. O'Keefe E, Kaplan E, Khoshnood K. *Preliminary Report: City of New Haven Needle Exchange Program*. New Haven, CT; Office of Mayor John C. Daniels; 1991.

57. Des Jarlais DC, Marmor M, Paone D, et al. HIV incidence among injecting drug users in New York City syringe-exchange programs. *Lancet* 1996; 348:987–991.

58. Hagan H, Des Jarlais DC, Friedman SR, et al. Reduced risk of hepatitis B and hepatitis C among injecting drug users participating in the Tacoma syringe exchange program. *Am J Public Health* 1995; 85:1531–1537.

59. MacGowan RJ, Brackbill RM, Rugg DL, et al. Sex, drugs and HIV counseling and testing: A prospective study of behavior-change among methadone maintenance clients in New England. *AIDS* 1997; 11:229–235.

60. Gibson DR, Wermuth L, Lovelle-Drache J, et al. Brief counseling to reduce AIDS risk in intravenous drug users and their sexual partners: Preliminary results. *Counselling Psychol Q* 1989; 2:15–19.

61. Sorensen JL, London J, Morales E. Group counseling to prevent AIDS. In: Sorensen JL, Wermuth L, Gibson DR, et al., eds. *Preventing AIDS in Drug Users and Their Sexual Partners*. New York: Guilford Press; 1991: 99–115.

62. Wermuth LA, Robbins R, Choi K. Reaching and counseling women sexual partners. In: Sorensen JL, Wermuth L, Gibson DR, et al., eds. *Preventing AIDS in Drug Users and Their Sexual Partners*. New York: Guilford Press; 1991:130–149.

63. Anderson JE, Cheney R, Clatts M, et al. HIV risk behavior, street outreach, and condom use in eight high-risk populations. *AIDS Educ Prev* 1996; 8:191–204.

64. Wiebel W, Jimenez A, Johnson W, et al. Positive effect on HIV seroconversion of street outreach intervention with IDU in Chicago: 1988–1992. International Conference on AIDS, 1993; Berlin, Germany.

65. Gibson DR, Kahn, JG. Maximizing the impact of needle exchange: The role of penetration and volume. North American Syringe Exchange Network Annual Meeting, April 1995; San Juan, Puerto Rico.

66. Gibson, DR. Prevention with injection drug users. In: Cohen PT, Sande MA, Volberding PA, eds. *The AIDS Knowledge Base*, 3rd ed. Boston: Little-Brown; 1997:925–930.

67. Centers for Disease Control and Prevention. *HIV/AIDS Surveillance Report* 1996; 8(1):8–12.

68. Rosenberg PS, Biggar RJ, Goedert JJ. Declining age at HIV infection in the United States. *N Engl J Med* 1994; 330:789–790. Letter.

69. Edlin BR, Irwin KL, Ludwig DD, et al. The Multicenter Crack Cocaine and HIV Infection Study Team: High-risk sexual behavior among young street-recruited crack cocaine smokers in three American cities: An interim report. *J Psychoactive Drugs* 1992; 24:363–371.

70. Kipke M, O'Connor S, Palmer R, et al. Street youth in Los Angeles: Profile of a group at high risk for human immunodeficiency virus infection. *Arch Pediatr Adolesc Med* 1995; 149:513–519.

71. Windle M. Substance use and abuse among adolescent runaways: A four-year follow-up study. *J Youth Adolesc* 1989; 18:331–344.

72. Yates GL, MacKenzie R, Pennbridge J, et al. A risk profile comparison of runaway and non-runaway youth. *Am J Public Health* 1988; 78:820–821.

73. Martinez T, Gleghorn A, Clements K, et al. A comparison of injection drug users and noninjection drug users from a street-based sample of substance abusing homeless and runaway youth. *J Psychoactive Drugs*, in press.

74. Kral AH, Molnar BE, Booth RE, et al. Prevalence of sexual risk behavior and substance use among runaway and homeless adolescents in San Francisco, Denver, and New York City. *Int J Sex Transm Dis AIDS* 1997; 8(2):109–117.

75. Hagan H, Des Jarlais DC, Friedman SR, et al. Risk of human immunodeficiency virus and hepatitis B virus in users of the Tacoma syringe exchange program. In: *Proceedings of the National Academy of Sciences Workshop on Needle Exchange and Bleach Distribution Programs*. Washington DC: National Academy Press; 1994:24–31.

76. Des Jarlais DC, Hagan HH, Friedman SR, et al. Maintaining low HIV seroprevalence in populations of injecting drug users. *JAMA* 1995; 274:1226–1231.

77. Des Jarlais DC, Casriel C, Friedman SR, et al. AIDS and the transition to illicit drug injection: Results of a randomized trial prevention program. *Br J Addict* 1992; 87:493–498.

78. Friedman SR, Des Jarlais DC, Ward TP. Overview of the history of the HIV epidemic among drug injectors. In: Brown BS, Beschner GM, eds. *Handbook on Risk of AIDS: Injection Drug Users and Sexual Partners*. Wesport, CT: Greenwood Press; 1993:3–15.

79. Vanichseni S, Des Jarlais DC, Choopanya K, et al. Condom use with primary partners among injecting drug users in Bangkok, Thailand and New York City, United States. *AIDS* 1993; 7:887–891.

80. Friedman SR, Jose B, Neaigus A, et al. Consistent condom use in relationships between seropositive injecting drug users and sex partners who do not inject drugs. *AIDS* 1994; 8:357–361.

81. Edlin BR, Irwin KL, Faruque S. Intersecting epidemics: Crack cocaine use and HIV infection among inner-city young adults. *N Engl J Med* 1994; 331:1422–1427.

82. Chaisson MA, Stoneburner RL, Hildebrandt DS, et al. Heterosexual transmission of HIV-1 associated with the use of smokable freebase cocaine (crack). *AIDS* 1991; 5:1121–1126.

83. Ekstrand ML, Coates TJ. Maintenance of safer sexual behaviors and predictors of risky sex: The San Francisco Men's Health Study. *Am J Public Health* 1990; 80:973–977.

84. Stall R, Ekstrand ML, Pollack L, et al. Relapse from safer sex: The next challenge for AIDS prevention efforts. *J Acquir Immune Defic Syndr* 1990; 3:1181–1187.

85. de Wit JFB, De Vroome EMM, Sandfort TGM, et al. Safer sexual practices not reliably maintained by homosexual men. *Am J Public Health* 1992; 82:615–616.

86. National Commission on AIDS. *The Twin Epidemics of Substance Use and HIV*. Washington, DC: The National Commission on AIDS; 1991.

87. Brettle RP. HIV and harm reduction for injection drug users. *AIDS* 1991; 5:125–136.

88. Des Jarlais DC, Friedman SR, Ward TP. Harm reduction: A public health response to the AIDS epidemic among injecting drug users. *Annu Rev Public Health* 1993; 14:413–450.

89. Des Jarlais DC. Editorial: Harm reduction—A framework for incorporating science into drug policy. *Am J Public Health* 1995; 85:10–12.

90. Heather N, Wodak A, Nadelmann E, et al., eds. *Psychoactive Drugs and Harm Reduction: From Faith to Science*. London: Whurr Publishers; 1993.

91. Harm Reduction Coalition. Statement of purpose, 1994. Harm Reduction Coalition, 3223 Lakeshore Ave., Oakland, CA 94610.

92. Ljungberg B, Christensson B, Tunving K, et al HIV prevention among injecting drug users: Three years of experience from a syringe exchange program in Sweden. *J Acquir Immune Defic Syndr* 1991; 4:890–895.

93. Ball A, Des Jarlais DC, Donoghoe M, et al. *Multi-Centre Study on Drug Injecting and Risk of HIV Infection.* Geneva: World Health Organization Programme on Substance Abuse; 1994.

94. Stimson GV. AIDS and injecting drug use in the United Kingdom, 1987–1993: The policy response and the prevention of the epidemic. *Soc Sci Med* 1995; 41:699–716.

95. Peak A, Sujato R, Maharjan SH, et al. Declining risk for HIV among injecting drug users in Kathmandu, Nepal: The impact of a harm-reduction programme. *AIDS* 1995; 9(9):1067–1070.

96. Hagan H, Des Jarlais DC, Purchase D, et al. The Tacoma Syringe Exchange. *J Addict Dis* 1991; 10:81–88.

97. Oliver K, Maynard H, Friedman SR, et al. Behavioral and community impact of the Portland syringe exchange program. In: *Proceedings of the Workshop on Needle Exchange and Bleach Distribution Programs.* Washington, DC: National Academy of Sciences; 1994:35–39.

98. Kaplan EH, Heimer R. HIV incidence among needle exchange participants: Estimates from syringe tracking and testing data. *J Acquir Immune Defic Syndr* 1994; 7:182–189.

9

Interventions for Sexually Active Heterosexual Women

ANN O'LEARY and GINA M. WINGOOD

INTRODUCTION

Women have been infected with human immunodeficiency virus (HIV) since the earliest days of the epidemic. Grethe Rask was the first woman now known to have died of acquired immunodeficiency syndrome (AIDS); the year was 1977.[1,2] However, despite their ongoing representation among HIV cases, little attention was paid to heterosexual women by the prevention research community until well into the second decade of the epidemic. This is unfortunate, because research conducted in other populations, for example, men who have sex with men, often generalizes poorly to situations encountered by women at risk through heterosexual encounters. There are two fundamental reasons for this. First, until the relatively recent availability of the female condom, men were in control of condom use: they wore the condoms. Second, in most cultures, women possess less power than men, particularly in sexual relationships and situations.[3–5] These facts, both of which will be discussed more fully below, have conspired often to render condom negotiation difficult for heterosexual women. The difficulty is more pronounced among those women who are at greatest risk of infection: the impoverished, the drug addicted, and those with abusive partners. However, a growing number of studies reporting positive risk reduction effects of behavioral prevention interventions is encouraging and suggests that many women possess or can develop skills to effectively reduce their risk of HIV infection. For other women, it may be necessary to identify new solutions to overcome the significant barriers that they face.

The present chapter will review the epidemiological and psychosocial research on HIV and women that has been conducted to date. We first review the factors that have been found to be associated with effective protection from HIV and other sexually transmitted diseases (STDs), as well as factors associated with risk behavior. Next, we will review the research on rigorously evaluated behavioral STD/HIV risk reduction interventions. Because commercial sex workers face unique challenges, and in light of space limitations, interventions targeting this population will not be reviewed; however, the interested reader is encouraged to pursue reading in this area. Finally, we will discuss some general limitations in our knowledge base and prevention arsenal and suggest some directions for future research.

ANN O'LEARY • Department of Psychology, Rutgers University, New Brunswick, New Jersey 08903.   GINA M. WINGOOD • Department of Behavioral Sciences and Health Education, Rollins School of Public Health, Emory University, Atlanta, Georgia 30322.

Handbook of HIV Prevention, edited by Peterson and DiClemente.
Kluwer Academic/Plenum Publishers, New York, 2000.

EPIDEMIOLOGY OF WOMEN AND AIDS

In the United States, the fastest growing sector of people with AIDS are women between 18 and 44 years of age. As of February 1995, the Centers for Disease Control and Prevention[6] (CDC) reported that 89,208 women had AIDS, accounting for slightly more than 15% of all AIDS cases nationally. Cumulative estimates, however, are misleading and underestimate the impact of the HIV epidemic on women. Time trend analysis, a more precise indicator of the changing dynamics of the HIV epidemic, suggests that nationally women comprise an increasingly larger proportion of AIDS cases. For instance, women accounted for 7% of AIDS cases in 1986, 10% during 1988, 23.1% during 1995, and 25.3% during 1996. Proportionally, the number of women with AIDS in 1996 was more than 3.6 times greater than the proportion of women with AIDS in 1986 (7%).[6]

As of December 1996, the majority of AIDS cases among women, 45%, are attributed to injection drug use, whereas 38% are attributable to heterosexual transmission. When considering only women 20–24 years of age, 53% of cases are attributed to heterosexual transmission, whereas only 30% are attributable to injection drug use. Over the course of the epidemic, from 1983 to 1996, the proportion of AIDS cases among women attributed to heterosexual contact has increased substantially, from 15 to 38%. The findings suggest that AIDS cases attributable to heterosexual transmission are increasing faster than any other exposure category.

Because several years generally pass between initial infection and the development of symptoms and AIDS diagnosis, and because AIDS diagnoses have been further delayed or prevented by recent treatment advances, AIDS trends lag far behind those of the epidemic of new infections.[7] Analysis of AIDS and HIV diagnoses from 1994 to 1997 indicate that the incidence of heterosexually transmitted infections among women has increased dramatically, with women representing 17% of AIDS diagnoses but 28% of HIV diagnoses.[8]

Among women diagnosed with AIDS in the United States, incidence rates are highest among African-American women and those living in the Northeast and metropolitan areas. However, the greatest increases in incidence between 1990 and 1995 occurred among women living in the rural South.[9]

CROSS-SECTIONAL AND LONGITUDINAL RESEARCH

The Significance of Consistent Condom Use among Women

A primary HIV prevention strategy for sexually active persons is to use condoms during every episode of sexual intercourse. Studies of sexually active persons demonstrate that condoms, when used correctly and consistently, effectively prevent the transmission of viral pathogens, including HIV. Consistent condom use is regarded as the primary outcome measure based on findings from prospective studies indicating that condoms, when used consistently, can provide a 70 to 100% reduction in the risk of HIV transmission.[10] In particular, findings from the European Study Group on Heterosexual Transmission of HIV observed no seroconversions among couples who used condom consistently, while among inconsistent condom users the seroconversion rate was significantly higher, 4.8 per 100 person-years.[11] Moreover, predictions based on mathematical modeling suggest that, irrespective of the number of sexual partners and the prevalence of HIV among potential sex partners, consistent condom use can substantially reduce the risk of sexually transmitted HIV infection relative to never or half-time condom use.[12] Thus, as empirical evidence supports the clinical and public health significance of consistent condom use for preventing HIV infection, future behavior change interventions should assess consistent condom use as a primary outcome measure for evaluating program efficacy. The authors have reviewed the studies that have empirically examined the correlates of consistent condom use among women.

Correlates of Consistent Condom Use

Perceived Attitudes and Beliefs

One study conducted among a community-recruited sample of African-American women ($N = 165$) examined the correlates of consistent condom use over a 3-month period.[13] Women who used condoms consistently were more than 7.5 times more likely to perceive having high self-control over using condoms and were more than 6.5 times more likely to have a high perceived control over the partner's use of condoms. Another study conducted among adolescent females recruited from a clinic noted that women who used condoms consistently were 6.5 times more likely to perceive that their partner preferred using condoms.[14]

Self-Efficacy

Self-efficacy is the level of confidence in one's ability to effect change in a specific practice.[15,16] Self-efficacy regarding sexual communication/negotiation is the confidence a women has in bargaining for safer sex in light of the social cost of such negotiations. While having low sexual communication self-efficacy has been associated with HIV-risk taking,[17] having a high sexual communication self-efficacy has been associated with being a consistent condom user. A study conducted among young African-American women recruited from a community-based setting noted that consistent condom users were 13 times more likely to have high sexual assertiveness self-efficacy.[13] One might expect communication self-efficacy to be a more important determinant for women than for men, in that women must convince men to wear condoms. A recent study of STD clinic patients provides evidence that this is the case: Among the results was a significant self-efficacy by gender interaction, indicating that self-efficacy was a significant predictor of condom use for women, but not for men.[18]

Partner Related

Because male partners must agree to condom use, partner characteristics and behavior patterns are pivotal in determining women's ability to protect themselves from HIV/STD. Several partner-related variables appear to be associated with being a consistent condom user. Specifically, women who perceive their partner as having a low commitment to the relationship[13] and women who are in shorter relationships, less than 3 months in duration,[14] are more likely to use condoms consistently. This later study noted that having a short relationship with a partner is an important predictor of condom use even when controlling for type of partner (main or casual) and the frequency of sexual intercourse. These findings suggest that women are more likely to use condoms early in a relationship with a new partner, but discontinue condom use they perceive that their partners are committed to the relationship and then continued condom use may threaten the stability of the relationship.

Pregnancy Related

While the desire to become pregnant may be associated with not using condoms,[19] one study conducted among African-American women noted that consistent condom users were 8.5 times less likely to desire pregnancy.[13] This suggests that in HIV prevention programs for women, addressing the dual concepts of HIV prevention and pregnancy prevention may be an effective means of enhancing condom use. On the other hand, when a woman does decide to become pregnant, she must be counseled in ways to do so with relative safety, for example, through joint HIV antibody testing with her partner.

Among women a high degree of individual compliance is necessary for condoms to be used consistently during sexual intercourse. For economically disadvantaged women, numerous behavioral, social, cultural, and gender-related factors may reduce their compliance with consistent condom use, and thus elevate their risk of HIV exposure.[20]

Contextualizing Women's Risk for HIV

HIV prevention research has excelled in identifying behaviors associated with risky sexual practices and transmission of HIV; however, behavioral variables often fail to provide insight into the influence of the pervasive cultural, sociodemographic, gender-specific, and relational factors that mediate risky sexual and drug related behaviors. When conducting research with women, it is important to understand their risk and HIV risk reduction efforts in a gender-specific manner. This means examining gender-related factors that are strongly associated with HIV sexual risk-taking practices including noncondom use (never having used a condom) and having multiple sexual partners (having more than one sexual partner). Clearly, understanding the social influences that shape sexual relationships for women is critical to the development and implementation of tailored and more efficacious programs designed to reinforce the adoption and maintenance of HIV preventive behaviors among women.[20]

Correlates of HIV-Related Sexual Risk Taking

While epidemiological data are informative with respect to quantifying the differential risk for STD/HIV infection, they provide less insight into the influence of cultural, gender-specific, and psychosocial factors that are the determinants of behavior. Thus reducing the risk of HIV infection among sexually active women requires the identification of factors associated with HIV-related sexual risk taking. This means examining factors associated with noncondom use (never having used a condom): having multiple sexual partners (having more than one sexual partner) or engaging in HIV sexual risk taking (a composite score of HIV risk taking including having multiple sexual partners and infrequent condom use). Understanding the influences that shape behavior is critical to the development and implementation of tailored and more efficacious programs designed to reinforce the adoption and maintenance of HIV preventive behaviors among women. Here we review the studies that have empirically examined the correlates of noncondom use and having multiple sexual partners among women using linear or logistic regression analyses.

Sociodemographics

Socioeconomic status (SES) is an important correlate of behavior that affects health, access to health services, the risk of disease, the risk of an adverse outcome once disease occurs, and mortality.[21,22] Socioeconomic factors exacerbating women's vulnerability to HIV are prevalent. Economic factors play an important role in enhancing women's risk of infection, as women having lower income levels[23] and women who are Aid to Families with Dependent Children (AFDC) recipients[24] are more likely not to use condoms. Additionally, African-

American and Latina women are 4 and 3.5 times less likely, respectively, to use condoms compared to white women.[17] This may be a result of ethnic minority women having less access to optimal and quality preventive care, including STD treatment. Further, compared to white women disenfranchised ethnic minority women may have more immediate survival concerns, such as obtaining money for food and shelter, that may hinder the implementation of protective health behaviors.[25]

A number of sociodemographic factors associated with having multiple sexual partners were reported in a nationally representative sample of 8450 women aged 15 to 44.[26] Women with multiple sex partners were almost 7 times more likely to have experienced their initial intercourse when they were younger than 16 years of age, were nearly 2.5 times more likely to report living in an urban residence, and were twice as likely to report having no religious affiliation. Sexual abuse in childhood has been found to predict HIV risk,[27–29] although the mechanisms are not fully understood. Additionally, several studies have illustrated that marital status is associated with HIV risk taking, with unmarried women being more likely to have multiple sexual partners.[26,30]

Perceived Beliefs and Attitudes

Beliefs associated with HIV-related sexual risk taking include: believing that condoms have a negative impact on sexual enjoyment,[17,23] feeling that using condoms is embarrassing,[23] perceiving oneself to be at risk for HIV[31] (this result is probably due to the fact that using condoms lowers perceptions of risk), perceiving that your partner will think you are unfaithful if you ask them to use a condom,[24] and having a negative attitude toward sex.[32]

Self-Efficacy

As described above, partner characteristics and characteristics of a particular relationship figure importantly into women's efficacy judgments. A woman's decision to negotiate condom use is based on her perceptions of the costs and benefits to a particular relationship and the relationship's role in the woman's economic, social and physical survival goals. Women's inability to negotiate condom use is one of the strongest correlates of never having used a condom.[17,23,24,32] A number of studies have reported that women with low levels of self-efficacy for using condoms[23] and being able to avoid HIV[32] also are more likely to engage in HIV-related sexual risk taking.

In fact, partners may be viewed in some cases as "barriers" to condom use, so that efficacy judgments are likely to vary, depending on partner characteristics. For example, a woman might possess strong confidence in her ability to persuade her new, sensitive partner to use a condom but lack confidence in her ability to do so with an abusive former partner. Assessment of self-efficacy to negotiate and achieve condom use should incorporate different levels of partner resistance.[33]

Partner-Related Influences

At the core of partner-related influences exacerbating women's HIV risk are the power inequities that exist between the sexes. Power inequalities in heterosexual relationships are evident in social norms dictating monogamy for women and not for men, men having control over condom use, and violence directed toward women as well as the threats of such victimization. Several studies have demonstrated that monogamous women, women who have one sexual partner and women who have a partner who is resistant toward using condoms[24] are nearly 4 and 3 times, respectively, less likely to use condoms.[17,24] Another study found that women who were monogamous in their relationships perceived themselves to be at less risk, had lower intentions to use condoms, and used condoms less.[34] Since most women who do become HIV-seropositive are infected by a primary partner, this is very unfortunate.[35,36] Other partner-related factors associated with HIV sexual risk taking include having a physically abusive partner,[37] having a sexually abusive partner,[4,38,39] and fearing partner victimization.[32,38] Because condom requests from women may be attributed by some men to female infidelity, and in light of the fact that sexual jealousy is a well-documented trigger for violence, such fears may be realistic. A recent study of male inmates demonstrated that those with a history of severe domestic violence were likely to view hypothetical condom requests from a main partner more negatively than their nonviolent counterparts, a reaction that was in turn associated with lower likelihood of compliance with the request and greater likelihood of responding coercively.[40] The potential importance of this finding is underscored by the fact that in this sample, one highly relevant to HIV risk, 37% of respondents reported severe levels of violence on the Modified Conflict Tactics Scale.

Cultural

Acculturation is the cultural learning and behavioral adaptation that takes place among individuals exposed to a new culture.[41] This concept has been repeatedly shown to modify significantly the effect of many health factors among Latin populations.[42] A telephone survey of 1592 Hispanic and 629 non-Hispanic white men and women aged 18–49, randomly selected from nine states in the northeastern and southwestern United States, found that Hispanic women who were moderately or highly acculturated were more likely to have multiple sexual partners, 4.9 and 8.4 times, respectively, than were less acculturated women.[42] Compared to less acculturated women, moderately or highly acculturated women, may be less likely to adhere to the traditional Latin culture that emphasizes the need for men to express their sexuality and for women to avoid such expression.[41,43]

A cultural factor that has been shown to affect African-American women's risk of HIV is their perception of the sex–ratio imbalance. For African-American women who are considering marriage, there are fewer marriageable men, that is, males who are heterosexual, employed, and not incarcerated, than there are marriageable females. Given this sex–ratio imbalance, African-American women may be more likely to tolerate objectionable behavior, whereas the male may feel less pressure to develop commitments, exhibit greater power within relationships, and be less likely to exert behavioral controls.[44,45]

Alcohol and Crack Cocaine

There are several theories that attempt to explain the relationship between alcohol use and high-risk sexual behavior. One interpretation is that alcohol is a sexual disinhibitor that may place individuals at greater risk of becoming infected with STDs, including HIV, through unsafe sex. Another interpretation is that chronic alcohol use may serve as a marker for individuals who tend to practice a constellation of high-risk behaviors.[46] Both theories stress the effects of alcohol use as influencing high-risk sexual behaviors. One study reported that daily use of alcohol use was associated with not using condoms,[47] while moderate use of alcohol was associated with having multiple sexual partners.[31,47]

Crack cocaine and the exchange of sex for drugs have emerged as major risk factors for HIV and HIV risk taking. Trading sex for drugs often involves having sex with multiple anonymous sex partners, thereby increasing a women's risk of HIV.[48] Further, giving oral sex in exchange for crack is associated with a high risk of HIV infection because crack use causes oral burns that may facilitate transmission.

Mental Health

Women, during the same years when they are at high risk of acquiring HIV infection, are also at high risk of being depressed. Prior research has demonstrated that among women, the time period from ages 25 to 45 is the time of the highest risk of depression.[49] One study reported that women between the age of 25 and 45 who reported a depressive symptomatology on the Center for Epidemiological Studies Depression Scale, scores > 16, were more likely to engage in HIV risk taking.[50]

Pregnancy Related

A study conducted among a clinic-recruited sample of adolescent women noted that women who consistently used oral contraceptives were half as likely to use condoms as those who did not. This suggests that this sample is using condoms as a birth control method and not for HIV prevention. In addition, another study noted that if one or both partners wished to conceive, they were less likely to use condoms.[19] While it is important to stress the importance of condom use for both pregnancy and HIV prevention, the desire to become pregnant may undermine conscientious use of condoms.

The Female Condom

Unfortunately, the female condom represents the only female-controlled contraceptive methods that is clearly effective against HIV. Although the first female condom was introduced in the 1920s, the female condom only recently has been approved for use in the United States and represents an important alternative to the male condom.[51,52] The female condom is an effective barrier to HIV.[51] A multisite study reported a 2.5% unintended pregnancy rate and no STDs for US women who used the female polyurethane condom consistently and correctly within a 6-month period.[53] There are several major advantages of the female condom over the male condom: greater control by the woman, it can be inserted prior to sexual intercourse, it protects a greater area of the vagina, and the female condom is less likely to break compared to the male condom.[54] There also are several potential disadvantages to use of the female condom: its relative high cost, its appearance, and its initial acceptance by women.[54,55] Further, because it is detectable by the partner, negative attributions, such as female infidelity, are just as likely to occur as when use of a male condom is requested. The development of nondetectable methods of protection, such as topical virucides, must remain a high research priority.[52]

PREVENTION

A number of behavioral risk reduction interventions for adult women at heterosexual risk have been evaluated.[56–58] These generally have been small-group skills-building interventions delivered to women recruited from health clinics and other venues in urban areas with significant HIV prevalence. Interventions tested to date have primarily promoted the use of male condoms as the method for HIV/STD risk reduction. Studies are reviewed here that compare an intervention to a control/comparison condition with sexual behavior change and/or biological (e.g., STD) outcomes for adult women at significant heterosexual risk of HIV/STD infection. Studies including male participants will be described in cases where gender effects were tested. In each case, methodological points relevant to study interpretability will be discussed.

Single-Session and Videotape Interventions for At-Risk Women

A number of studies have evaluated brief, single-session informational risk reduction interventions. Single-session interventions can be advantageous in their ability to capitalize on fleeting opportunities for intervention, for example, by targeting patients in waiting rooms of STD treatment facilities. However, by virtue of their brevity, such interventions are limited in the amount of individualized skill building they can confer.

A program of research conducted by Nyamathi and colleagues[59,60] has evaluated brief sexual risk reduction interventions for impoverished women in homeless shelters and drug treatment centers in southern California. Interestingly, these interventions target coping and distress as well as drug use and sexual risk (multiple partners–condom use does not appear to be a focus). One large-scale study[59] compared a single-session "traditional" HIV risk reduction intervention with a "specialized" intervention providing HIV education, risk reduction skill building, and referral to other resources needed by the individual woman ($N = 858$). HIV antibody testing was provided to all women. Unfortunately, the treatment groups differed at baseline with women in the traditional group exhibiting greater distress, better HIV knowledge, and less problem-focused coping. The report is not clear in describing randomization procedures, although it appears that all women in a given site received the same intervention (suggesting that site was the unit of randomization, although it was not the unit of analysis). A further methodological concern is that the assessment and educational programs were administered by the same individuals (nurses), possibly increasing demand for socially desirable responding. At a 2-week follow-up, intervention effects were tested by examining time by treatment group interactions and repeated measures analysis of covariance (ANCOVAs) in which baseline values of the dependent variable and site were controlled. While significant improvements were apparent at follow-up among participants in both treatment conditions for every behavioral and psychological variable measured except one (problem-focused coping), significant treatment group by time interactions were obtained for knowledge, emotion-focused coping, and multiple sex partners. For these factors, improvements were greater for traditional intervention recipients. This finding was unexpected, but may have been due to the more diffuse focus in the specialized intervention. The finding of reduced reports of multiple partners is difficult to evaluate because condom use was not assessed.

A subsequent study designed specifically for Latina women compared the same two interventions in a quasi-experimental design in which randomization occurred by site.[60] Again, baseline differences existed between the groups for a number of demographic variables and drug use. At the 2-week follow-up, no differences between groups in risk reduction were observed, although again women in both groups improved on all measures except problem-focused coping. These results are difficult to interpret, as it is possible that all subjects were responding to demand.

Patients seeking care for STD other than HIV are at considerable risk for HIV infection for a variety of reasons, not the least of which is that STD diagnosis can be considered a proxy measure for unsafe sexual behavior.[61] For this reason, numerous studies have targeted patients in the publicly funded STD clinics that serve low-income communities.[62] One study compared one-session videotaped interventions designed to differentially affect skills and self-efficacy among low-income African-American women.[63] Women were randomized to view one of three risk reduction videotapes. One contained information only; one information plus modeling of risk reduction behaviors (i.e., negotiation sequences were presented); and the third provided the former two components but also created opportunity for cognitive rehearsal of the modeled behaviors by the participant (i.e., the woman practices in her mind negotiating safer sex with her partner). All three tapes contained a recommendation for condom use. Participants were assessed for changes in self-efficacy and a variety of behaviors 1 month later. As predicted by the investigators, self-efficacy rose the least in the information-only condition and the most in the information plus modeling plus rehearsal condition. In terms of actual behavior change, the rehearsal group reported buying more condoms and talking more to friends about HIV than the information-only group; however, no differences emerged for actual reduction of risk, that is, using condoms, number of partners, or number of partners using condoms, or even reports of any one of these.

It is generally believed that interventions for members of ethnic minority groups must be culturally tailored to be acceptable, credible, and effective. A study by Kalichman and colleagues[64] was designed to test this assertion experimentally. It sought to evaluate single-session videotaped interventions for African-American women recruited from housing projects in Chicago. One Public Health Service videotape provided HIV information delivered by two white men and one white woman; another gave the same information but presented by African-American women; and the third was similar to the second but with the addition of culturally relevant contextual information. A 2-week follow-up assessment was conducted by interviewers who were blind to participant treatment condition, with 72% of participants retained. Women who had received the culturally tailored tape reported greater concern about AIDS and were more likely at follow-up to have received an HIV antibody test, to have talked with friends about AIDS, and to request condoms. However, no differences between groups were obtained for seeking HIV information or trying to use condoms. Results of this study suggest that cultural relevance and sensitivity may have beneficial effects, even in the context of an intervention lacking sufficient intensity to achieve behavior change.

Surprisingly little research has explored the potential for health care providers to serve as sexual risk behavior change agents. In one study, however, peer educators were compared with health care providers for their effectiveness in delivering brief informational interventions. Participants were young women seeking care in an inner-city health clinic.[65] Both interventions were very brief; the provider one lasted at most 10 minutes. The interventions were evaluated with a series of Likert scale items. At a 1-month follow-up, no effects of either intervention were observed. However, among a subset of participants who were very sexually active (reporting intercourse more than once/week), reports of the difficulty of requesting condom use decreased significantly, as did their self-reported frequency of vaginal intercourse. To examine differences between the two treatment modalities, a series of treatment group by time interactions was performed. Results of these analyses indicated that the interventions were not differentially effective in changing behavior. It should be noted that the significance of these findings is limited by severe attrition, resulting in a follow-up retention rate of only 45%.

A recent study delivered a single-session intervention to low-income women and compared its effects with those of an HIV informational session that controlled attention.[66] This intervention combined elements of motivational enhancement and skill building. While the sample size was relatively small ($N = 74$), the randomization was successful and the study achieved excellent retention (92%) at the 3-month follow-up. At this time, women receiving the intervention reported significantly greater increases in condom use (from 22 to 66%) relative to comparison condition participants (27 to 43%), and fewer unprotected intercourse occasions in the prior 90 days (from 26 to 8 vs. 25 to 17). Confidence in the effects achieved by this intervention is strengthened by the methodological superiority of this study.

Multiple-Session Skill-Building Interventions for At-Risk Women

Interventions designed to build skills and self-efficacy in condom use, sexual negotiation, self-control, and problem-solving are included in this section. While such interventions are more costly on a per capita basis, they may have more power to enable behavior change, and thus may be cost-effective if delivered to very highly at-risk women.

A small-group cognitive–behavioral intervention was delivered to women receiving methadone maintenance by Schilling and colleagues.[67,68] The five-session intervention provided training of condom use and negotiation skills and was compared with a single-session informational control. Participants were Latina (64%) and African-American (36%) women, and the study was conducted in 1988. At 2 weeks postintervention, intervention participants reported significant increases in condom use, measured on a four-point Likert scale, although number of risk encounters was not assessed and number of sex partners did not change. While no differences between groups were found in a behavioral assessment of assertiveness–social skills at posttest, intervention participants did perceive themselves as better able to control their HIV risk. Frequency of condom use remained significantly higher among intervention participants than controls at a 15-month follow-up.[67] However, other intervention effects lost significance, and surprisingly skills intervention participants endorsed stronger belief in the role of "luck" in HIV prevention. The 32% attrition rate obtained at the follow-up limits confidence in these findings, although retained participants differed from those lost to follow-up only in their lower likelihood of injecting drugs at baseline.

Continuing their program of research among drug-using women, El-Bassel and colleagues[69] delivered a skill-building supportive intervention to women incarcerated in a correctional facility. Women responded to posted notices or were referred by jail staff. Eligibility criteria included projected release within 10 weeks, and drug use at lease three times per week prior to incarceration. At baseline, almost half the sample reported sexual abstinence or consistent condom use. Participants were randomized to receive either three 2-hour HIV informational sessions or to a very intensive intervention consisting of 16 2-hour skills-building sessions. The latter intervention also focused on building non-drug-using social support networks. Both interventions were delivered to small groups of women. The present report provided follow-up data for 1 month postintervention. At that time point, retention was 70%. Logistic regression analyses were performed with the dependent variable dichotomized into maintaining or improving safer sex practices versus getting worse or remaining unsafe. Treatment condition did not contribute significantly to this variable, but a marginally significant trend emerged when controls were added for marital status and number of sessions attended, although the rationale for this latter control was not given and is difficult to imagine. The intensive intervention group increased their positive coping skills; this effect was marginally significant. Surprisingly, though, the intensive intervention was not more effective than information alone on increasing women's self-efficacy to achieve condom use. In discussing this finding, the authors point out that it may take longer follow-up for women's experiences to produce self-efficacy enhancement.

Another more recent study also targeted drug-using women.[56] Participants in this study were women entering court-ordered inpatient treatment for chemical dependence; most were heavy users of alcohol and crack cocaine. Known HIV-seropositive women were excluded from analysis. This study obtained a participation rate of 69%. All patients in the facility received 3 hours of HIV education; this intervention comprised the control condition. Participants in the behavioral skills training (BST) condition received an additional four sessions that provided skill building for sexual negotiation and condom use. A randomized block design was used to avoid contamination between the treatment conditions. Self-administered questionnaires assessing risk behavior and a variety of possible intervention mediators were augmented by behavioral skills assessments at baseline, postintervention, and at a 2-month follow-up. Retention at the follow-up assessment point was only 49%. However, among the remaining participants, women receiving BST exhibited significantly improved prevention attitudes and more positive expected partner reactions relative to control participants, evidenced as significant group by time interactions. In addition, BST participants exhibited improved skills for sexual communication and condom use. With respect to sexual behavior, improvement was observed in both groups over time in number of partners, frequency of risk acts, and number of drugs used. However, no differences between treatment groups emerged for these variables; a significant treatment effect was obtained only for proportion of intercourse acts during which a condom was used (from 36% to 50%).

A study by Kelly and colleagues[70] evaluated a five-session intervention designed to enhance HIV awareness and provide ample opportunity for skill building. In this study, inner-city women attending a primary care clinic who met stringent risk criteria were randomized to receive either this intervention or an attention control focusing on other health promotion issues. Risk behavior was evaluated at baseline and at a 3-month follow-up. Many participants were not available at follow-up, with retention rates of 54% and 44% in the treatment and control conditions, respectively. This attrition was handled via imputation of missing data, using follow-up data for study completers similar in age, education, and STD history. It is not clear from the report, however, how treatment condition of completers compared with those of the participants lost to follow-up whose data theirs replaced. Results indicated that the intervention was effective in significantly reducing the number of unprotected intercourse episodes (from 14 to 11.7 in the treatment group), and percentage of occasions on which condoms were used (from 26% to 56% in the treatment group), although not in reducing number of sex partners in the previous 3 months (from 2.3 to 1.7 in the experimental group). Behavioral skill assessments were conducted in this study; the intervention produced a significant effect on two indexes of communication requiring self-control (postponing sex until condom obtained and refusing sex without a condom), but not on two indexes of assertively negotiating condom use. This well-designed study provides evidence that women can respond effectively to intensive cognitive–behavioral skill-building interventions.

A similar study tested a four-session intervention against a health promotion attention control and a no-intervention control among single pregnant inner-city women.[71] The intervention included modeling and practice for negotiation skill building, as well as cognitive imagining of negative (AIDS) and positive (prevention) outcomes to build motivation. Again, some statistically significant effects were obtained, although it should be noted that analyses were conducted only for participants who completed at least three of four intervention sessions, a point we shall return to. Frequency of condom and spermicide use, assessed with a four-point scale, changed significantly among treated women postintervention, from 2.93 at baseline to 3.86 at follow-up. However, it is impossible to tell from the report how much of this effect was due to condom use and how much to spermicide use. The treatment group showed significantly greater improvement than the no-intervention group at an immediate postintervention assessment; it did not differ from the attention control at this time point; and specific tests of intervention effects at the 3 month mark are not reported. However, an ANCOVA in which baseline level was used as the covariate produced a nonsignificant treatment group by time (postintervention to follow-up) interaction, suggesting maintenance of change. Number of intercourse events did not change significantly, and number of unprotected encounters was not reported (but in theory should have been reduced if condom use increased). Redemption of condom coupons increased significantly in both the AIDS prevention and health promotion groups but did not differentiate the groups. In summary, while this study suggests modest intervention effects for condom–spermicide use, the failure to perform an intention-to-treat analysis represents a serious threat to study interpretability. It is not clear whether the same standard for inclusion—attendance at three of four intervention sessions—was applied to the attention control; it could not have been applied to the no-treatment control. Inasmuch as more frequent attenders are likely to be differentially skilled and motivated for behavior change, comparisons with the no-intervention control are almost certainly biased. Further, women who are better able to change their behavior are likely to find the intervention more appealing, and thus to show better attendance, suggesting the possibility of bias in all comparisons. It is impossible to tell from the report the magnitude of this problem, as it is unclear what percentage of randomized participants were in fact included in the analyses.

Another randomized trial targeting young African-American women compared a theoretically derived social skills intervention with a control for demand (one session of HIV education) and a delayed-treatment control.[72] Women responded to recruitment materials and street outreach; those reporting the recent use of crack cocaine or injection drugs were excluded. The peer-led social skills intervention comprised five 2-hour sessions that included ethnic and gender pride, risk sensitization and building skills for assertive sexual communication, condom use, and sexual self-control through cognitive rehearsal. The primary outcome measure was consistent condom use. Differences between treatment groups were identified at baseline; these included duration of relationship with partner and income and were adjusted in outcome analyses. At the 3-month follow-up, attrition of 28% was largely accounted for by relocation out of the community, but was very low in the social skills condition (9.4%) and especially high (42.5%) in the delayed-treatment condition. Results indicated that the social skills intervention was associated with significant increases in consistent condom use (from 35% to 47% of participants) relative to the delayed-treatment control (22% to 29%). In addition, social skills participants demonstrated significantly improved coping and self-control skills and communication skills and reported improved partner normative beliefs regarding condoms. While the significance levels for differences between the social skills intervention and the demand control condition are not reported, analyses indicated that the latter did not differ significantly from the delayed treatment condition.

Carey and colleagues[73] recently completed another study targeting low-income women, but used a different intervention approach. In addition to the types of skill-building described in connection with many of the studies described above, this intervention provided a motivational enhancement component drawn from substance use intervention research. Women were randomized to receive this four-session intervention or to a wait-list control. Risk behavior and mediators were assessed at baseline, 3 weeks postintervention, and at a 3-month follow-up. Although some women did not attend any intervention sessions, they were not excluded from analyses on this basis. However, analysis was restricted to participants who had undergone at least one postintervention assessment. This criterion produced a loss of 10 experimental and 11 control participants (out of totals of 53 and 49, respectively). Data missing from one of the two postintervention assessments were imputed based on baseline and single postintervention data. Nonnormal variables were transformed to maximize normality. Results indicated that those receiving the intervention reported increased risk sensitization, stronger intentions to practice safer sex, more communication with partners (3-week time point only), and frequency of unprotected vaginal intercourse compared with control women. This last effect was significant only at the 3-week time point. The authors present effect size data, based on mediator as well as risk variables at the 3-week assessment point, for their own study and for previous studies of women. These data indicate the improved effectiveness of the intervention approach incorporating motivational enhancement.

Individuals with severe and persistent mental illness (SMI) are a group that has been severely affected by HIV. In a recent study, Weinhardt and colleagues[74] evaluated an intervention specifically designed for women with SMI. Twenty women receiving outpatient mental health care were randomized either to a 10-session intervention focusing on training assertiveness skills or to a wait-list control condition. The interventions were conducted daily during 2 consecutive weeks and combined risk feedback, HIV information, and extensive communication skill building for assertive condom request negotiation. Behavioral skills assessments for sexual assertiveness were conducted. Assessments were administered at baseline and immediately, 2 months, and 4 months postintervention. Women who had received the intervention were found to have significantly better sexual assertion skills at all follow-up time points and improved knowledge at the posttest and 2-month time points. They also reported more instances of protected intercourse at the 2-month but not the 4-month assessments; no significant differences were obtained for frequency of unprotected intercourse. However, the differences were in the expected direction and approached significance ($P < .06$) at the 2-month point.

Null results were reported for a seven-session intervention delivered to STD clinic patients.[75] In this study, 472 participants (195 of whom were women) were randomized to receive either an intensive seven-session intervention or a brief HIV information control. A 90-minute interview assessing risk behavior and several social cognitive theory condom-related mediators was conducted at baseline and 3 months after the intervention. Substantial attrition— 28%—occurred; unfortunately, retention was greater in the control condition (83%) than the intervention condition (70%). Differential attrition showing this pattern is suggestive that intervention nonresponders may have self-selected out of the follow-up. However, this issue is moot. While participants in both conditions reported improved self-efficacy and outcome beliefs as well as reduced risk after the intervention, no differences between the groups was apparent for any of these factors. It is thus impossible to know which of several possibilities accounts for the changes observed over time: (1) participants were engaging in socially desirable responding due to experimental demand; (2) even the brief informational intervention was effective in changing behavior; or (3) the lengthy interview was reactive and actually changed behavior. No interaction between gender and treatment condition was found for any outcome, suggesting that women and men responded similarly to the interventions.

Community-Level Intervention

All of the interventions described in this chapter were delivered to small groups or individuals, with the exception of a recent multisite study conducted by Sikkema and colleagues.[76] Community-level interventions represent a cost-effective way to reach larger numbers of individuals and may be particularly empowering for women. In this study, interventions were delivered to women living in 18 low-income housing developments in five US cities. Housing developments were randomized in matched pairs either to receive the intervention or to receive packets with HIV informational brochures, free condoms, and order forms to obtain additional condoms. The interventions included small group workshops and community events, delivered by resident-nominated opinion leaders. Assessment of HIV risk behavior was conducted in all housing developments at baseline and one year. Of the 1,265 women surveyed at baseline, 690 were available at follow-up and constituted a longitudinal cohort of women. The proportion of women reporting any unprotected intercourse in the previous two months changed from 50% at baseline to 38% at follow-up for intervention women; corresponding figures for control women were 50% and 46%. Percentage of intercourse occasions for which a condom was used also increased among intervention women; both of these treatment effects were significant. Corroborating these results were significant effects on having a condom at home or on her person, and scores on an AIDS knowledge measure. The authors acknowledge the possibility of bias in the longitudinal sample, causing uncertainty regarding generality of findings. Nonetheless, this first community-level intervention is promising for such approaches, possibly superior to individual and small-group intervention in terms of cost-effectiveness, sustainability, and generalization of empowerment to other community issues.

Studies Comparing Theoretical Approaches to Intervention

As this review makes apparent, most intervention studies have compared a single intervention with multiple components with some sort of control condition. If the intervention proves superior to the control in changing risk behavior, it is difficult to know which intervention components might have been necessary or sufficient. Two studies have actually randomized women to different active intervention arms to compare more focused intervention strategies for effectiveness.

Most of the interventions described above included skill building in communication to enhance women's ability to negotiate condom use with partners. Another skill domain with relevance to sexual risk behavior is self-control or self-management. Skills can be developed for identifying and managing antecedents of risk behavior so that difficult situations can be avoided, which may obviate the need for negotiating with a male partner. Thus, negotiation and self-control are separable skill domains that may affect behavior change differently. A study by Kalichman and colleagues[77] compared these approaches in a factorial design: Women were randomized to receive either communication skills training, self-management skills training, a combination of the two, or an educational/risk sensitization control. The design controlled both for attention—all interventions were delivered in four sessions of the same length—and demand—as each contained a recommendation for condom use. Measures included sexual risk behavior and mediation behaviors such as actually communicating with partners and avoiding antecedents such as use of drugs or alcohol prior to sex. Assessments were conducted at baseline, postintervention, and at 3 months postintervention. Twenty-eight percent of participants dropped out after a single intervention session and did not undergo follow-up assessment in an intention-to-treat analysis. The report does not include information regarding which arms these women had been randomized to; however, it appears that the first session was quite similar across the four groups, suggesting the likelihood that attrition from them was similar. Results at the 3-month follow-up provided partial support for study hypotheses. Women who had received the communication skills training reported more conversations with partners about condoms and more frequent refusal of unprotected sex (although the greatest frequency was obtained in the educational control condition). Regarding sexual risk behavior, women receiving the combined skills intervention reported the fewest unprotected intercourse acts. However, no differences emerged for proportion of protected acts, suggesting that avoidance of sex accounts for the former finding. This study suggests that both sets of skills must be in place for women to be successful in reducing their HIV risk.

Another recent study compared interventions driven by three different theoretical orientations delivered to low-income, African-American women in Mississippi.[78] The theories were social learning theory (SLT), social cognitive theory (SCT), and the theory of gender and power (TGP). A wait-list control was also included. In developing and delivering the gender and power intervention, care was taken to foster discussion but not to provide modeling or practice (i.e., skill-building techniques were avoided). While the SLT intervention provided modeling of skills, only the SCT intervention prompted participants to practice the skills themselves. Each intervention was delivered in six 90- to 120-minute sessions. For ethical reasons, the wait-list participants were given an intervention following the first postintervention assessment, so that subsequent comparisons are for the three intervention groups. Strengths of this study included a large sample ($N = 363$) and very low attrition even at a year postintervention. In this study, 18% of women assigned to one of the intervention arms failed to attend the first session and were dropped from the study. As predicted, both of the skill-building interventions produced greater increases in communication and condom use skills, relative to the other two conditions. Percentage of intercourse occasions during which condoms were used was greater at the immediate postintervention time point for all intervention conditions relative to the control (increasing from 37 to 44%). Women in the intervention conditions did not differ, but condom use gains were maintained at 6 months (54%) and 1 year (49%). It is of considerable interest that a non-skills-based intervention, based on the TGP, was equally effective in changing behavior, although presumably via different mechanisms. It is possible, however, that discussion in the TGP groups included reports of previously successful risk reduction strategies women had used. A secondary analysis conducted at 6 and 12 months revealed that women who had formed a new relationship since the intervention were significantly more likely to be using condoms (68%). This result highlights the relative difficulty that women may experience attempting to initiate condom use in an ongoing relationship.

Studies Evaluated with Biological Outcomes

All the intervention studies described above were evaluated via self-reported sexual behavior. Unfortunately, self-reports can suffer limitations in reliability due to memory inaccuracy and desire to "please" the investigators. While underreporting of stigmatized behaviors is a widespread phenomenon,[79] in the context of an intervention trial it can be particularly problematic.[80] This is because demand to report behavior change may be greater among those who received the intervention (or the more intensive intervention, or the one focusing more directly on the dependent variable being assessed). This differential demand can produce spurious positive intervention effects. Thus, recent studies often have assessed the incidence of other STDs, reasoning that the behavior changes that reduce the likelihood of HIV infection (e.g., condom use) also reduce the likelihood of infection by other sexually transmitted pathogens. Thus, STD incidence constitutes an objective index of behavior change.

Most studies that have employed biological STD outcomes have been conducted, wholly or primarily, in publicly funded STD clinics.[81] Patients seeking care in these clinics tend to have high rates of reinfection, providing statistical power to detect effects, and these clinics routinely perform diagnostic tests for STD of the sort needed for outcome evaluation. One early study delivered three brief interventions to male and female patients in public STD clinics.[82] In this study, all patients in the clinic waiting room on a given day were randomized to receive one of the three interventions followed by a psychosocial assessment, or to undergo assessment only: (1) condom skills, which provided a brief condom use demonstration; (2) social influences, which provided the condom, assertion of condom popularity (normative information), and eroticization of condoms; and (3) distribution of condoms, also accompanied by the condom demonstration. Outcomes included postintervention condom attitudes and behavioral intentions and STD (re)infection in the subsequent 6–9 months, identified through tracking clinic medical charts. Women who had received the condom distribution reported significantly stronger intentions to use condoms than control women; but while male participants receiving condom skills were reinfected significantly less than control men, women demonstrated no such effect. Further, behavioral intention and attitudes failed to correlate with STD diagnoses, a common finding in HIV/STD behavioral research.[80] Results of this study appear to suggest that very brief interventions that do not provide individualized skill building may be ineffective for women, even at intensity levels that enable behavior change in men. Another later study obtained similar results.[83] Participants ($N = 399$) were randomized to receive four 1-hour individual counseling sessions based on behavioral theory or to receive standard STD counseling (about 15 minutes). Participants were assessed at 3 and 5 months following the intervention. Unfortunately, retention was poor in this study, with 65% returning at 3 months and 60% at 5 months. While STD incidence did not differ significantly between the intervention and control groups, a self-reported behavior effect was obtained for men. Women displayed no such effect.

Two national multisite studies evaluating behavioral interventions for high-risk men and women and employing STD incidence to evaluate them have been completed recently.[84,85] These studies are important because of their size, their cross-site consistency of effects, and their use of biological STD data to supplement self-reported reductions in risk behavior.

Project RESPECT randomized STD patients in five inner-city sites to receive one of three individual interventions delivered by clinic staff.[84] Entry criteria included age over 14 years, unprotected intercourse within the previous month, willingness to receive an HIV antibody test, and seronegative test result. Altogether, 5758 patients, 2476 of them female, were enrolled. This number represents 44% of those eligible. Participants in the education condition received two brief informational messages; those in HIV prevention counseling condition were given two counseling sessions aimed at enhancing risk awareness and negotiating a behavior change step; a third condition, enhanced counseling, provided four sessions driven by the theory of reasoned action. Participants received interviews regarding their risk behavior at baseline and 3, 6, 9, and 12 months following the intervention. They also received biological screening for three STDs (syphilis, chlamydia, gonorrhea) and HIV at each assessment point. While attrition by the 12-month assessment was high (34%), 86% of participants completed at least one follow-up. Results for self-reported behavior indicated significantly higher levels of consistent condom use among enhanced and HIV prevention conditions compared to the educational one at 3-month point; by 6 months enhanced and HIV prevention participants had significantly fewer STDs than their educational counterparts. Neither the behavioral nor biological effects were significant at 12 months. Results were similar for men and women.

The National Institute of Mental Health (NIMH) Multisite HIV Prevention Trial tested a seven-session intervention against a one-session HIV informational control at seven inner-city sites.[85] Participants were men and women recruited in STD clinics and women meeting stringent risk criteria recruited from health service organizations. The small-group intervention provided HIV information, risk sensitization, and skill building for condom use, negotiation, and self-control. Interviews concerning risk behavior, the social cognitive theory mediators that formed the basis for the intervention, and STD symptoms were conducted at baseline and at 3, 6, and 12 months postintervention. For participants recruited in STD clinics, data on

STD during the follow-up period were extracted from clinic charts. At the 12-month assessment point, all participants gave urine samples for the detection of chlamydia and gonorrhea. Results indicated that consistent condom use/abstinence was reported by significantly more intervention than control participants at all follow-up points. While effects for overall STD based on chart review did not significantly distinguish groups, men in the intervention group received gonorrhea diagnoses half as often as men in the control condition. In addition, self-reported symptoms, which were correlated with chart diagnoses, were significantly less frequent among intervention participants than controls. Point prevalence (at 12 months) of chlamydia and gonorrhea were not significantly different between groups. A nonsignificant gender by treatment group interaction suggests that the intervention was not differentially effective for men and women. Further, the social cognitive theory factors, self-efficacy, and relevant outcome expectancies were shown to mediate the intervention effect.[85]

Another single-site study obtaining significant STD effects with fewer methodological limitations has recently been reported.[86] In this study, over 500 women, all of minority ethnicity (Mexican American and African American), were randomized to receive a small-group cognitive behavioral intervention delivered in four sessions for a total of 12–16 hours, or to a standard STD counseling control. Participants were followed for 1 year and were assessed for chlamydia and gonorrhea at each assessment point. Retention was excellent, 89%, at the 1-year follow-up. Incidence of infection was significantly lower among those receiving the more intensive intervention compared to controls both at 6 months (11% versus 17%) and 12 months (17% versus 27%). This excellent study provides particularly compelling evidence for the effectiveness of behavioral intervention in reducing sexually transmitted disease and by extension sexually transmitted HIV infection.

SUMMARY AND CONCLUSIONS

Taken together, these studies are moderately encouraging in their promise for AIDS prevention among women at risk. Results are most impressive in studies using a no-treatment or wait-list control condition; when controls for attention or demand are used, nonsignificant results are often obtained. Many studies do not report critical information, such as participation rates or when randomization was performed, making it difficult to evaluate and compare studies.[80] Very few studies reviewed here used follow-up periods longer than 2–4 months, and even those interventions that demonstrated effectiveness at early postintervention assessment points tended to lose effectiveness at the later ones.

It also seems clear that more intensive interventions, that is, interventions that devote more time to each individual participant including skill building, are more effective than briefer, single-session ones. This is not surprising in light of women's greater need for the skills discussed above. Indeed, a study of college students[87] found that men were able to respond effectively to a low-intensity intervention, but women's behavior did not change and their self-efficacy decreased relative to controls. This result may be interpreted as resulting from the low level of individualized skill building provided by this low-intensity intervention.

However, these studies do illustrate that many inner-city women can reduce their behavioral risk for HIV infection after intensive training in negotiation and condom use skills, particularly if they are not in stable ongoing relationships. Thus, it is important that interventions found to be effective in the studies reviewed here be disseminated for at-risk women in affected communities.

Evidence is clear that it is more difficult for women to achieve condom use in an ongoing stable relationship. Unfortunately, many (probably most) women who have become infected globally have been infected by a primary partner.[35,36] In most cultures (although to varying degrees), male infidelity is sanctioned while female infidelity is stigmatized and punished. At the same time, women encounter many difficulties in trying to negotiate consistent condom use with primary partners. Condoms can be taken as indications of female infidelity or disease, and the male partner may correctly perceive that he is himself not at risk of infection from his primary partner. Further, couples in stable relationships may wish to conceive children. It is imperative that the prevention research community test other options for women in this situation, such as joint antibody testing and condom use with secondary partners or the use of condom request messages that may avoid negative partner reactions.[89] A more detailed discussion of this issue can be found in O'Leary.[90]

Methodological Issues: The Problem of Attrition

Virtually every study reviewed here that required multiple contacts with participants suffered significant attrition. Many of these studies presented data showing that retained participants did not differ significantly from those lost at follow-up on baseline demographic or risk variables. However, it seems likely that other factors (e.g., personality factors; inability to respond to intervention) may have been unmeasured sources of bias. Attrition that occurs prior to randomization threatens external validity, while attrition occurring afterward threatens internal validity.[80] The NIMH Multisite study chose to maximize internal validity by randomizing individuals only after they had demonstrated significant commitment to the study and had appeared to receive the first session of the intervention. This strategy was effective, in that retention of its very low-income participants was excellent: 90% for health service organization women and 86% for STD clinic women. It is critically important that future studies strive to maximize retention, perform intent-to-treat analyses, and use conservative imputation techniques as needed to replace missing data. It is particularly important that every effort be made to prevent differential attrition by treatment condition, which may result from differential experimental demand. Both the differential demand and differential attrition can create artefactual positive intervention effects (see O'Leary et al.[80]).

Conclusions

While behavioral interventions have shown promise for women, it is clear that we have not resolved all the barriers that at-risk women face.[7,80,89] We must continue to work with women to develop effective ways to help them to avoid the risk of HIV and other STD. At the same time, it will be important that we begin to address the economic, cultural, and sociopolitical issues that underlie the difficulty many women face in their efforts to protect themselves. These include poverty, power imbalances associated with gender, and inadequate services to prevent and treat drug addiction, domestic violence, and childhood sexual abuse.

ACKNOWLEDGMENTS.   Work on this chapter was supported by grants MH48013 from the National Institute of Mental Health to the first author and was completed while she was a visiting scientist at the Centers for Disease Control and Prevention. This chapter was completed with support from the Center for Mental Health Research on AIDS, NIMH R01MH55726 and R01MH54412 to the second author. The authors wish to thank Rich Wolitski for comments on an earlier draft of the manuscript.

REFERENCES

1. Corea G. *The Invisible Epidemic: The Story of Women and AIDS*. New York: HarperCollins; 1992.
2. Shilts R. *And the Band Played On*. New York: Penguin Books; 1987.
3. Amaro H. Love, sex and power: Considering women's realities in HIV prevention. *Am Psychol* 1995; 50: 437–447.
4. Zierler S, Krieger N. Reframing women's risk: Social inequalities and HIV infection. *Annu Rev Public Health* 1997; 18:401–436.
5. Mantell JE, Karp GB, Ramos SE, et al. Women, power and negotiating condoms: A new perspective in understanding HIV prevention behavior. Unpublished manuscript. New York: Columbia University; 1998.
6. Centers for Disease Control and Prevention. Mid-year edition. *HIV/AIDS Surveillance Report*. Atlanta, GA: CDC; 1996.
7. O'Leary A, Jemmott LS. General issues in the prevention of AIDS in women. In: O'Leary A, Jemmott LS, eds. *Women at Risk: Issues in the Primary Prevention of AIDS*. New York: Plenum Press; 1995:1–12.
8. Centers for Disease Control and Prevention. Diagnosis and reporting of HIV and AIDS in states with integrated HIV and AIDS surveillance—United States, January 1994–June 1997. *Morb Mortal Wkly Rep* 1998, 47:309–314.
9. Wortley PM, Fleming PL. AIDS in women in the United States. *JAMA* 1997; 278:911–916.
10. Roper WL, Peterson HB, Curran JW. Commentary: Condoms and HIV/STD prevention—clarifying the message. *Am J Public Health* 1993; 83:501–503.
11. De Vincenzi I. A longitudinal study of human immunodeficiency virus transmission by heterosexual partners. *N Engl J Med* 1994; 331:341–346.
12. Fineberg HV. Education to prevent AIDS: Prospects and obstacles. *Science* 1988; 239:592–596.
13. Wingood GM, DiClemente RJ. Gender-related correlates and predictors of consistent condom use among African-American women: A prospective analysis. *Int J STD AIDS* 1997; 8:1–7.
14. Plichta SB, Weisman CS, Nathanson CA, et al. Partner-specific condom use among adolescent women clients of a family planning clinic. *J Adolesc Health* 1992; 13:506–511.
15. Bandura A. Social cognitive theory and exercise of control over HIV infection. In: DiClemente RJ, Peterson J, eds. *Preventing AIDS. Theories and Methods of Behavioral Interventions*. New York: Plenum Press; 1994:25–59.
16. Bandura A. *Self-Efficacy: The Exercise of Control*. New York: WH Freeman; 1997.
17. Catania JA, Coates TJ, Kegeles S, et al. Condom use in multi-ethnic neighborhoods of San Francisco: the population-based AMEN (AIDS in multi-ethnic neighborhoods) study. *Am J Public Health* 1992; 82:284–287.
18. LoConte J, O'Leary A, Labouvie E. Psychosocial correlates of HIV-related sexual behavior in an inner-city STD clinic. *Psychol Health* 1997; 12:589–601.
19. Adler NE, Tschann JM. Conscious and preconscious motivation for pregnancy among female adolescents. In: Lawson A, Rhode DL, eds. *The Politics of Pregnancy: Adolescent Sexuality and Public Policy*. New Haven, CT: Yale University Press; 1993:144–158.
20. Wingood GM, DiClemente RJ. Cultural, gender and psychosocial influences on HIV-related behavior of African-American female adolescents: Implications for the development of tailored prevention programs. *Ethn Dis* 1992; 2:381–388.
21. Adler NE, Boyce T, Chesney MA, et al. Socioeconomic inequalities in health: No easy solution. *JAMA* 1993; 269:3140–3145.
22. Pappas G, Queen S, Hadden W, Fisher G. The increasing disparity in mortality rates between socioeconomic groups in the United States, 1960 and 1986. *N Engl J Med* 1993; 329:103–109.
23. Peterson JL, Grinstead OA, Golden E, et al. Correlates of HIV risk behaviors in black and white San Francisco heterosexuals: The population-based AIDS in Multiethnic Neighborhoods (AMEN) study. *Ethn Dis* 1992; 2: 361–370.
24. Wingood GM, DiClemente RJ. Partner influences and gender-related factors associated with noncondom use among young adult African-American women. *Am J Commun Psychol* 1998; 26:29–53.
25. Mays VM, Cochran SD. Issues in the perception of AIDS risk and risk reduction activities by Black and Latino/Latino women. *Am Psychol* 1988; 43:949–957.
26. Seidman S, Mosher W, Aral S. Women with multiple sexual partners: United States, 1988. *Am J Public Health* 1992; 82(10):1388–1394.
27. Cunningham RM, Stiffman AR, Dore P, Earls F. The association of physical and sexual abuse with HIV risk behaviors in adolescence and young adulthood: Implications for public health. *Child Abuse Neglect* 1994; 18:233–245.
28. Wyatt GE. The relationship between child sexual abuse and adolescent sexual functioning in Afro-American and white American Women. *Ann NY Acad Sci* 1990; 528:111–122.

29. Zierler S, Feingold L, Laufer D, et al. Adult survivors of childhood sexual abuse and subsequent risk of HIV infection. *Am J Public Health* 1991; 81:572–575.
30. Grinstead OA, Faigeles B, Binson D, Eversley R. Sexual risk for human immunodeficiency virus infection among women in high-risk cities. *Fam Plann Perspect* 1993; 25:252–256.
31. Sikkema KJ, Heckman TG, Kelly JA, et al. HIV risk behaviors among women living in low-income, inner-city housing developments. *Am J Public Health* 1995; 86:1123–1128.
32. Harlow LL, Quina K, Morokoff PJ, et al. HIV risk in women: A multifaceted model. *J Appl Biobehav Res* 1993; 1:3–38.
33. Forsyth AD, Carey MP. Measuring self-efficacy in the context of HIV risk-reduction: Research challenges and recommendations. *Health Psychol* 1998; 17:559–568.
34. St. Lawrence JS, Eldridge GD, Reitman D, et al. Factors influencing condom use among African American women: Implications for risk reduction interventions. *Am J Community Psychol* 1998; 26:7–28.
35. Carpenter CJ, Mayer KH, Stein MD, et al. Human immunodeficiency virus infection in North American women: Experience with 200 cases and a review of the literature. *Medicine* 1991; 70:307–325.
36. Marmor M, Krasinski K, Sanchez M, et al. Sex, drugs, and HIV infection in a New York City hospital outpatient population. *J Acquire Immunodefic Syndr* 1990; 3:307–318.
37. Wingood GM, DiClemente RJ. Effects of having a physically abusive partner on the condom use and sexual negotiation practices of young adult African-American women. *Am J Public Health* 1997; 87:1016–1018.
38. Kalichman SC, Williams EA, Cherry C, et al. Sexual coercion, domestic violence, and negotiating condom use among low-income African American women. *J Women Health* 1998; 7:371–378.
39. Wingood GM, DiClemente RJ. Rape among African-American women: Sexual, psychological and social correlates predisposing survivors to STD/HIV. *J Women Health* 1988; 7:77–84.
40. Neighbors CJ, O'Leary A, Labouvie E. Domestically violent and non-violent male inmates' evaluations and responses to their partner's requests for condom use: Testing a Social-Information Processing model. *Health Psychol* 1999; 18:427–431.
41. Pavich EG: A Chicano perspective on Mexican culture and sexuality. *J Soc Work Hum Sex* 1986; 4:47–65.
42. Marin B, Gomez CA, Hearst N. Multiple heterosexual partners and condom use among Hispanics and non-Hispanic whites. *Fam Plann Perspect* 1993; 25:170–174.
43. Vasquez-Nuttal E, Romero-Garcia I, DeLeon B. Sex roles and perceptions of femininity and masculinity of Hispanic women. *Psychol Women Q* 1987; 11:409–425.
44. Gasch H, Fullilove MT, Fullilove RE. "Can do" thinking may enable safer sex. *Multicultural Inquiry Res AIDS Q Newsletter* 1990, 4:5–6.
45. Wingood GM, DiClemente RJ. Understanding the role of gender relations in HIV prevention research. *Am J Public Health* 1995; 85:592.
46. Leigh BC, Stall R. Substance use and risky sexual behavior for exposure to HIV: Issues in methodology, interpretation, and prevention. *Am Psychol* 1993; 48:1035–1045.
47. Wingood GM, DiClemente RJ. The influence of psychosocial factors, alcohol, drug use on African-American women's high risk sexual behavior. *Am J Prev Med* 1998; 15:54–60.
48. DeHovitz JA, Kelly P, Feldman J, et al. Sexually transmitted diseases, sexual behavior, and cocaine use in inner-city women. *Am J Epidemiol* 1994; 140(12):1125–1134.
49. Weissman M. Advances in psychiatric epidemiology: Rates and risks for major depression. *Am J Public Health* 1987; 77:445–451.
50. Orr ST, Celentano DD, Santelli J, Burwell L. Depressive symptoms and risk factors for HIV acquisition among black women attending urban health centers in Baltimore. *AIDS Educ Prev* 1994; 6(3):230–236.
51. Centers for Disease Control and Prevention. Barrier protection against HIV infection and other sexually transmitted diseases. *Morb Mortal Wkly Rep* 1993; 42:589–591,597.
52. Institute of Medicine. *Contraceptive Research and Development: Looking to the Future.* Harrison PF, Rosenfield A, eds. Washington, DC: National Academy Press; 1996.
53. Farr G, Gabelnick H, Sturgen K, Dorflinger L. Contraceptive efficacy and acceptability of the female condom. *Am J Public Health* 1994; 84:1960–1964.
54. Gollub EL. Women-centered prevention techniques and technologies. In: O'Leary A, Jemmott LS, eds. *Women at Risk: Issues in the Primary Prevention of AIDS.* New York: Plenum Press; 1995:43–82.
55. Eldridge GD, St. Lawrence JS, Little CE, et al. Barriers to condom use and barrier method preferences among low-income African American women. *Women Health* 1995; 23:73–89.
56. Eldridge GD, St. Lawrence JS, Little CE, et al. Evaluation of an HIV risk reduction intervention for women entering inpatient substance abuse treatment. *AIDS Educ Prev* 1997; 9(A):62–76.

57. Ickovics JR, Yoshikawa H. Preventive interventions to reduce heterosexual HIV risk for women: Current perspectives, future directions. *AIDS* 1998; 12(suppl. A):S197–S208.

58. Wingood GM, DiClemente RJ. HIV sexual risk reduction interventions for women: A review. *Am J Prev Med* 1995; 12(3):209–217.

59. Nyamathi AM, Flaskerud J, Bennett C, et al. Evaluation of two AIDS education programs for impoverished women. *AIDS Educ Prev* 1994; 6:296–309.

60. Nyamathi AM, Leake BL, Flaskerud J, et al. Outcomes of specialized and traditional AIDS counseling programs for impoverished women of color. *Res Nurs Health* 1993; 16:11–21.

61. Aral SO, Wasserheit JN. Interactions among HIV, other sexually transmitted diseases, socioeconomic status, and poverty in women. In: O'Leary A, Jemmott LS, eds. *Women at Risk: Issues in the Primary Prevention of AIDS*. New York: Plenum Press; 1995:13–41.

62. O'Donnell LN, San Doval A, Duran R, O'Donnell C. Video-based sexually transmitted disease patient education: Its impact on condom acquisition. *Am J Public Health* 1995; 85:817–822.

63. Maibach E, Flora J. Symbolic modeling and cognitive rehearsal: Using video to promote AIDS prevention self-efficacy. *Community Res* 1993; 20:517–545.

64. Kalichman SC, Kelly JA, Hunter TL, et al. Culturally tailored HIV-AIDS risk-reduction messages targeted to African-American urban women: Impact on risk sensitization and risk reduction. *J Consult Clin Psychol* 1993; 61:291–295.

65. Quirk ME, Godkin MA, Schwenzfeier E. Evaluation of two AIDS prevention interventions for inner-city adolescent women. *Am J Prev Med* 1993; 9:21–26.

66. Belcher L, Kalichman S, Topping M, et al. A randomized trial of a brief HIV risk reduction counseling intervention for women. *J Consult Clin Psychol*, 1998; 66:856–861.

67. El-Bassel N, Schilling RF. 15-month follow-up of women methadone patients taught skills to reduce heterosexual HIV transmission. *Public Health Rep* 1992; 107:500–504.

68. Schilling RF, El-Bassel N, Schinke SP, et al. Building skills of recovering women drug users to reduce heterosexual AIDS transmission. *Public Health Rep* 1991; 106:297–304.

69. El-Bassel N, Ivanoff A, Schilling RF, et al. Preventing AIDS in drug-abusing incarcerated women through skills building and social support: Preliminary outcomes. *Soc Work Res* 1995; 19:131–141.

70. Kelly JA, Murphy DA, Washington CD, et al. The effects of HIV/AIDS intervention groups for high-risk women in urban clinics. *Am J Public Health* 1994; 84:1918–1922.

71. Hobfoll SE, Jackson AP, Lavin J, et al. Reducing inner-city women's AIDS risk activities: A study of single, pregnant women. *Health Psychol* 1994; 13:397–403.

72. DiClemente RJ, Wingood GM. A randomized controlled trial of a community-based HIV sexual risk reduction intervention for young adult African-American females. *JAMA* 1995; 274:1271–1276.

73. Carey MP, Maisto SA, Kalichman SC, et al. Enhancing motivation to reduce the risk of HIV infection for economically disadvantaged urban women. *J Consult Clin Psychol* 1997; 65:531–541.

74. Weinhardt LS, Carey MP, Carey KB, Verdecias N. Increasing assertiveness skills to reduce HIV risk among women living with a severe and persistent mental illness. *J Consult Clin Psychol* 1999; 66:680–684.

75. O'Leary A., Ambrose T, Raffaelli M, et al. Effects of an AIDS risk reduction program on sexual risk behavior of low-income STD patients. *AIDS Educ Prev* 1998; 10:483–492.

76. Sikkema KJ, Kelly JS, Winnett RA, et al. Outcomes of a randomized community-level HIV prevention intervention for women living in 18 low-income housing developments. *Am J Public Health*, in press.

77. Kalichman SC, Rompa D, Coley B. Experimental component analysis of a behavioral HIV-AIDS prevention intervention in inner-city women. *J Consult Clin Psychol* 1996; 64:687–693.

78. St. Lawrence JS, Wilson TE, Eldridge GD, et al. Evaluation of community-based interventions to reduce low income, African American women's risk of sexually-transmitted diseases: A randomized controlled trial of three theoretical models. Unpublished manuscript. Jackson, MS: Jackson State University; 1998.

79. Smith LB, Adler N, Tschann JM. Underreporting sensitive behaviors: The case of young women's willingness to report abortion. *Health Psychol* 1998; 18:37–43.

80. O'Leary A, DiClemente RJ, Aral SO. Reflections on the design and reporting of STD/HIV behavioral intervention research. *AIDS Educ Prev* 1997; 9(A):1–14.

81. Bhave G, Lindan CP, Hudes ES, et al. Impact of an intervention on HIV, sexually transmitted diseases, and condom use among sex workers in Bombay, India. *AIDS* 1995; 9(suppl):S21–S30.

82. Cohen DA, Dent C, MacKinnon D, Hahn G. Condoms for men, not women: Results of brief promotion programs. *Sex Transm Dis* 1992, 19:245–251.

83. Boyer CB, Barrett DC, Peterman TA, Bolan G. STD and HIV risk in heterosexual adults attending a public STD

clinic: Evaluation of a randomized controlled behavioral risk-reduction intervention trial. *AIDS* 1997; 11: 359–367.

84. Kamb ML, Fishbein M, Douglas JM, et al. Efficacy of risk-reduction counseling to prevent human immunodeficiency virus and sexually transmitted diseases: A randomized controlled trial. *JAMA* 1998; 280:1161–1167.

85. The NIMH Multisite HIV Prevention Trial. The NIMH Multisite HIV Prevention Trial: Reducing sexual HIV risk behavior. *Science* 1998; 280:1889–1894.

86. The NIMH Multisite HIV Prevention Trial. Social Cognitive Theory Mediators of Behavior Change in the NIMH HIV Prevention Trial, under review.

87. Shain RN, Piper JM, Newton ER, et al. A randomized, controlled trial of a behavioral intervention to prevent sexually transmitted disease among minority women. *N Engl J Med* 1998; 340:93–100.

88. O'Leary A, Jemmott LS, Goodhart F, Gebelt J. Effects of an institutional AIDS prevention intervention: Moderation by gender. *AIDS Educ Prev* 1996; 8:49–61.

89. Neighbors CJ, O'Leary A, Labouvie E. Responses of male inmates to primary partner requests for condom use: Effects of attributions, message content, and domestic violence history. Under review.

90. O'Leary A. Preventing HIV infection in heterosexual women: What do we know? What do we need to learn? *Appl Prevent Psychol* 1999; 8:257–263.

10

Interventions to Reduce HIV Transmission in Homosexual Men

MICHAEL W. ROSS and JEFFREY A. KELLY

An understanding of any intervention to reduce the impact of an infectious disease always rests on three domains: an understanding of the biology of the infectious agent, an understanding of the epidemiology of the disease, and an understanding of the behavioral contribution to infection or disease progression. In the case of human immunodeficiency virus (HIV), the lack of a cure or vaccine at present means that in terms of biology there is little option to intervene except to reduce HIV disease progression. In the case of epidemiology, the misuse of the term "risk group" damaged early prevention efforts by focusing on identity rather than behavior. Nevertheless, epidemiology still makes a significant contribution to HIV prevention by highlighting the geographic and behavioral areas to target. However, it is the behavioral and contextual factors in all groups that best define the most appropriate areas for targeting preventive efforts and addressing interventions. There is an extensive literature on the behavioral and social factors associated with HIV transmission risk and we have chosen only a few of these to illustrate each domain of potential intervention.

In the beginning of the HIV epidemic, the term "homosexual" was used to define risk, ignoring the fact that being homosexual (the identity) was not a risk factor in itself, but that particular sexual *behaviors* that were part of homosexual (and heterosexual) sex were. More recently, the term "men who have sex with men" further emphasizes that it is the behavior, rather than the self-identification as homosexual, that may confer the risk. Now, we recognize that not all sexual behaviors that occur between men can transmit HIV, and that for some, such as unprotected oral sex, the risk is generally lower than for unprotected anal intercourse. In this chapter, we will review the literature which describes the attitudes, beliefs, behaviors and situations which lead to risk in men who have sex with men, and describe the interventions which are effective in reducing those risks.

RISKS AMENABLE TO INTERVENTION IN GAY AND BISEXUAL MEN

Behavior Change

Behavior that puts homosexual men at risk includes unprotected anal intercourse and to a lesser extent unprotected oral intercourse and brachioproctic sex ("fist fornication"). Mutual

MICHAEL W. ROSS • WHO Center for Health Promotion Research and Development, School of Public Health, University of Texas, Houston, Texas 77225. *JEFFREY A. KELLY* • Center for AIDS Intervention Research, Medical College of Wisconsin, Milwaukee, Wisconsin 53202.

Handbook of HIV Prevention, edited by Peterson and DiClemente.
Kluwer Academic / Plenum Publishers, New York, 2000.

masturbation and frottage (rubbing bodies together) convey minimal if any risk, and thus a major series of interventions focus on either protecting risky acts through consistent condom use or changing to acts of no risk. However, there are also cultural (and thus also ethnic) differences in preferred acts. In a pre-acquired immunodeficiency syndrome (AIDS) study of gay men in Australia, Sweden, Finland, and Ireland, Ross[1] found that the more well-developed the gay subculture, the more complex the homosexual activity and the greater the amount of anal intercourse. Studying gay and bisexual behavior in over 12,000 men in eight European countries, Bochow et al.[2] noted major similarities in risk behaviors but also striking differences in strategies of risk management. They reported that, as Ross[1] had previously found, mutual masturbation followed by fellatio were the most common activities, with less than 40% engaging "always" or "often" in anal intercourse with steady partners (and less than 20% with casual partners). Unprotected anal intercourse with a partner of different or unknown HIV serostatus in the past year ranged from a low of 16% in Denmark and the United Kingdom to a high of 35% in East Germany (25% in West Germany). About half of these risky acts were with a stable partner. Bochow et al.[2] also report that the proportion of men who use ineffective risk reduction strategies such as "selective" strategies (avoiding particular places such as bathhouses, or persons such as those frequenting the gay subculture) is low (2–9%). "Protective" strategies are effective in protecting against HIV transmission, such as condom use or avoidance of anal intercourse, and ranged from over 80% who reported condom use with casual partners in anal intercourse in Switzerland to less than 60% in East Germany.

In addition to cultural differences, there also are differences in risk behavior between exclusively homosexual and bisexual men. Heckman et al.[3] studied over 1300 men in gay bars in the United States and found that bisexual men had lower intentions to use condoms in their next anal intercourse and had more oral sex occasions and partners than exclusively gay men. One third of bisexual men reported unprotected anal intercourse, and 17% had multiple unprotected anal sex partners in the past 2 months; higher figures than exclusively gay men. These data suggest that strategies to reduce risk may involve either a move to low-risk activities or to protection of higher-risk activities, depending on the cultural values associated with such changes. Interventions that do not take into account geographic and cultural differences in homosexual behaviors are unlikely to be as effective as tailored programs.

Risk Situations

In determining possible points of intervention, one of the areas that may be amenable to modification is the situation or context of risk. Risk situations may include bathhouses, bars, dance parties, and bedrooms. Situation is important in that affects, attitudes, beliefs, and behaviors may be context specific, as may substance use. Further, the context itself may contribute to risk: availability of condoms, darkness, time constraints, risk of police detection or other danger. Coxon[4] calls a subset of these the "3D theory": "It was dark, I was drunk, and I didn't have a condom" (p. 172). The issue of state- and context-dependent learning may also be a contributor: skills and knowledge learned in one context may not be recalled in another, since the situation may act as a learning cue.[5] Indeed, the situation may interact with cognitions, affects, and partners to account for a substantial proportion of the variance of risk. Kelaher et al.[6] used situational vignettes, the seven variables of which were randomly presented on a laptop computer to gay men in bars and bathhouses. They found that they could explain over one third of the variance of unprotected anal intercourse using the variables of attraction to partner, condom availability, and perceptions of attractiveness to partner.

Supporting the importance of situation, Sacco and Rickman[7] studied 267 gay and bisexual men in the United States. They found that variation in condom use for anal sex could be substantially accounted for in the preference of the partner for condom use. The receptive partner's preference influenced condom use decisions to a greater extent than that of the insertive partner, and the HIV serostatus of the respondent and partner interacted in that those with discordant serostatus used condoms the most, those with concordant serostatus the least. These data confirm that the interpersonal situation plays an important role in sexual risk. Interventions that target the physical situation and the interpersonal situation (particularly communication-enhancing strategies in the latter case) may be effective in reducing HIV transmission.

Risk Cognitions

Similar interpersonal data on risk in serodiscordant couples are reported by Remien et al.[8] In a qualitative study of 15 Latino and non-Latino male couples in the United States, they found that the major barriers to safe sex included lack of perception of risk from oral sex, with repeated previous seronegative tests being considered a justification for not using condoms and an indication that previous activities are not risky. This is a fallacious rationalization that is often equated with the simplistic view that HIV is invariably transmitted in unsafe activity, rather than it being a "lottery." Repeated unsafe episodes followed by negative tests only serve to reinforce this fallacy. Remien et al.[8] also reported avoidance of the topic of safer sex, length of the relationship (familiarity and length of time in the relationship leading to a sense of protection) as leading to unsafe behavior, along with cultural beliefs (the Latinos tending to see anal penetration as being a basic, indispensable component of male sexual behavior).

Lowy and Ross[9] looked at the "folk construction" of sexual risk in gay men and found that epidemiological constructs were transformed into personal risk concepts. Men used several categories of signifiers of risk: age, appearance, diction, and HIV knowledge, along with epidemiological factors. This epidemiological fallacy takes variables that in a large population may be associated with lower risk of HIV infection, such as few partners, being the insertive partner in anal intercourse, being in a stable relationship, and past history of infrequent anal intercourse, and translates them into individual risk data. Along with emotional needs and sexual arousal, these are transformed into pseudo-epidemiological models of risk to determine the actual risk of each potential partner. Lowy and Ross[9] found that rather than the absolutes of "safe," "safer," and "unsafe" sex, men created their own cognitive schema of safety gradients by extrapolating epidemiological data and principles and applying them to individual cases.

Cognitions that are associated with risk behavior are thus central to understanding the continued transmission of HIV. Gold and colleagues[10–12] looked at the rationalizations and thought processes associated with unprotected anal intercourse in Australian gay men. Respondents were asked to recall a sexual encounter in which they had engaged in this risk behavior and a safe encounter. Of the sample of 250, 30% had known that they were HIV-infected. Over 90% of the sample reported at least one of these groups of self-justifications: reactions to being in a negative mood state; being already infected and having nothing to lose; getting "what you can while you can"; dislike of condoms; the resolution to withdraw before ejaculation, used with a partner whom the respondent did not know well; and confidence in oneself and a desire to demonstrate confidence in the partner. The mood state variables showed that in the unsafe encounter, the older respondents had been in a better mood at the start of the evening in the unsafe encounter and the younger respondents in a more negative mood, emphasizing the importance of risk affects. For the uninfected men, the major self-justification involved inferring from perceptible characteristics (healthy looking) that the partner was uninfected, or because he was not using a condom, he must be uninfected. Unfortunately, this same act was used by those already infected to infer that the partner was also infected.

Attitudes and beliefs associated with risk and safety have been the focus of extensive research in gay and bisexual men. In a test of the theory of reasoned action, Fishbein et al.[13] found that attitude was the best variable explaining intention to adopt 15 sexual practices, whereas Ross and McLaws[14] found that subjective norms were the significant factor explaining intention to use condoms. Cochran et al.[15] found both attitudes and subjective norms significantly explained intention to adopt safe sex recommendations. Ross and McLaws[14] suggested that the stage of development of the epidemic may influence whether norms or attitudes played the more dominant role in intention to engage in safe behavior. However, Godin et al.[16] in a Canadian study found that perceived behavioral control, as hypothesized in the theory of planned behavior, along with personal normative belief and perceived subjective norm, was the best predictor of intention to use condoms. Further, perceived behavioral control was the best predictor of having sex without anal intercourse. Godin et al.[16] concluded that interventions in gay and bisexual men should attempt to increase perception of behavioral control. Cognitive change interventions have been the most common, largely because of the measurability and modifiability of attitudes and beliefs.

Attitudes toward Condom Use

Attitudes toward condoms and condom use have been reviewed by Ross,[17,18] who found that the major dimensions of attitudes toward condoms in this population were seeing condoms as unerotic and unreliable; level of protection from infection; availability; interruption of sex; and having a responsibility to use and comfort in using condoms. In a longitudinal study of factors that predicted condom use in gay men, Ross[19] found that a more assertive and forceful personality style was associated with increased condom use, probably through making raising condom use with sexual partners easier. Further, he found that beliefs in the ability of condoms to protect from infection and greater availability were also associated with increases in use over 6 months. Variables associated with lack of change to safer sex included dysphoric mood state and level of psychological distress. In a Canadian study, Godin et al.[16] also found that in men with HIV disease, the best predictor of safe sex practices was degree of perceived behavioral control over condom use, along with a perceived responsibility to use condoms. The importance of attitudes toward changes in sexual practices (including condom use) was further confirmed by Fishbein et al.,[13] who found in a multisite study in the United States that attitude was the best factor explaining intention to adopt these behaviors.

In a criticism of both the "relapse" and "negotiated safety" accounts of unsafe sex, Coxon[4] reports on sexual diary studies of homosexual men in the United Kingdom. He argues that the role of cognitive processes, decision, negotiation, consideration, and reasoning is overstressed and that the avoidance of condoms is often as much a matter of waiting for the partner to object as it is a prenegotiated condition. He suggests that those who come closest to the ideal of choice, responsibility, and negotiation are those already HIV-seropositive. Cognitions and rational calculus, then, should not be the only target of interventions. Offir et al.[20] looked at inconsistent HIV prevention among gay men and found that participants engaged in a process of cognitive distortion to maintain consistency between perceptions of their inconsistent preventive behavior and themselves as low-risk individuals. In such cases, they suggest, strategies to make individuals aware of their cognitive dissonance and rationalizations may be the most effective form of intervention.

Social Context

In considering characteristics of gay and bisexual men that are amenable to modification to reduce HIV risks, the influence of the social and societal context must also be considered. Ross[21] has summarized the macrocontextual influences on behavior and notes that in health care and health behaviors the most disadvantaged individuals are those most likely to have the fewest treatment options and the worst access to care. Where homosexual behavior is stigmatized or criminalized, this will impact care seeking, the level of admitting to the source of the infection, and the level of anonymity of contacts. For example, Sinclair and Ross[22] noted lower levels of sexually transmitted diseases (STDs) in homosexual men in states that had decriminalized homosexuality compared with those that had not. More recently, Ross and Rosser[23] developed a measure of internalized homophobia and found that length of longest relationship, disclosure of sexual orientation, proportion of time spent with gay people, and HIV serostatus were all significantly associated with level of internalized homophobia. There are clear links between discrimination, prejudice, HIV risk behaviors, and HIV infection, and interventions to reduce risk must target, through legal and policy modifications and community interventions, the societal contexts that lead to internalized homophobia and to risks associated with lack of contact with subcultures that promote safety.

Norms

Norms associated with changing behavior to safer sex may be related to perceptions of normative behavior or to actual contact with subcultures that encourage safer sex. Thus, social supports and contacts with gay subcultures or satellite cultures are central. Reviewing the concept of the "gay subculture," Ross et al.[24] suggested that this can be traced through a series of informal and formal stages from smaller rural areas at one extreme to the internationally known gay "ghettos" at the other. The development of a gay community and family of choice (as compared with a "family of origin"[25]) provides structures for the development and reinforcement of norms supportive of safer sex. Turner et al.[26] suggest that integration into gay communities may be a critical variable in safer sexual behaviors. Joseph et al.[27] found in a longitudinal study that time socializing with other gay men, degree to which respondents were "out," social participation with other gay men, and a positive attitude toward one's sexual identity predicted lower sexual risk over the short term (6 months), although it had no apparent impact over 1½ years; Adib et al.[28] also found that absence of peer support led to relapse to unsafe sex. Also in the United States, Seibt et al.[29] found that an acculturation measure of membership of gay organizations and level of gay community reading material were significantly associated with higher levels of anal condom use.

Acculturation to the gay subculture, social support, and subjective norms emphasizing safer sex all appear to have an association with safer sexual behavior, although the mechanisms are unclear. Folkman et al.,[30] however, reported that subjects in their study in San Francisco who used sex to cope with stressful situations reported unprotected anal intercourse more often than those who sought social support and who engaged in spiritual activities. They suggested that social aspects of coping, which would require the availability of social supports and interaction with such supports rather than a coping style that involved keeping things to oneself, are important in promoting and maintaining safer sex. Interventions that increase or promote social supports and emphasize safer sex norms, combined with other interventions, are thus likely to decrease risk.

Relapse to Unsafe Sex

Failure to maintain safe sex (referred to here as "relapse") unfortunately occurs, although frequently it is episodic rather than consistent. Adib et al.,[28] in a 2-year follow up in a Chicago cohort, found that 45% of their sample maintained safe practices and 47% relapsed (reported unprotected receptive anal intercourse) at least once. This pattern was repeated for unprotected insertive anal intercourse. There were no significant differences between men in monogamous and nonmonogamous relationships. Relapse in the context of partners of concordant serostatus and in mutually monogamous relationships has very different implications for HIV transmission compared with casual and serodiscordant (or seroincognizant) relationships. Data on casual relationships suggest that there are consistent factors associated with unsafe sex. Van de Ven et al.[31] found that those who had had less contact with the HIV epidemic were engaged in a more extensive range of anal practices, a belief that withdrawal was safe, and less favorable attitudes toward condoms. Less favorable attitudes toward condoms have been found in previous studies; de Wit et al.[32] in the Netherlands also noted negative attitudes toward condoms and lower self-efficacy as being associated with lower condom use.

In a qualitative study of gay men's accounts of unsafe sex in the United Kingdom, Boulton et al.[33] found four distinct categories of motives. One of the most common was expressed in the language of emotional needs and drives: Boulton et al. note that experiences such as love, pleasure, and erotic sensations have yet to find a proper place in our explanatory frameworks. Second, accounts of the "calculus of risk" suggested that participants considered a variety of factors such as previous seronegative tests, sexual histories as reported by the partner, situation of partner, and sexual activities and decided that there was virtually no risk of HIV transmission in the encounter. Third, the social meanings attached to condom use were barriers: Particularly in regular relationships, condom use implied lack of trust. Finally, lapses in control were a feature of accounts: These tended to emphasize mitigating circumstances like being carried away in the heat of the moment, sex while emotionally distressed, the influence of alcohol and drugs, and blaming the partner. These accounts emphasize the potential fragility of perceived control over behavior and the ease with which cognitions can be overridden by affects.

HIV Transmission within Couples

As already noted, different levels of analysis may apply to regular and casual partners and their risk behaviors. In Remien and co-workers'[8] study of serodiscordant couples, accidents of passion occurred in much the same way as in casual relationships, although risk perceptions may be the most significant variable acting in regular relationships. Bosga et al.[34] studied differences between gay men who practiced unprotected anal intercourse in the Netherlands and found that the majority of men who engaged in risky behaviors within a primary relationship did not subjectively appraise those behaviors as risky. Even when some of these men did not know their partner's HIV serostatus, they did not consider the behavior to be risky because they were optimistic and believed that others were at greater risk than themselves. This optimistic bias appears to be a significant factor in risk behavior,[35] and *risk perceptions* should be a major focus of interventions to reduce risk. They also found that those with fewer friends who had HIV/AIDS and those who had never knowingly had an HIV-seropositive partner underestimated risk, suggesting that past confrontation with AIDS in close friends was a trigger to more accurate risk perception. In contrast, those who had had unprotected anal intercourse with casual partners were more aware of the risks and had more accurate risk perception.

Alcohol and Drugs

There has been a great deal of speculation about the role of alcohol and drugs in unsafe behavior. Paul et al.[36] reported a 32% increase in frequency of unprotected anal intercourse in their San Francisco sample of gay and bisexual substance abusers and that two thirds of their sample were "always" intoxicated during unprotected anal intercourse. Stall et al.[37] found that men who used three or more drugs during sexual activity were more than four times more likely to engage in risky sexual behavior in a bathhouse or bar setting than those who did not combine drugs. However, Weatherburn et al.,[38] in a sexual diary study in the United Kingdom, found that while 30% of their sample used alcohol in sexual encounters, there was no statistically significant difference between alcohol users and nonusers in the prevalence of risky sex. Supporting this, in those who used alcohol, there was no dose–response effect with quantity of alcohol and sexual safety. Thus, while multiple substance users may be at higher risk than nonusers, other factors may account for or interact with substance use. Lewis and Ross,[39] in a major qualitative study of gay circuit (dance) parties in Australia, found that substance use and unsafe sex were often associated with a desire to escape from a stigmatized everyday reality that included homonegative environments, fear of HIV/AIDS and the pervasiveness of HIV infection and risk in their subculture, and a desire to celebrate their sexuality in a "safe" context. Paradoxically, this safe context also could provide a context in which unsafe behavior could occur, often aided by cognition and affect-altering substances and "magical" thinking. However, when one looks at samples of injecting drug users and within them compares gay, bisexual, and heterosexual men, the homosexual men exhibit the safest sexual behaviors, followed by bisexual men, with heterosexual men being the least safe. There was little overlap between safety in sexual behavior and safety in drug-using behavior, suggesting the importance of considering other risks besides the sexual for HIV transmission in gay men.[40] While the data on alcohol and drug use as risk factors for unsafe sex suggest that they may function as contextual markers rather than risks as such, drugs as disinhibitors may be a useful focus of interventions. However, both drugs and unsafe sex are more likely behaviors resulting from an underlying trait: sensation seeking. Kalichman et al.[41] found it predicted HIV risk behavior in homosexual men, and even with substance use controlled for, sexual adventurism and sensation seeking were major predictors of unsafe sexual behavior.

The research on factors that are associated with unsafe sexual behavior in men who have sex with men identifies a number of variables that are susceptible to intervention. Probably the most effective interventions are those that target multiple domains—at levels of legal and policy issues, community interventions, and of the individual—and in the domains of risk cognitions, risk situations, risk behaviors, social support and norm development, substance use, and interpersonal interactions and communication skills.

RISK REDUCTION INTERVENTIONS FOR GAY AND BISEXUAL MEN

The gay community was first affected by the HIV epidemic and, in many Western and developed countries, remains the population most harshly affected by AIDS. There is a long history of HIV prevention activities focused toward gay and bisexual men. Many innovative, grassroots HIV prevention programs originated in the gay communities of urban AIDS epicenters and continue to be undertaken as service programs designed to meet local needs. Increasingly and as a result of the AIDS Community Planning Process initiated by the Centers for Disease Control and Prevention (CDC),[42] states, jurisdictions, and organizations that receive CDC funds also have been encouraged to develop programs informed by findings of HIV behavioral research and to carry out prevention approaches for which there is a scientific basis of support. In the remainder of this chapter, we will review and summarize results of research trials of HIV prevention interventions with gay and bisexual men, including both face-to-face interventions and community-level intervention approaches. We then will discuss some new and emerging issues in HIV prevention efforts that will require attention in the next generation of HIV prevention interventions for men who have sex with men (MSM).

Face-to-Face and Individual-Focused HIV Prevention Interventions for Gay and Bisexual Men

Face-to-face interventions are undertaken with persons in the context of individual counseling, groups, or workshop programs. The intent of these approaches is to assist individuals in making and maintaining reductions in the risk level of their sexual behavioral practices. A variety of theoretical perspectives have been used to conceptualize HIV risk reduction interventions, including social–cognitive theory,[43] the theory of reasoned action,[44] and AIDS-specific behavioral change theories.[45,46] Regardless of differences in their theoretical underpinnings, face-to-face interventions studied in research trials with gay men share a number of common characteristics. Most combine risk education with exercises to promote positive attitudes toward safer sex, encourage persons to understand and problem solve ways to change their current patterns of high-risk behavior, teach risk reduction behavioral skills such as condom use and safer sex negotiation, and provide reinforcement and support for behavior change efforts.

The earliest controlled trials evaluating face-to-face risk reduction interventions for gay and bisexual men were reported in studies published by Valdiserri et al.[47] and Kelly et al.[48] In the Valdiserri et al.[47] study, 450 men were recruited and followed after being randomly assigned to attend one of two HIV risk reduction workshop programs. One was a safer sex education program that conveyed information about AIDS, provided instruction about risk behavior and safer sex practices, and corrected misconceptions about AIDS. The second program provided the same information but added role-play, psychodrama, and group activities intended to help participants practice safer sex negotiation skills, to induce norms to "legitimize" safe sex, and to encourage personal problem solving to adopt safer sex practices. Risk behavior interviews were conducted with all participants at baseline and at 6- and 12-month points following program participation. Men who had attended the skills building workshops increased their condom use by 44%, relative to only a 11% change for men who had attended the educational program alone.

The Kelly et al.[48] project examined the effects of a longer and more intensive intervention consisting of 12 75-minute small-group sessions. A sample of 104 men were recruited from a variety of gay community venues and, following a baseline risk assessment, were randomly assigned to the intervention or to a delayed-intervention comparison group. Intervention sessions, which included 8 to 15 participants and were led by two group facilitators, addressed risk education; skills training and practice exercises in areas such as sexual negotiation, assertiveness, and condom use; risk reduction self-management and problem-solving skills training focused on identifying and changing the manner in which current "triggers" to high-risk behavior are handled; and group discussion concerning pride, self-esteem, relationship development, and responsibilities to protect oneself and others from HIV.

At an 8-month follow-up point, all participants were readministered risk assessment measures. Participants who received the group intervention, relative to control group members, increased their levels of condom use (from an average of 23% of anal intercourse occasions in the past 4 months at baseline to 77% of intercourse occasions at follow-up) and decreased in their mean frequency of unprotected anal intercourse occasions (from 7.8 occurrences in the past 4 months at baseline to 0.7 occurrences at follow-up). In a later 16-month follow-up of individuals who completed the intervention, 60% had maintained their avoidance of high-risk sexual practices.[49] Those who resumed engaging in unprotected anal intercourse were younger, had more extensive high-risk behavior histories prior to program participation, and were more likely to believe that risk for HIV infection is due to chance or luck. Finally, the same intervention, but in a more abbreviated seven-session format, was offered to men who had formerly been in the original study's comparison group. Behavior change effects comparable in magnitude were found following participation in this briefer program.[50]

The interventions just described enrolled samples that were composed of predominantly white men. Several more recent investigations have examined the impact of similar group or workshop programs for ethnic minority MSM. Peterson and colleagues[51] enrolled a sample of 318 African-American MSM recruited from community venues in San Francisco and, following baseline risk behavior assessment, randomly assigned the men to a single 3-hour risk reduction workshop, a triple program of these 3-hour workshops, or a waiting-list control group. The workshops included risk education, sexual assertiveness and negotiation skill training exercises, activities to strengthen behavior change commitment, and discussion intended to foster positive self-identity and support as an African-American MSM. Follow-up risk behavior assessments were undertaken 12 and 18 months following program participation. Control group members showed little change in the riskiness of their sexual behavior practices, and participants in the single workshop showed evidence of only modest change. In contrast, men who had attended the three-workshop program exhibited considerable risk behavior change, including reductions in the percentage of men reporting any unprotected anal intercourse in the past 6 months (from 45% at baseline to 20% at 18-months follow-up).

Choi and colleagues[52] evaluated the impact of a single 3-hour risk reduction workshop program for Asian and Pacific Islander gay or bisexual men. The workshop included components similar to those of the other programs discussed earlier, including safer sex education, sexual negotiation skills training, exercises to eroticize safer sex, and activities intended to promote positive identity as an Asian and Pacific Islander MSM. The effectiveness of the program was evaluated by comparing 152 men randomly selected to receive the intervention with 106 waiting-list control group members at baseline and at a 3-month follow-up point. Relative to controls, men in the intervention condition reported having fewer male sexual partners in the past 3 months at follow-up (mean = 3.9) than at baseline (mean = 6.4), but did not change significantly in their rates of unprotected anal intercourse. However, post hoc analysis broken down by Asian and Pacific Islander ethnic subgroups revealed that Chinese and Filipino participants only reduced their frequency of high-risk sexual acts at follow-up.

Conclusions Regarding the Effectiveness of Face-to-Face Research-Based HIV Prevention Interventions for Gay Men

The studies just reviewed all employed randomized outcome designs, the most rigorous experimental methodology for determining the effects of an intervention. Although tailored in many cases to meet the risk, cultural, and ethnic identity issues of different subgroups of gay or bisexual men, all the interventions evaluated in these studies have much in common with one another including a focus that moves beyond risk education and promotes the development of positive attitudes and intentions toward safer sex; behavioral skills needed to enact risk reduction behavior changes; risk reduction problem-solving and self-management skills; and positive appraisals of self-identify, self-esteem, and relationship goals. Relative to study participants who did not immediately receive intervention or who attended AIDS education sessions alone, men who received small-group or workshop interventions showed reductions in sexual risk behavior at follow-up across the different projects. In some studies, the magnitude of behavior change found at follow-up was related to duration and intensity of intervention,[51] and more intensive interventions often produced greater levels of behavior change. Clearly, this body of research has established the positive impact for gay men of culturally tailored sexual risk reduction interventions based on social–cognitive principles.

At the same time, all these studies relied on samples of participants who were willing to attend risk reduction programs of considerable intensity. Since all the studies recruited volunteers from the community, one does not know what proportion of MSM will not volunteer to attend programs of these kinds, nor whether the samples in these studies constitute groups representative of the MSM community or instead are persons highly motivated and "ready" for change. Most of the research summarized here was conducted during the period from the mid-1980s to the early 1990s. It may be the case that gay men were less knowledgeable about AIDS and more eager to learn how to reduce risk for contracting HIV. Interest in attending workshop and small-group programs may now be lower, at least among some persons. If true, this would argue against "freestanding" intensive HIV workshop programs for gay men but for the integration of these approaches in service programs for at-risk MSM. Examples of these programs include "coming out" programs, mental health and substance use treatment programs for MSM, service programs for street youth, and HIV workshops conducted in outreach fashion within social venues that serve MSM.

Finally, although intensive in nature, face-to-face interventions can be cost-effective when offered to men at high risk for contracting HIV, in part because of the considerable magnitude of risk behavior change produced by the interventions. Two of the interventions, those by Valdiserri et al.[47] and Kelly et al.,[48] have been subjected to formal cost-effectiveness analyses.[53,54] In both cases, the interventions were estimated to avert HIV infections at a cost well within the standards considered not only cost-effective but actually cost-saving to society.

Community-Level HIV Prevention Interventions for Gay and Bisexual Men

In contrast to face-to-face programs that involve work with individuals, community-level HIV approaches attempt to bring about reductions in the level of risk behavior within entire populations or particular population subsets. To achieve their objective of promoting population-level risk behavior reduction, community interventions frequently attempt to bring about changes in safer sex knowledge, attitudes, intentions, and peer norms among members of the entire target population.

The earliest published examples of controlled community-level HIV prevention research interventions directed toward gay and bisexual men were reported by Kelly and colleagues[55,56] and involved interventions undertaken with men patronizing gay bars in three small cities in the southern United States. In this research, men entering bars were surveyed concerning their sexual practices in the past 2 months to establish baseline levels of risk in each city. Following baseline data collection on population risk characteristics, an intervention was initiated in one of the three cities, with the other two cities serving as controls. The intervention, based on Rogers' diffusion of innovation theory,[57] relied on bartenders and other key informants to observe and identify persons who appeared to be opinion leaders within their social network in the bars. Diffusion of innovation theory postulates that opinion leaders exist in all community populations, and because they are popular and well-liked these opinion leaders can model and endorse behavior standards that diffuse throughout the population and create new peer norms. Opinion leaders were defined as persons who were popular, well-liked, and frequently interacted with MSM in the bars. Persons nominated by bartenders and others as key opinion leaders were then contacted; told that, because of their popularity, they could help others make behavior changes to reduce the threat of AIDS in their community; and invited to attend a series of four group meetings to learn how to communicate effective HIV prevention conversational messages to others with whom they interacted. Between 8 and 15% of the persons present in a bar on a "typical" weekend were opinion leaders recruited for the training.

In the four-session program, key opinion leaders were taught characteristics of effective health communication messages and how to have conversations in which they recommended and personally endorsed the desirability of making specific behavior changes to reduce HIV risk and were asked to practice role-plays of conversations they could have with friends or acquaintances. Following each weekly training session, each opinion leader agreed to have conversations with between four and ten men, and outcomes of the conversations were always reviewed in the next week's group session. In effect, the intervention recruited and engaged persons already popular in their social networks to become active and visible risk reduction behavior change advocates to their own friends and acquaintances.

An initial study examined the impact of the intervention by repeating risk behavior surveys of all men entering the intervention city's bars 3 and 6 months following the intervention and compared population behavior changes with the behavior found among men in the two control cities surveyed at the same points.[55] This initial study revealed that the percentage of intervention city male bar patrons who reported engaging in any unprotected anal intercourse in the past 2 months declined from 37 to 28%, a reduction of 25% from baseline levels. There was a 30% decrease in the percentage of men reporting any unprotected receptive anal intercourse. No change was found over time in the risk behavior patterns of men in control city bars. In a follow-up study, the intervention was then extended to each of the two former control cities.[56] Following the points when the intervention was implemented in each of these cities, risk behavior surveys were repeated, with results that replicated the population risk behavior shifts found in the original intervention city.

More recently, a larger-scale trial of the same intervention was completed in eight small US cities, four of which received the intervention and four of which were control cities.[58] This study extended the earlier research because it included more cities in different regions of the country, determined population risk behavior levels 1 year following intervention, compared the effects of the popular opinion leader intervention against a traditional AIDS education campaign undertaken in the control cities, and obtained data on condom-taking patterns in study city bars to corroborate population members' risk behavior change self-reports. Between baseline and 1-year follow-up, significant reductions were found in mean frequency of unprotected anal intercourse episodes reported by men in the intervention cities (from 1.7 occurrences in the past two months at baseline to 0.6 occurrences at follow-up), and the percentage of population members anal intercourse occasions protected by condoms increased from 45 to 67%. Rates of condom taking from free dispensers in intervention city bars increased by 65%. No significant changes occurred in the study's four control cities over the same period of time.[58]

Kegeles and colleagues[59] also have examined the impact of a community-level risk reduction intervention focused on young gay men. Two small cities were studied in this trial, one of which received an intervention and one of which served as a control. In the intervention city, a core group of about 15 men were recruited to provide leadership to a program that entailed three components: (1) peer outreach in which safer sex messages were diffused to others in a manner similar to that used in the Kelly et al.[55,56,58] projects just described; (2) small-group, 3-hour risk reduction workshops similar to workshop programs described earlier in this chapter; and (3) a safer sex educational material distribution focused in venues that served young gay men in the community. The entire program lasted for 8 months.

The Kegeles et al.[59] study was evaluated by examining changes in risk behavior of cohorts of men longitudinally followed from baseline to a 1-year postintervention. Reductions were found in the proportion of intervention city cohort members who reported any unprotected anal intercourse in the past 2 months, from 41% at baseline to 30% at the follow-up point. Changes in behavior were found for men who had sex in both primary and nonprimary relationships, although rates of unprotected anal intercourse declined more among men with casual partners than among men who had steady boyfriends.

Conclusions Regarding the Effectiveness of Research-Based Community HIV Prevention Interventions for Gay and Bisexual Men

In contrast to intensive interventions that encourage risk reduction behavior change with individual men being counseled face-to-face, community-level programs have shown success in promoting norm and risk behavior changes within larger gay community populations. Although the magnitude of risk reduction produced by community-level interventions is often somewhat smaller than that produced by the very intensive face-to-face programs described earlier, community-level approaches can reach a much greater number of persons. By creating peer norms and supports favoring safer sex, community interventions may be able to help persons maintain behavior change better than approaches that work with the individuals in isolation but do not change peer group norms. In population segments where safer sex is not yet an accepted peer norm, community approaches can have considerable potential impact. Further, the interventions reviewed here all engaged members of the target population to deliver intervention activities to their peers. Such approaches are likely to be culturally appropriate in the community and may be more sustainable than HIV preventions carried out by external agents.

At the same time, behavioral research on community-level HIV risk reduction interventions is still in its early stages; there have been only a small number of controlled community-level interventions for gay and bisexual men. All these interventions have examined the risk behavior of individual population members as outcomes. Community-level interventions also imply that community structures, organizations, and capacity should be targeted for change. Examples of desirable "superindividual" outcomes might include an increase in the number, range, and quality of HIV prevention services for MSM offered by existing service organizations; improved health, social, and HIV risk reduction services for persons with HIV infection; and decreases in indicators of homophobia. The extent to which community-level HIV prevention interventions can influence such community capacity and structural characteristics that are also likely to mediate HIV risk has not yet been explored.

Issues That Will Need To Be Addressed in the "Next Generation" of HIV Prevention Interventions for Gay and Bisexual Men

Many gay and bisexual men have made substantial and impressive changes in their sexual practices in response to AIDS. In this context, individuals who remain at risk may have special prevention needs and require "new generation" HIV prevention programs to meet those needs. There are several areas in which more advanced HIV prevention approaches are especially important:

1. *Young MSM, and especially young men of color, continue to contract HIV infection at unacceptable rates.* A number of HIV seroprevalence, seroincidence, and risk behavior studies indicate that young gay men, and particularly young minority men, remain vulnerable to HIV infection.[60–62] Most HIV prevention research studies have enrolled participants and have evaluated the effectiveness of interventions with samples composed of men considerably older than the MSM groups who are now most vulnerable to new infections. To direct efforts to the MSM population segments now at greatest risk, it will be necessary to develop interventions that better address risk issues faced by gay youth and also to issues faced by young MSM of color.

2. *Adherence to safer sex recommendations is much lower in affectionate than casual relationships.* Research undertaken with both gay men and heterosexuals consistently indicates higher rates of condom use in sexual encounters with casual partners than with affectionate partners.[12,63] Further, it appears that a key determinant of condom nonuse in affectionate relationships is less the result of an objective appraisal of few partner risk than it is liking, knowing, and holding affectionate feeling toward the partner or simply having had sex before with that same individual.[64,65] The dynamics of introducing and maintaining safer sex in affectionate relationships may be considerably different than the dynamics of condom use in casual relationships and may require new prevention approaches and messages. Further, although consistent condom use is usually the public health objective of HIV prevention efforts, some MSM who have primary relationships are not willing to use condoms with their primary partners. More research is needed to identify interventions and risk reduction strategies appropriate within affectionate relationships. These may include not only the encouragement of condom use but also mutual HIV serostatus testing, adoption of safer sex with any nonprimary partners, and similar strategies of informed decision making by persons in affectionate relationships.

3. *The association of HIV risk behavior with other coexisting problems such as alcohol use, drug use, and homelessness requires the development of more specialized risk reduction interventions for these groups of MSM.* It has long been known that MSM with heavy alcohol and drug use patterns also are more likely to engage in high-risk sex, even though the reasons for this association are still not fully understood.[66] Similarly, street youth, homeless youth, and other disenfranchised MSM are at particularly high risk.[67] For these groups, HIV prevention approaches tailored to address not only sexual risk behavior but also the contextual problems that surround it, such as problem drinking, other substance use, and unmet social service needs, may be especially important. To date, there have been few reports in the literature of such tailored HIV prevention interventions for MSM.

4. *Risk behavior reduction interventions are needed for HIV-seropositive MSM who continue to engage in unprotected sex.* Most HIV prevention interventions reported to date in the literature appear primarily oriented toward helping HIV-seronegative persons avoid contracting infection. While the same behavior changes made by seropositive persons will result in reduced likelihood of HIV transmission to others, HIV-seropositive MSM who continue to engage in unprotected sexual activities may confront issues that require interventions tailored to their special needs. Research indicates that most persons who learn of their positive HIV serostatus make changes to protect others.[68] However, some HIV-positive MSM report continued high-risk transmission acts.[61,69] These patterns have been related to the presence of coexisting substance use problems, mental health and coping difficulties, poor access to health

and social services, difficulty in disclosing serostatus to others, and other problems.[69] Greater attention is now needed to the development of risk behavior change maintenance interventions for those HIV-seropositive MSM who have had difficulty refraining from unprotected sexual behavior.

SUMMARY

The most effective interventions to reduce risk will be those that are aimed at variables that can be modified and that cover all the possible domains from the macro- to the microsituation. Those that incorporate multiple factors—attitude change, communication skills, modification of norms and social supports, modification of situations and larger policy settings, community involvement and outreach, role modeling, increase in self-efficacy and behavioral control, and limitation of substance use—and that use theories of behavior change with demonstrated efficacy will be the most effective. As Hart[70] has commented, peer education has considerable appeal in terms of its intellectual, financial, and emotional attractiveness; it is not only fashionable, but also supported by evidence. It is clear from the data presented here that interventions can reduce risk behavior significantly and over substantial periods of time. However, effective targeting and tailoring of interventions is necessary to maximize change and the extension of interventions from individual to community level will be needed to bring them to larger population groups.

REFERENCES

1. Ross MW. *Psychovenereology*. New York: Praeger; 1986.
2. Bochow M, Chiarotti F, Davies P, et al. Sexual behaviour of gay and bisexual men in eight European countries. *AIDS Care* 1994; 6:533–549.
3. Heckman TG, Kelly JA, Sikkema KJ, et al. Differences in HIV risk characteristics between bisexual and exclusively gay men. *AIDS Educ Prev* 1995; 7:504–512.
4. Coxon APM. *Between the Sheets: Sexual Diaries and Gay Men's Sex in the Age of AIDS*. London: Cassell; 1996.
5. Jenkins JJ. Remember that old theory of memory? Well, forget it!. *Am Psychol* 1974; 29:785–795.
6. Kelaher MA, Ross MW, Rohrsheim R, et al. Dominant situational determinants of sexual risk behaviour in gay men. *AIDS* 1994; 8:101–105.
7. Sacco WP, Rickman RL. AIDS-relevant condom use by gay and bisexual men:the role of person variables and the interpersonal situation. *AIDS Educ Prev* 1996; 5:430–443.
8. Remien RH, Carballo-Diéguez A, Wagner G. Intimacy and sexual risk behavior in serodiscordant male couples. *AIDS Care* 1995; 7:429–438.
9. Lowy E, Ross MW. "It'll never happen to me": Gay men's beliefs, perceptions and folk constructions of sexual risk. *AIDS Educ Prev* 1994; 6:467–482.
10. Gold RS, Skinner MJ. Situational factors and thought processes associated with unprotected intercourse in young gay men. *AIDS* 1992; 6:1021–1030.
11. Gold RS, Skinner MJ, Grant PJ, Plummer DC. Situational factors and thought processes associated with unprotected intercourse in gay men. *Psychol Health* 1991; 5:259–278.
12. Gold RS, Skinner MJ, Ross MW. Unprotected anal intercourse in HIV-infected and non-HIV-infected gay men. *J Sex Res* 1994; 31:59–77.
13. Fishbein M, Chan DK-S, O'Reilly K, et al. Attitudinal and normative factors as determinants of gay men's intentions to perform AIDS-related sexual behaviors: A multi-site analysis. *J Appl Soc Psychol* 1992; 22:999–1011.
14. Ross MW, McLaws M-L. Subjective norms about condoms are better predictors of use and intention to use than attitudes. *Health Educ Res* 1992; 7:335–339.
15. Cochran SD, Mays VM, Ciarletta J, et al. Efficacy of the theory of reasoned action in predicting AIDS-related risk reduction among gay men. *J Appl Soc Psychol* 1992; 22:1481–1501.

16. Godin G, Savard JM, Kok G, et al. HIV seropositive gay men: Understanding adoption of safe sex practices. *AIDS Educ Prev* 1996; 8:529–545.
17. Ross MW. Attitudes toward condoms and condom use: A review. *Int J STD AIDS* 1992; 3:10–16.
18. Ross MW. Attitudes toward condoms as AIDS prophylaxis in homosexual men: Dimensions and measurement. *Psychol Health* 1988; 2:291–299.
19. Ross MW. Psychological determinants of increased condom use and safer sex in homosexual men: A longitudinal study. *Int J STD AIDS* 1990; 1:98–101.
20. Offir JT, Fisher JD, Williams SS, Fisher WA. Reasons for inconsistent AIDS-preventive behaviors among gay men. *J Sex Res* 1993; 30:62–69.
21. Ross MW. AIDS and the new public health. In: Waddell C, Petersen A, eds. *Just Health*. Melbourne: Churchill Livingstone; 1994:323–335.
22. Sinclair KCP, Ross MW. Consequences of decriminalisation of homosexuality: A study of two Australian states. *J Homosex* 1986; 12:119–127.
23. Ross MW, Rosser BRS. Measurement and correlates of internalized homophobia: A factor analytic study. *J Clin Psychol* 1996; 52:15–21.
24. Ross MW, Fernández-Esquer ME, Seibt A. Understanding across the sexual orientation gap: Sexuality as culture. In: Landis D, Bhagat R, eds., *Handbook of Intercultural Training*, 2nd ed. Beverly Hills: Sage; 1995: 414–430.
25. Weston K. *Families We Choose: Lesbians, Gays, Kinship*. New York: Columbia University Press; 1991.
26. Turner HA, Hays RB, Coates TJ. Determinants of social support among gay men: The context of AIDS. *J Health Soc Behav* 1993; 34:37–53.
27. Joseph JG, Adib SM, Koopman JS, Ostrow DG. Behavioral change in longitudinal studies: Adoption of condom use by homosexual/bisexual men. *Am J Public Health* 1991; 80:1513–1514.
28. Adib SM, Joseph JG, Ostrow DG, et al. Relapse in sexual behavior among homosexual men: A 2-year follow-up from the Chicago MACS/CCS. *AIDS* 1991; 5:757–760.
29. Seibt AC, Ross MW, Freeman A, et al. Relationship between safe sex and acculturation into the gay subculture. *AIDS Care* 1995; 7(suppl 1):S85–S88.
30. Folkman S, Chesney MA, Pollack L, Phillips C. Stress, coping, and high-risk sexual behavior. *Health Psychol* 1992; 11:218–222.
31. Van de Ven P, Campbell S, Kippax S, et al. Factors associated with unprotected anal intercourse in gay men's casual partnerships in Sydney, Australia. *AIDS Care* 1997; 9:637–649.
32. de Wit JBF, van Griensven GJP, Kok G, Sandfort TGM. Why do homosexual men relapse into unsafe sex? Predictors of unprotected anogenital intercourse with casual partners. *AIDS* 1993; 7:1113–1118.
33. Boulton M, McLean J, Fitzpatrick R, Hart G. Gay men's accounts of unsafe sex. *AIDS Care* 1995; 7:619–630.
34. Bosga MB, de Wit JBF, de Vroome EMM, et al. Differences in perception of risk for HIV infection with steady and non-steady partners among homosexual men. *AIDS Educ Prev* 1995; 7:103–115.
35. Weinstein N. Perceptions of personal susceptibility to harm. In: Mays VM, Albee GW, Schneider SF, eds. *Primary Prevention of AIDS: Psychological Approaches*. Newbury Park, CA: Sage; 1989:142–167.
36. Paul JP, Stall R, Davis F. Sexual risk for HIV transmission among gay/bisexual men in substance abuse treatment. *AIDS Educ Prev* 1993; 5:11–24.
37. Stall R, McKusick L, Wiley J, et al. Alcohol and drug use during sexual activity and compliance with safe sex guidelines for AIDS: The AIDS Behavioral Research Project. *Health Educ Q* 1986; 13:359–371.
38. Weatherburn P, Davies PM, Hickson FCI, et al. No connection between alcohol use and unsafe sex among gay and bisexual men. *AIDS* 1993; 7:115–119.
39. Lewis LA, Ross MW. *A Select Body: The Gay Dance Party Subculture and the HIV/AIDS Pandemic*. London: Cassell; 1995.
40. Ross MW, Wodak A, Gold J, Miller ME. Differences across sexual orientation on HIV risk behaviours in injecting drug users. *AIDS Care* 1992; 4:139–148.
41. Kalichman SC, Johnson JR, Adair V, et al. Sexual sensation seeking: Scale development and predicting AIDS-related behavior among homosexually active men. *J Person Assess* 1994; 62:385–397.
42. Valdiserri RO, Pultman TV, Curran JW. Community planning: A national strategy to improve HIV prevention programs. *J Community Health* 1995; 20:87–100.
43. Bandura A. Perceived self-efficacy in the exercise of control over AIDS infection. In: Mays VM, Albee GW, Schneider SF, eds. *Primary Prevention of AIDS: Psychological Approaches*. Newbury Park, CA: Sage; 1989: 128–141.
44. Fishbein M, Ajzen I. *Belief, Attitude, Intention, and Behavior: An Introduction to Theory and Research*. Reading, MA: Addison-Wesley; 1975.

45. Catania JA, Kegeles S, Coates TJ. Towards an understanding of risk behavior: An AIDS risk reduction model (ARRM). *Health Educ Q* 1990; 17:53–72.
46. Fisher JD, Fisher WA. Changing AIDS risk behavior. *Psychol Bull* 1992; 111:455–474.
47. Valdiserri RO, Lyter DW, Leviton LL, et al. AIDS prevention in homosexual and bisexual men: Results of a randomized trial evaluating two risk reduction interventions. *AIDS* 1989; 3:21–26.
48. Kelly JA, St. Lawrence JS, Hood HV, Brasfield TL. Behavioral intervention to reduce AIDS risk activities. *J Consult Clin Psychol* 1989; 57:60–67.
49. Kelly JA, St. Lawrence JS, Brasfield TL. Predictors of vulnerability to AIDS risk behavioral relapse. *J Consult Clin Psychol* 1990; 59:163–166.
50. Kelly JA, St. Lawrence JS, Betts R, et al. A skills training group intervention to assist persons in reducing risk behaviors for HIV infection. *AIDS Educ Prev* 1990; 2:24–25.
51. Peterson JL, Coates TJ, Catania JA, et al. Evaluation of an HIV risk reduction intervention among African American homosexual and bisexual men. *AIDS* 1996; 10:319–325.
52. Choi KH, Lew S, Vittinghoff E, et al. The efficacy of brief group counseling in HIV risk reduction among homosexual Asian and Pacific Islander men. *AIDS* 1996; 10:81–87.
53. Holtgrave DR, Kelly JA. The cost-effectiveness of an HIV prevention intervention for gay men. *AIDS Behav* 1997; 1:173–180.
54. Pinkerton SD, Holtgrave DR, Valdiserri RD. Cost-effectiveness of HIV prevention skills training for men who have sex with men. *AIDS* 1997; 11:347–357.
55. Kelly JA, St. Lawrence JS, Diaz YE, et al. HIV risk behavior reduction following intervention with key opinion leaders of a population: An experimental community-level analysis. *Am J Public Health* 1991; 81:168–171.
56. Kelly JA, St. Lawrence JS, Stevenson LY, et al. Community AIDS/HIV risk reduction: The effects of endorsement by popular people in three cities. *Am J Public Health* 1992; 82:1483–1489.
57. Rogers E. *Diffusion of Innovations*. New York: Free Press; 1983.
58. Kelly JA, Murphy DA, Sikkema KJ, et al. Randomized, controlled community-level HIV prevention intervention for sexual-risk behavior among homosexual men in US cities. *Lancet* 1997; 350:1500–1505.
59. Kegeles SM, Hays RB, Coates TJ. The Mpowerment Project: A community-level HIV intervention for young gay men. *Am J Public Health* 1996; 86:1129–1136.
60. Hays RB, Kegeles SD, Coates TJ. High HIV risk-taking among young gay men. *AIDS* 1990; 4:901–907.
61. Lemp GF, Hrozawa PM, Givertz D, et al. Seroprevalence of HIV and risk behaviors among young homosexual and bisexual men: The San Francisco/Berkeley Young Men's Survey. *JAMA* 1994; 272:449–454.
62. Osmond DH, Page K, Wiley J, et al. HIV infection in homosexual and bisexual men 18 to 29 years of age: The San Francisco Young Men's Health Study. *Am J Public Health* 1994; 84:1933–1937.
63. Silvestre AJ, Lyter DW, Valdiserri RO, et al. Factors related to seroconversion among homosexual and bisexual men after attending a risk education session. *AIDS* 1989; 3:147–150.
64. Ku LC, Sonnenstein FL, Pleck JH. The dynamics of young men's condom use during and across relationships. *Fam Plann Perspect* 1994; 26:246–251.
65. Williams SS, Kimble DL, Covell NH, et al. College students use implicit personality theory instead of safer sex. *J Appl Soc Psychol* 1992; 22:921–933.
66. Leigh BC, Stall R. Substance use and risky sexual behavior for exposure to HIV: Issues in methodology, interpretation, and prevention. *Am Psychol* 1993; 48:1035–1045.
67. Rotheram-Borus MJ, Rosario M, Meyer-Bahlburg HFL, et al. Sexual and substance use acts of gay and bisexual male adolescents in New York City. *J Sex Res* 1994; 31:47–57.
68. Higgins DL, Galavotti C, O'Reilly K, et al. Evidence for the effects of HIV antibody counseling and testing on risk behaviors. *JAMA* 1991; 226:2419–2429.
69. Robins AG, Dew MA, Davidson S, et al. Psychosocial factors associated with risky sexual behavior among HIV-seropositive gay men. *AIDS Educ Prev* 1994; 6:482–492.
70. Hart GJ. Peer education and community based HIV prevention for homosexual men: Peer led, evidence based, or fashion driven? *Sex Transm Infect* 1998; 74:87–89.

11

HIV Prevention among African-American and Latino Men Who Have Sex with Men

JOHN L. PETERSON and ALEX CARBALLO-DIÉGUEZ

INTRODUCTION

Public health data indicate that the incidence of acquired immunodeficiency syndrome (AIDS) among racial and ethnic minority men who have sex with men (MSM) has been disproportionately high among African-American and Hispanic men in the United States.[1] AIDS cases due to male-to-male sexual contact account for 39% of AIDS cases among African Americans and 43% among Hispanic Americans.[2] Also, cross-sectional and cohort studies among these ethnic minority men have revealed they have maintained elevated levels of high-risk sexual behavior.[3–8] These data suggest that more effective human immunodeficiency virus (HIV) prevention programs are needed among homosexual and bisexual racial and ethnic minority men to achieve the significant reductions in HIV transmission reported among white gay and bisexual men.[9] However, notable differences between white and nonwhite MSM increase the difficulty to provide effective intervention programs to minority men. The emphasis on HIV transmission among minority heterosexuals diverts attention from the substantial route of HIV transmission through male-to-male sexual activity. Also, the opportunity for HIV prevention with minority MSM is greatly diminished by the influence of prejudice and discrimination toward nonwhite MSM by both minority culture and mainstream gay culture. Finally, these efforts are hampered by the lack of sufficient prevention research to guide further development of community programs. Despite these obstacles, such evidence is urgently needed to help provide directions for HIV prevention among minority MSM populations.

CROSS-SECTIONAL STUDIES WITH AFRICAN-AMERICAN MSM

There are few data on HIV risk reduction among African-American MSM. Among the few studies available, however, several sociocultural, psychosocial, and situational factors have been found associated with HIV high-risk sexual behavior among African-American MSM. These factors include sexual orientation; social background; perceived risk, beliefs about social norms, behavioral consequences, and perceived control; sociosexual contexts; and resources for social support.

JOHN L. PETERSON • Department of Psychology, Georgia State University, Atlanta, Georgia 30303. *ALEX CARBALLO-DIÉGUEZ* • HIV Research Center, New York, New York 10032.

Handbook of HIV Prevention, edited by Peterson and DiClemente.
Kluwer Academic/Plenum Publishers, New York, 2000.

In one study, Peterson et al.[5] examined factors associated with HIV high-risk behaviors among African-American gay and bisexual men ($N = 250$) in San Francisco, Oakland, and Berkeley. Respondents were recruited from bars, bath houses, and adult bookstores and through African-American newspapers, health clinics, and personal referrals of study participants. It was found that unprotected anal intercourse was strongly associated with marginal status, such as low income, payment for sex, or being an injection drug user, and with discomfort about public disclosure of one's homosexual behavior. Mays[6] reported similar effects of social class (e.g., income, education, and employment) on HIV risk behaviors in a multisite sample ($N = 889$) of African-American gay and bisexual men.

This study by Peterson et al.[5] also found an association between perceived norms and unprotected anal intercourse. Those men who were more likely to use condoms had stronger beliefs that condom use was the social norm among their peers in the community. Moreover, the results failed to demonstrate an association between race-related beliefs about the AIDS epidemic and HIV high-risk sexual behavior. The data further showed that these men's expectations about the positive or negative effect of safe sex practices are associated with unprotected anal intercourse. Those men who were more likely to use condoms had more positive expectations about using them. Last, this study found that the perceived self-efficacy to use condoms was strongly associated with condom use among African-American MSM. Men who had stronger beliefs that they could practice safe sex were more likely than others to use condoms.

A study by McKirnan et al.[7] and Stokes et al.[8] provides data on correlates of HIV risk behavior among their sample ($N = 536$) of bisexually active African-American men. Participants were recruited from bars, print advertisements, community outreach, and personal referrals by respondents. Results showed that those men who had engaged in male–male sexual contact were more likely than others to report their self-identity as bisexual rather than homosexual. Even after controlling for sociodemographic background, African-American bisexual men were still more likely to have exchanged money or drugs for sex. This study found that the setting in which men met their sexual partners is a strong predictor of high-risk sexual behavior. Men who met their potential partners in bars were more likely to have engaged in high-risk sexual behavior than those men who met their partners through friends; this finding was unaffected by differences in alcohol consumption between meeting locales.

CROSS-SECTIONAL STUDIES WITH LATINO MSM

As with African-American men, there is a scarcity of empirical studies on the sexual risk behavior of Latino MSM. The available studies have reported several individual, contextual, and developmental factors related to unprotected sex in Latino MSM. These factors include attitudes toward condoms, risk perceptions, substance use, emotional relationship with the sexual partner, sexual self-identity, socioeconomic status, history of childhood sexual abuse, perceived stigmatization of homosexuality, history of harassment, and victimization.

In an exploratory study of Puerto Rican MSM, Carballo-Diéguez and Dolezal[10] found that the sexual self-identity of MSM (i.e., gay, bisexual, straight, or drag queen) was significantly associated with different types of sexual behavior, as well as different levels of unprotected receptive anal sex. The further from mainstream norms the individual felt himself (the more female-identified), the more likely he was to engage in receptive anal sex and to do so without a condom. The authors also found that men with a history of childhood sexual abuse were more likely than nonabused men to engage in receptive anal sex and to do so without protection.[11] In terms of the most frequently cited obstacles to condom use, the authors found them to be dislike of condoms, low risk perception, trust in and emotional connection with the partner, unavailability and inconvenience of condom use, lack of control, and indifference.[12]

This study of Puerto Rican MSM also found that those men who had both lovers and one-night stands ($N = 67$) were more likely to have unprotected anal sex (both receptive and insertive) with their lovers regardless of their HIV status. The qualitative data of the study were analyzed together with the qualitative data from a subsequent study of male couples of mixed HIV status (one partner being HIV-positive and the other one HIV-negative) that took place between 1994 and 1996. Focusing only on the Puerto Rican men involved in serodiscordant partnerships who participated in the study, Carballo-Diéguez et al.[13] found that among coupled men the wish for unrestricted sexual pleasure and intimacy and trust and love for the partner often overpowered concerns about HIV transmission.

A more recent work by Carballo-Diéguez et al.[14] focused on a comparative study between 80 Colombian, 80 Dominican, 80 Puerto Rican, and 67 Mexican MSM residing in New York City at the time of the study. Three quarters of the men had been born outside the continental United States and had moved to the United States at an average age of 20. The results of this study by Carballo-Diéguez et al.[14] and Carballo-Diéguez[15] showed that men in these groups felt highly stigmatized. For example, only a few of them reported ever hearing the only two Spanish terms that do not connote stigmatization of homosexuals ("de ambiente" and "entendido"). Most of the participants could only refer to themselves in Spanish by using derogatory terms, including the ever-popular "loca" (crazy woman). Terms like "partido" (cracked), "dañado" (damaged), and "mujercita" (little woman) were reported to be frequently used both by homosexuals and nonhomosexuals. Most of the participants reported heavy familial pressure to conform to traditional masculine behavior and continuous fear of being thrown out of their homes if their sexual orientation was discovered. One out of three participants had been sexually initiated by a man at least 4 years their senior when they were 12 years old or younger, and one out of five respondents felt physically or emotionally damaged by the experience. Those few who disclosed the abuse to family members were generally asked to conceal the information in order to safeguard the family's good name.

During adolescence and adulthood, many of the participants who had lived in Latin America had been detained by uniformed or nonuniformed policemen who had extorted money from them. Those who had not had this direct experience lived in fear of it, knowing that it had happened to their friends. Some participants reported being taken to mental health practitioners who attempted conversion therapies, using electric shocks to create negative associations to masculine erotic stimuli. All these experiences took place in environments where no positive gay role models were available, much less any organized gay community. Hence, participants revealed, with poignant intensity, their experiences of stigmatization, discrimination, harassment, and victimization. These experiences resulted in traumatic sequelae that hampered adult self-protective behavior. When these Latino MSM moved to the United States, especially to cities with established gay enclaves like New York and San Francisco, they experienced a sense of release and liberation. However, they quickly became aware that they had joined a discriminated-against Latino minority, and that within the Latino community, they were still subject to prejudice.

Other investigators also have studied the factors related to unprotected sex in Latino MSM. Díaz et al.[16] studied 159 English-speaking Latino MSM recruited in Tucson, Arizona. They found that those men who practiced unprotected intercourse with nonmonogamous partners reported lower annual income and were less educated than those who used protection. The authors found that two cognitive variables—behavioral intentions and perceptions of self-efficacy and self-control—and two behavioral variables—sex under the influence of alcohol and/or drugs and sex in public environments—were the most important correlates of HIV risk. Interestingly, Díaz et al. emphatically caution against overinterpreting unprotected sex in Latino MSM as a result of self-regulatory, volitional processes:

> It is possible that the internalization of sociocultural factors—such as internalized homophobia, inability to publicly acknowledge homosexuality, and the consequent anxiety raised by same-sex encounters—so prevalent in the socialization of Latino men, might promote the observed incongruence between behavioral intentions and actual sexual behaviors. The task at hand is thus to develop new culturally sensitive models to explain the fact that unsafe sexual behavior tends to occur after a breakdown of self-regulatory processes, when internalized socio-cultural factors such as homophobia, sexual shame, and closet issues (rather than a self-formulated plan of action) regulate the expression of sexual behavior. (pp. 427–428)

In a study of 200 Mexican gay and bisexual men in the Mexico-US border city of Juárez, Ramírez et al.[17] found that unprotected anal intercourse was significantly more frequent among individuals who were older, had blue-collar occupations (factory workers), met their sexual partners in the streets (rather than in bars), or had a history of at least one sexually transmitted disease (STD). In a study of San Francisco Latino gay–bisexual males, Sabogal et al.[18] explored the reasons associated with the high rate of unprotected anal sex (35%) in the sample. Those reasons, ranked in order of endorsement, were: feeling very aroused, not having condoms available, being in love, thinking that the sexual partner looked healthy, being under the influence of drugs or alcohol, their partner refusing to use condoms, and having seroconcordant status.

Taken together, studies among African-American and Latino MSM suggest the pervasive disempowerment experienced by these men as both ethnic and sexual minorities. These men grew up and often continue to live in harsh environments where their lifestyles and emotional inclinations are subject to critique and even persecution. They adopt survival systems that focus on immediate gratification, pushing away health-related concerns and more distant goals. It is not surprising that HIV prevention messages are less successful among minority MSM than among mainstream white MSM to achieve the desired behavior changes.

PREVENTION AMONG AFRICAN-AMERICAN AND LATINO MSM

Given the few cross-sectional studies among minority MSM, the absence of documented effective prevention interventions for Latinos and the existence of only one random control intervention among African Americans may be expected. This does not mean that there are not a number of local initiatives, especially undertaken by community organizations, that attempt to prevent HIV transmission among minority MSM. However, their effectiveness still needs to be demonstrated. The one evaluated intervention with African-American MSM produced significant reductions in HIV risk behavior over an 18 month follow-up.[19] Results showed that participants in the triple-session intervention greatly reduced their frequency of unprotected anal intercourse in comparison to the single-session group and control group.

HIV prevention programs directed at Anglo white gay men have relied on cognitive behavioral theory and have been based on skills-building approaches.[20–22] These programs have had demonstrated effectiveness among the post-Stonewall gay community that had well-established social institutions, places of reunion, symbols of self-identification (flags, triangles), traditions (gay parade), press, literary and artistic movements, positive role models, and secure financial resources.

Minority MSM are generally not in the same position of comparative privilege enjoyed by white gay males. The AIDS epidemic found minority MSM not only with considerably fewer financial resources but also struggling under the double stigma of being minority and homosexual, as well as with limited social organization. For this reason, when minority investigators and community-based organizations attempted to develop prevention programs for minority MSM, they quickly saw the necessity of raising consciousness regarding the circumstances of disempowerment, marginalization, and ostracism that MSM felt in their social milieu and to foster a reaction to this disempowerment in order to help them gain pride in their ethnicity and sexual orientation, decrease internalized homophobia, and achieve a sense of gay community.

In awareness of this reality, the intervention study with African-American MSM included an entire session dedicated to group discussion of the participants' dual-identity process— being black and being gay—along with a discussion of benefits, disadvantages and consequences.[19] Similarly, Fundación SIDA of Puerto Rico,[23] in their prevention program "No lo Dejes Caer," also included a discussion about acceptance and validation of participants' feelings about their sexual choices and analysis of the place of homosexuality within the historical and cultural context of Puerto Rico. Díaz,[24] in his prevention program in the Mission district of San Francisco, "Hermanos de Luna y Sol," also focused on two similar goals: to promote participants' awareness about the difficulties involved in their dual-minority status, that is, the issues about being gay–bisexual in a homophobic–machista culture or an ethnic minority in a racist society, and to promote a sense of bonding and community among persons who have experienced similar types of oppression in their lives.

Those small-group skills-building interventions developed for Anglo white men and the one for African-American men that have been successful when evaluated appear to share several common features.[19,22,25] They all involved peers teaching peers, took place in the environments commonly frequented by the target population, and were embedded in the men's normal life routines. Parker[26] states:

> While changes in behavior which will reduce the risk of HIV infection are of course the ultimate goal of all intervention activities, it is important to remember that AIDS prevention programs almost never intervene directly at the level of the behavior. On the contrary, to the extent that they intervene at all, they normally do so at the level of social and cultural representations—at the level of the subjective and inter-subjective meanings which people hold about their behaviors. In short, they try to change the ways in which people think about and conceive of sexual relations, HIV-related risk, and so on, in the hopes that these changes will enable both individuals and communities to take decisions and make choices that will in fact effectively reduce the risk of HIV infection. (p. 64)

Based on these experiences, it appears that an effective prevention program for Latino MSM should seek to elicit the participants' own strategies for preventing HIV transmission and within their social, cultural, and semantic realities.[27,28] Some initiatives currently underway that focus on personal and community empowerment have been designed within this framework.[14,28] However, their effectiveness still needs to be evaluated. Similarly, interventions for African-American MSM are more likely to be effective if they are informed by the psychological, social, and situational context of these men's lives.[29,30]

CONCLUSIONS

It is evident that more effective HIV interventions need to be developed and evaluated among the two largest populations of minority MSM: African Americans and Latinos.

Typically, the few interventions tested have relied on individual-level approaches. However, the stigma of homosexuality reduces the ability to access many of these men in hidden populations because of their fear of being publicly identified. Those men who are more likely to attend small-group skills-building interventions are probably more open about their sexual behavior and more likely to self-identify as gay. If so, then they constitute only a minority proportion of African-American and Latino MSM in need of HIV prevention. Hence, other approaches are required to reach the larger majority of nonwhite MSM who do not identify as gay and who are bisexual.

Diffusion interventions offer a prominent strategy to reach the larger segment of minority MSM than individual-level approaches.[31] These interventions are intended to promote behavior change through the adoption of new reference group norms within people's social networks. Peer outreach provides a valuable way in which to diffuse messages through these men's networks. Peer outreach approaches in sexual venues offer useful opportunities to reach some minority MSM who engage in high-risk sexual behavior. The social settings most prominent among these venues include bars, parks, public restrooms, private house parties, and the sex industry. These situations represent the social contexts in which many MSM meet eligible and potential sexual partners. Condom distribution and prevention messages delivered by peers and opinion leaders of men in these social situations may prove to be effective strategies.

However, beyond sexual venues, interventions must include more traditional institutions in minority communities that provide opportunities for peer outreach. Major institutions, such as churches, offer potentially useful sources to recruit and provide HIV prevention because of the high number of MSM involved in them. However, these institutions rarely have included MSM in their responses to HIV prevention in minority communities. The perception of homosexuality as a sin poses a formidable obstacle to churches as a possible resource to provide HIV prevention to MSM. This perception often leads to an intolerance of same-sex behavior within the larger church population. This intolerance may explain why data showed that few African-American MSM seek help regarding their HIV risk behavior from their family or clergy.[32] Social opposition is needed that can lead to a more hospitable reception toward African-American and Latino MSM by Protestant and Catholic churches. Hence, prevention approaches are warranted that can increase the community capacity of minority institutions to provide HIV prevention to MSM.

Innovative social marketing campaigns are needed that deliver HIV prevention messages for MSM along with messages for minority heterosexual men. Broadcast and print media provide useful channels to disseminate messages to minority MSM as members of the general minority population. Beyond awareness, these social marketing campaigns need to provide information about other resources regarding help-seeking for HIV prevention. Other social marketing approaches may include use of the novella, video technology, and the internet to reach minority MSM. These approaches can take advantage of media to disseminate culturally appropriate prevention messages that can be tailored to the respective audience of MSM in minority populations.

As we near the third decade of the HIV pandemic, the Centers for Disease Control estimates that the majority of HIV cases will eventually occur among ethnic minority populations.[33] Sizable proportions of these HIV cases are likely to be among African-American and Latino MSM. Substantially more effective interventions are required to reduce the rate of HIV transmission in these minority men. The interventions will need to offer the possibility of reaching broader populations of MSM if they are to be effective. Also, they should be based on rigorous public health and behavioral science data to support their development, implementation, and evaluation. However, currently there is inadequate research available to assist such efforts with HIV prevention in these populations. Unless more successful prevention efforts are achieved, there is little likelihood that the HIV epidemic will substantially change among African-American and Latino MSM in the United States.

REFERENCES

1. Centers for Disease Control. Update: Trends in AIDS among men who have sex with men-United States, 1989–1994. *Morb Mortal Wkly Rep* 1995; 44:401–404.
2. Division of HIV/AIDS. *Surveillance Report*. Atlanta, GA: Centers for Disease Control; December 1997.
3. Carballo-Diéguez A, Dolezal C. Contrasting types of Puerto Rican men who have sex with men (MSM). *J Psychol Hum Sex* 1994; 6:41–67.
4. Doll LS, Peterson LR, White CR, et al. Homosexually and nonhomosexually identified men who have sex with men: A behavioral comparison. *J Sex Res* 1992; 29:1–14.
5. Peterson JL, Coates TJ, Catania JA, et al. High-risk sexual behavior and condom use among gay and bisexual African-American men. *Am J Public Health*, 1992; 82:1490–1494.
6. Mays VM. High-risk HIV-related sexual behaviors in a national sample of US black gay and bisexual men. Paper presented at the IXth International Conference on AIDS. Berlin, Germany, June 1993.
7. McKirnan DJ, Stokes JP, Doll L, Burzette RG. Bisexually active men: Social characteristics and sexual behavior. *J Sex Res*, 1995; 32:64–75.
8. Stokes JP, McKirnan DJ, Burzette RG. Sexual behavior, condom use, disclosure of sexuality, and stability of sexual orientation in bisexual men. *J Sex Res*, 1993; 30:203–213.
9. Choi KH, Coates TJ. Prevention of HIV infection. *AIDS* 1994; 8:1371–1389.
10. Carballo-Diéguez A, Dolezal C. Contrasting types of Puerto Rican men who have sex with men (MSM). *J Psychol Hum Sex*, 1994; 64:41–67.
11. Carballo-Diéguez A, Dolezal C. Association between history of childhood sexual abuse and adult HIV-risk sexual behavior in Puerto Rican men who have sex with men. *Child Abuse Neglect Int J* 1995; 19:595–605.
12. Carballo-Diéguez A, Dolezal C. HIV risk behaviors and obstacles to condom use among Puerto Rican men in New York City who have sex with men. *Am J Public Health*, 1996; 86:1619–1622.
13. Carballo-Diéguez A, Remien R, Dolezal C, Wagner G. Unsafe sex in Puerto Rican MSM primary relationships. *AIDS Behav* 1997; 1:9–17.
14. Carballo-Diéguez A, Dolezal C, Nieves L, Diaz F. Latino men who have sex with men (MSM). Abstract of the XXVI International Congress of Psychology. *Int J Psychol* 1996; 31:521.5.
15. Carballo-Diéguez A. The challenge of staying HIV-negative for Latin-American immigrants. *J Gay Lesbian Soc Serv* 1998; 8:61–82.
16. Díaz RM, Stall RD, Hoff C, et al. HIV risk among Latino gay men in the southwestern United States. *AIDS Educ Prev* 1996; 8:415–429.
17. Ramirez J, Suarez E, de la Rosa G, et al. AIDS knowledge and sexual behavior among Mexican gay and bisexual men. *AIDS Educ Prev*, 1994; 6:163–174.
18. Sabogal F, Sandlin G, Reyes R, et al. Hombres Latinos "gay" y bisexuales: Una comunidad de alto riesgo del VIH/SIDA. *Rev Latino Am Psicol* 1992; 24:57–69.
19. Peterson JL, Coates TJ, Catania J, et al. Evaluation of an HIV risk reduction intervention among African-American homosexual and bisexual men. *AIDS* 1996; 10:319–325.
20. Bandura A. Social cognitive theory and the exercise of control over HIV infection. In: DiClemente RD, Peterson J, eds. *Preventing AIDS: Theories and Methods of Behavioral Interventions*. New York: Plenum Press; 1994: 25–59.
21. Fishbein M, Chan DKS, O'Reilly K, et al. Factors influencing gay men's attitudes, subjective norms, and intentions with respect to preforming sexual behaviors. *J Appl Soc Psychol* 1993; 23:417–438.
22. Kelly J, St. Lawrence J, Hood H, Brasfield T. Behavioral interventions to reduce AIDS risk activities. *J Consult Clin Psychol* 1989; 57:60–67.
23. United States Conference of Mayors. HIV prevention programs targeting gay/bisexual men of color. *HIV Educ Case Stud* 1996; 8:3–11.
24. Diaz R. *Latino Gay Men and HIV: Culture, Sexuality and Risk Behavior*. London and New York: Routledge; 1998.
25. Kelly J, St. Lawrence J, Betts R., et al. A skills training group intervention to assist persons in reducing risk behaviors for HIV infection. *AIDS Educ Prev* 1990; 2:24–35.

26. Parker RG. Behaviour in Latin American men: Implications for HIV/AIDS interventions. *Int J STD AIDS* 1996; 7:62–65.

27. Carballo-Diéguez A. The challenge of staying HIV-negative for Latin-American immigrants. *J Gay Lesbian Soc Serv* 1998; 8:61–82.

28. Morales J. Intervention reducing HIV risk for gay/bisexual Latinos. Oral presentation at the First International Congress of the National Latino/A Lesbian and Gay Organization (LLEGO). San Juan, Puerto Rico; 1997.

29. Beeker C, Kraft JM, Peterson JL, Stokes JP. Influences on sexual risk behavior in young African-American men who have sex with men. *J Lesbian Gay Med Assoc* 1998; 2:59–67.

30. Stokes JP, Peterson JL. Homophobia, self-esteem, and risk for HIV among African-American men who have sex with men. *AIDS Educ Prev* 1998; 10:278–292.

31. Kelly JA, St. Lawrence JS, Stevenson Y, et al. Community AIDS/HIV risk reduction: The effects of endorsements by popular people in three cities. *Am J Public Health*, 1992; 82:1483–1489.

32. Peterson JL, Coates TJ, Catania JA, et al. Help-seeking for AIDS high-risk sexual behavior among gay and bisexual African American men. *AIDS Educ Prev*, 1995; 7:1–9.

33. Centers for Disease Control and Prevention. *HIV Prevention Update to the Congressional Black Caucus.* Washington, DC: CDC; March 1998.

12

HIV Prevention in Developing Countries

JULIA DAYTON and MICHAEL H. MERSON

Although a serious concern all over the world, the acquired immunodeficiency syndrome (AIDS) epidemic is concentrated and has the most severe health, social, and economic consequences in developing countries. Averting additional cases of infection in these countries therefore is a critical priority. This chapter first discusses the epidemiology of human immuno-deficiency virus (HIV) in developing countries and reviews prevention interventions that have been shown to be effective in reducing HIV transmission. It then provides guidance for setting prevention priorities. The last section has an agenda for research on HIV prevention in developing countries.

EPIDEMIOLOGY OF HIV IN DEVELOPING COUNTRIES

General Epidemiology

UNAIDS[1] estimates that by the end of 1997 a total of 42.3 million adults and children worldwide had been infected by HIV. About 11.7 million of these individuals have already died from AIDS, and 30.6 million are still living with HIV. Over 90% of those living with HIV are in developing countries (Table 1). About 5.2 million adults and 590,000 children are believed to have acquired HIV during 1997, and almost all of these were in living developing countries.[1]

HIV is a sexually transmitted disease (STD) that mostly affects adults in the prime of life—ages 15 to 49 years old. As with other STDs, as the epidemic matures, the average age of infection decreases; this is already occurring in sub-Saharan Africa, as in the United States. HIV is mainly transmitted by sex or other direct contact with bodily fluids of an infected person. Most adult transmission in the developing world is by heterosexual sex, though transmission by sex between men occurs to some extent in all countries. The second most important mode of transmission is by the sharing of unsterilized needles and syringes among injection drug users (IDUs), which is predominant in many countries in Asia, in Brazil and Argentina, and in Eastern Europe. Parenteral transmission also can occur by blood transfusion or medical injection, but these account today for a relatively small percentage of total transmission. Mother-to-child transmission is a third mode of transmission. It is presently most common in sub-Saharan Africa, the region with the greatest number of HIV-infected women, where as many as 15 to 20% of HIV infections may occur by this route.[2]

JULIA DAYTON and MICHAEL H. MERSON • Department of Epidemiology and Public Health, Yale University School of Medicine, New Haven, Connecticut 06511.

Handbook of HIV Prevention, edited by Peterson and DiClemente.
Kluwer Academic / Plenum Publishers, New York, 2000.

Table 1. Estimated Number of People
Living with AIDS Worldwide, 1997[a]

People with HIV or AIDS	Regional total
Developing world	
Sub-Saharan Africa	20.8 million
South and Southeast Asia	6 million
Latin America	1.3 million
East Asia and Pacific	440,000
Caribbean	320,000
North Africa and Middle East	210,000
Eastern Europe and Central Asia	150,000
Industrialized world	
North America	860,000
Western Europe	530,000
Australia and New Zealand	12,000

[a]SOURCE: UNAIDS, 1997.[1]

How the Epidemic Spreads

The extent to which an infectious disease spreads in a population depends on its *reproductive rate*, or the average number of susceptible people infected by an infected person over his or her lifetime.[3] In order for an epidemic to grow, its reproductive rate must be treater than 1. The larger the reproductive rate, the more rapidly it will spread. The amount of time a person remains infectious, his or her risk of transmission per sexual contact and the rate of acquisition of new partners all affect the reproductive rate of any STD, including HIV. Biological, behavioral, and economic factors influence these three variables.

Biological Factors

Recent evidence suggests that the average probability of transmission from an infected person to a noninfected person (called *infectivity*) is greatest during two periods of high viral load. The first is during primary infection, which occurs during the time between exposure to HIV and the appearance of HIV antibodies. The second is when the person is in the advanced stages of the disease and has developed AIDS (as indicated by a low CD4 T-lymphocyte count).[4] Untreated STDs also increase the risk of HIV transmission. Genital ulcer disease increases the risk of HIV transmission per sexual exposure 10 to 50 times for male-to-female transmission and 50 to 300 times for female-to-male transmission,[5] and nonulcerative STDs (chlamydia and gonorrhea) increase the risk two- to fivefold.[6] Simulations of the initial 10 years of the HIV epidemic in rural Uganda indicate that over 80% of HIV infections can be attributed to STDs.[7] Male circumcision also has been shown to have a protective effect against HIV transmission.[4]

Behavioral Factors

The rate of partner change, the number of concurrent partners, and mixing patterns influence the reproductive rate. Both the average rate of partner change in the society and the variation across individuals have an influence on the dynamic of the epidemic.[8] The greater the number of partners, the faster the spread of HIV. In almost all societies, most individuals have few sexual partners during their lifetime and a small number of individuals have many partners. But even a very small group of people with many partners may be enough to sustain the epidemic and gradually spread it to the rest of the population. Recent evidence suggests that the number of concurrent partners is more important than the total number of sexual partners, a finding that has important implications for prevention messages.[9] The more mixing between high-risk individuals (those with many partners) and low-risk individuals (those with few sexual partners), the faster the epidemic will spread in the general population.[10] This occurs, for example, in countries with an active commercial sex industry.

Economic Factors

Poverty, which is endemic in many developing countries, also may increase transmission. For women, being impoverished may make them more vulnerable and less effective in negotiating safe sex with partners, or they may be more likely to engage in sex work. For men, poverty may motivate them to migrate for work, putting them at risk for having more sexual partners while away from the family. Empirical analysis by the World Bank of national-level aggregate data supports these hypotheses.[8]

Factors that accompany economic growth, particularly improved infrastructure and increased travel, may facilitate the spread of the epidemic. One reason is that an open economy facilitates the movement of individuals, and countries with larger immigration populations tend to have more severe HIV/AIDS epidemics, all else being equal. Economic growth also may contribute to a shift from more conservative to more liberal social attitudes, which may lead to greater individual freedom and more risky sexual activity. In regression analysis of aggregate national-level data, the percentage of the population that is Muslim, a proxy for social conservatism, was associated with statistically significant lower rates of HIV infection.[8]

Women Are at Greater Risk Than Men

Although globally more men than women have been infected with HIV (with the exception of sub-Saharan Africa), new infections are increasing faster among women. Women also are becoming infected at a younger age than men.[11] Biological, behavioral, and social factors explain these gender differences. With sexual transmission, HIV is more easily transmitted from men to women than from women to men.[12] Young women and girls are particularly vulnerable, possibly due to more cervicovaginal fragility or other biological features related to the lack of genital maturity. Females also are more likely than males to have nonsymptomatic STDs and, since these STDs are likely to go untreated, have an elevated risk for HIV infection. Social factors, such as lack of control over the conditions under which they have sex, also can contribute to increases in HIV. This applies to a spectrum of sexually active females, from sex workers (SWs) to monogamous, married women.[11] A recent study from India found that the HIV prevalence rate among monogamous, married women (a group previously thought to be at low risk) is increasing dramatically. Since sexual contact with their only partner was the only risk factor significantly associated with HIV infection, the report concluded that these women are likely being infected by their spouses.[13]

Impact on Health and Life Expectancy

AIDS causes a large share of mortality in developing countries: by the end of 1997, a total of 9 million adults and 2.7 million children had died since the beginning of the epidemic.[1] By

Table 2. Causes of Death from Infectious
Diseases in the Developing World,
Adults Aged 15–59, 1990–2020[a]

1990	Percent	2020	Percent
Tuberculosis	51.4	Tuberculosis	54.7
Respiratory	10.0	HIV	37.1
HIV	8.6	Respiratory	2.6
Malaria	5.4	Malaria	1.3
Other	23.5	Other	4.4

[a]SOURCE: Murray and Lopez.[14]

1990, AIDS was the third leading cause of adult death in the developing world (following tuberculosis and other infectious diseases), but its share of mortality is growing much faster than any other type of disease (Table 2).[14] In African countries with the most severe epidemics, over half of adult mortality is already attributed to AIDS.[15] It has been estimated that HIV will be the second largest contributor to prime-age adult death in developing countries by the year 2020, accounting for over one third of adult deaths from infectious disease.[14]

The HIV epidemic is also decreasing life expectancy rates in developing countries, reversing the important gains made in recent decades. In Zimbabwe, life expectancy in 1998 is almost 25 years shorter than it would have been in the absence of the epidemic (Fig. 1). In Côte d'Ivoire and South Africa it is 10 years shorter, and in Brazil it is already 7 years shorter.[16] AIDS also is expected to reduce population growth rates in many countries, although it is not expected to cause negative growth or an absolute decline in population size.

Stages of the Epidemic

There is wide variation in patterns of the epidemic across countries and regions of the developing world. A useful way to compare the epidemic in different countries is according to two broad criteria: first, the extent of HIV infection among groups of people who engage in high-risk behavior, and second, whether the infection has spread to populations assumed to

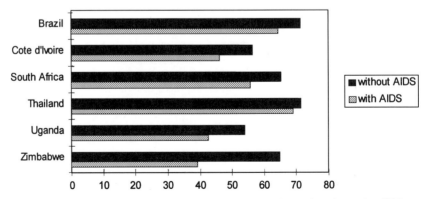

Figure 1. Effect of AIDS mortality on life expectancy at birth, selected countries, 1998.

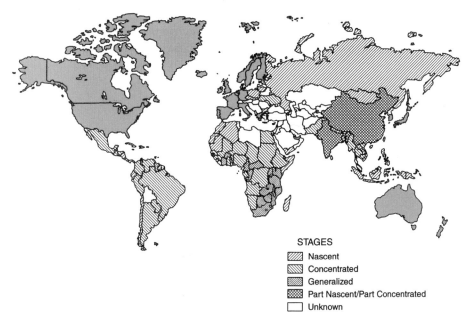

STAGES
▨ Nascent
▧ Concentrated
▦ Generalized
▩ Part Nascent/Part Concentrated
☐ Unknown

Figure 2.   Stages of the AIDS epidemic in developing countries. SOURCE: World Bank, 1997.

practice lower-risk behavior. Based on these criteria, the World Bank recently delineated a typology of "stages" of the epidemic (Fig. 2)[8]:

- Nascent: HIV prevalence is less than 5% in all known subpopulations presumed to practice high-risk behavior.
- Concentrated: HIV prevalence has surpassed 5% in one or more subpopulations presumed to practice high-risk behavior, but prevalence among women attending urban antenatal clinics is still less than 5%.
- Generalized: HIV prevalence has surpassed 5% in one or more subpopulations at high risk and among women attending urban antenatal clinics.

Sub-Saharan Africa has been hardest hit by the HIV pandemic, with 20.8 million people living with HIV/AIDS at the end of 1997. There were over 3.4 million new adult infections in 1997, the most for any region. In addition, mother-to-child transmission resulted in 530,000 newly infected children, about 90% of the world total in 1997.[1] Heterosexual transmission accounts for over 90% of all HIV infections in the region. As the epidemic matures, the average age of those contracting HIV has been decreasing and rates of newly acquired HIV are highest among young women (and to a lesser extent, young men) aged 15–24.[17]

At least 19 countries in this region have generalized epidemics. This includes most countries in southern Africa, where HIV is currently spreading fastest, probably due to ease of transportation and recent economic growth. In South Africa, the epidemic exploded in the early 1990s, as indicated by an increase in the prevalence among urban antenatal clinic attendees from 4.2% in 1991 to almost 9% in 1994. In Harare, Zimbabwe, 32% of pregnant women were infected as of 1995, and in Francistown, Botswana, 43% of pregnant women tested were HIV-positive in 1997.[1] The West African countries of Côte d'Ivoire, Benin, Burkina Faso, and Guinea-Bissau also have generalized epidemics, but HIV rates appear to be stabilizing in this region.

The AIDS epidemic also is generalized in most countries in East Africa, which was one of the first areas to suffer from AIDS. It accounts for only 15% of the region's population but over 50% of the HIV infections.[18] There is evidence that prevalence is declining in at least one East African country, Uganda, particularly among young people living in urban areas. A few sub-Saharan African countries—Cape Verde, Madagascar, Mauritania, Mauritius, and Somalia—are still at the nascent stage of the epidemic.

In South and Southeast Asia, 6.4 million persons are estimated to be living with HIV, and infection rates are increasing most rapidly in this region. Most countries in the region, including China, India, and Malaysia, have concentrated epidemics.

Levels of infection and modes of transmission vary greatly across the region. Often several epidemics occur concurrently in a single country. Genetic typing procedures have shown that there is little overlap in the epidemics among SWs and IDUs.[1] This is the situation in Thailand, where the AIDS epidemic is particularly well-documented. In Bangkok the prevalence among IDUs rose from 1% in late 1987 to over 30% 8 months later.[19] In parallel to the epidemic among IDUs, HIV was transmitted among SWs and their clients, and then to the general population.[18] By mid-1993, the prevalence was 35% among IDUs, 29% among brothel-based SWs, and 1% among pregnant women.[20] After 1993, the overall epidemic is thought to have declined, as reflected by a decrease in prevalence among young army conscripts, as discussed later in the chapter.

There are two major epidemics in China, where the government estimates that up to 200,000 people were living with HIV/AIDS at the end of 1996. One epidemic is among IDUs, who are mostly in the southwest region of the country. About 70% of all reported AIDS cases are among IDUs in the Yunnan Province,[21] and HIV prevalence in this population is estimated at 80%.[22] The other, newer epidemic is among heterosexuals, mainly along the increasingly prosperous eastern seaboard. Although rates in this region are still thought to be low, even among those at high risk, two factors suggest that HIV infection may be on the rise. First, STD rates are rising rapidly. Second, there has been large-scale migration and an increase in prostitution associated with the free-trade zones and economic reforms more generally.

In India, prevalence rates in some populations are over ten times those in neighboring China. Although surveillance is limited, between 3 and 5 million people were estimated to be infected by 1997, making India the country with the greatest number of HIV-infected persons.[1] The male-to-female ratio of reported cases id 5–1, with most female cases being SWs, although this figure may be unreliable due to underreporting. There are multiple epidemics in India, concentrated in three epicenters: Maharashtra State, Tamil Nadu State, and the northeastern states. In 1997, Maharashtra accounted for about half of all reported AIDS cases. Here the epidemic began among SWs and their clients but now has spread to the general population. In 1996, 2.4% of pregnant women in Mumbai (formerly Bombay) were infected.[1] In Tamil Nadu, where 22% of AIDS cases were reported in 1997, sexual transmission is also the primary mode of transmission, including sex between men. In the Northeast, transmission is mainly by needle sharing among IDUs. Manipur State alone reported 6% of the AIDS cases in 1997, all among IDUs.[23] Some drug clinics in this region reported HIV prevalence rates as high as 73% in 1996.[1] The epidemic is predicted to spread by heterosexual sex to the general population in all regions of India, following the pattern in other Asian countries.

In Cambodia, HIV is spreading rapidly and has already reached 40% prevalence among SWs and 2–3% of the 15- to 49-year-old population in 1997. Vietnam and Myanmar also are seeing a rapid surge on HIV prevalence rates. In Myanmar, infection among SWs increased from 4% in 1992 to over 20% in 1996, and two thirds of IDUs and about 2% of pregnant women were found infected in 1996.[1] In Vietnam, the epidemic is concentrated among IDUs: HIV prevalence was 11% in IDUs, 0.7% in SWs, and 0.04% in pregnant women 1997.[22]

The epidemic is nascent in other countries of the region, such as the Philippines, Indonesia, and Singapore. It is not clear why the epidemic has not spread more widely in these countries, which appear to have similar risk factors to those with more severe epidemics: the virus has been there for several years and sex work is common. One possible explanation regards differences in the commercial sex industry. Recent evidence suggests that the intensity of epidemics associated with SWs is primarily determined by the daily and weekly number of sex partners (clients) per sex worker, the frequency of use of commercial sex by men, and the rate of regular condom used in commercial sex. In at least two countries with low rates of HIV infection, Indonesia and the Philippines, it is thought that there are fewer customers per sex worker and a smaller percentage of men engaging in commercial sex.[23] Countries like the Philippines, Bangladesh, and Indonesia also have much less intravenous drug use. Another potential explanation for the low rates in Indonesia is the widespread availability of STD treatment.

In Latin America, about 1.3 million people are estimated to be living with HIV. More than half of the countries in Latin American have concentrated epidemics, including both Brazil and Mexico. Haiti and Guyana have generalized epidemics, and six other countries have nascent epidemics. In several countries of the region, including Brazil, Mexico, and the countries of the Southern Cone (Argentina, Chile, Paraguay, and Uruguay), HIV infections were initially concentrated among men who have sex with men and IDUs.[18] Although data are scarce for both these population groups, one study estimated that as many as 30% of Mexican men who have sex with men may be infected. Rates among IDUs vary from 5 to 11% in Mexico to close 50% in Argentina and Brazil.[1] More recently, heterosexual transmission has become predominant and now accounts for 80% of all HIV transmission in adults. This share ranges from 64% in Brazil to 93% in the Andean region (Bolivia, Colombia, Ecuador, Peru, and Venezuela).[21]

In the Caribbean, most transmission early in the epidemic also was by sex between men, but heterosexual transmission is now the primary mode of transmission. HIV rates are generally higher here than in other parts of Latin America. In Haiti, HIV prevalence increased from 2% in 1989 to 5% of the adult rural population in 1994.[21] In 1993, over 8% of pregnant women were HIV-positive.[1] In the Dominican Republic, HIV prevalence rates were also high in 1993: 11% among SWs and 1.2% in pregnant women.[21]

Reliable data about the epidemic are scarce in most countries of Eastern Europe and the Former Soviet Union, but what are available suggest that most countries have nascent epidemics. The exception is Ukraine, where the epidemic is concentrated due to a prevalence as high as 70% among IDUs.[1] There are signs, however, that the epidemic is spreading quickly in this region. The Russian Federation Health Ministry recently reported over 1500 new cases of HIV infection in 1996, a tenfold increase over 1995, and officials estimate that reported infections represent no more than 10% of the true figures.[24] Increasing incidence rates among IDUs in some of the major cities, like those in Ukraine, suggest that the epidemic may be spreading rapidly among this group in other countries as well. The potential for spread by sexual transmission also exists, as STD rates also are increasing dramatically in many countries. Between 1994 and 1995, syphilis incidence rates nearly doubled in the Russian Federation and Belarus and tripled in Kazakhstan.[21]

Although data are weak for North Africa and the Middle East, the existing data suggest that the epidemic is in the nascent stage in these regions. There is evidence, however, of rapid transmission among drug users in Bahrain and Egypt[8] and among SWs in Djibouti.

According to the World Bank, half the population of developing countries—2.3 billion people—live in areas where the epidemic is still nascent. Most live in a handful of countries, including China, India, Indonesia, and the Philippines. Another one third live in developing countries where the epidemic is concentrated but not yet generalized. There is still hope therefore of preventing a generalized epidemic in many places, but it is imperative to act quickly to prevent further HIV transmission.

EVALUATION OF HIV/AIDS PREVENTION INTERVENTIONS IN DEVELOPING COUNTRIES

The goal of HIV prevention is to minimize the number of new HIV infections. This suggests the need to focus prevention interventions on individuals who are likely to transmit HIV infection to many others, that is, those with many sexual or needle-sharing partners. Behavioral research in developing countries has identified several groups who are at particularly high risk: SWs and their clients, IDUs, truck drivers, fisherman, the military, men who have sex with men, and people with STDs. Collecting information about the incidence and prevalence among high-risk populations and about their characteristics and behaviors is a critical first step in HIV prevention.

Three broad approaches to prevention can be applied: (1) influencing individuals to engage in less risky behavior; (2) STD treatment; and (3) altering the larger social and policy environment in which people live. The first two approaches have been the most widely implemented in all countries, but the third approach, which involves structural and environmental changes, could potentially affect change on a much larger scale.

Behavioral Change at the Individual Level

We recently reviewed published evaluations of prevention interventions in developing countries (Table 3). We first examined the effectiveness of interventions that aim to change individual behavior, including condom promotion and voluntary counseling and testing. Condom promotion interventions significantly increased condom use rates when targeted to high-risk groups, such as SWs. In most of the studies we reviewed, condom use rates increased at least twofold when evaluated 6 months after program implementation. One study also showed that easy accessibility to condoms (either by free distribution or sale) was important for increasing condoms use.

We found that the effectiveness of voluntary counseling and testing (VCT) programs in

Table 3.   Interventions for HIV Prevention
in Developing Countries[a]

	Number of studies
Behavioral change	
Targeted condom promotion	6
Communitywide risk reduction	3
School-based education	2
Harm reduction among IDUs	3
Voluntary counseling and testing	12
STD treatment with or without condom promotion	6
Structural and environmental interventions	5

[a]SOURCE: Merson et al.[54]

preventing HIV transmission was mixed and depended on the population being studied. It was most effective in increasing and sustaining condom use, as well as maintaining low sero-conversion rates in uninfected partners, when directed at discordant couples. Condoms were used more consistently when the man was the HIV-negative partner, suggesting that the effectiveness of programs promoting condom use depended on its acceptance by the male partner. In other situations, such as when only one sexual partner receives VCT or among childbearing women, the effectiveness of VCT remains unclear and more evaluation is needed.

The evidence was also inconclusive as to whether behavior change as a result of VCT varies according to serostatus and more careful assessment is also needed in this area. A recent evaluation of a large VCT program in Uganda showed that those who learned they were HIV-positive were more likely to abstain from sexual activity, whereas HIV-negative clients resumed sexual activity but became more faithful to their steady partners and used condoms consistently.[25] Childbearing women who participated in studies in Zaire and Rwanda also differed in behavior according to serostatus: The women who knew they were seropositive were more likely to use condoms and had lower fertility rates than women who were seronegative. A study of childbearing women in Kenya, however, found no significant differences according to serostatus in use of oral contraceptives, condoms, or pregnancy rates 1 year after VCT.

Few studies have evaluated behavior change interventions directed at other risk groups in developing countries, such as IDUs, men who have sex with men, and youth. The only evaluation of a harm reduction program in a developing country was of a program in Kathmandu, Nepal, which distributed sterile injecting equipment and educated IDUs in its use. The program resulted in significant declines in self-reported unsafe injecting practices and a maintained low HIV seroprevalence.[26] Likewise, there was only one evaluation of an intervention for youth, which was a school-based education program for Tanzanian primary school students. Students who participated in the program had significantly higher scores than nonparticipants on a range of self-reported outcome measures regarding AIDS awareness, subjective norms, and intention to engage in sexual intercourse.[27]

STD Treatment: Alone and Combined with Targeted Condom Promotion

We also examined the effectiveness of STD treatment and interventions that combined STD treatment with condom promotion. The most convincing evidence of the effectiveness of STD treatment has come from a randomized, controlled trial in Mwanza, Tanzania. The intervention of provided community-based STD care (including training of primary health care workers in STD syndromic case management, making available effective antibiotics, and promoting health-care-seeking behavior by those infected) and reduced HIV incidence by 42% after 2 years.[28] This reduction was the result of a reduction in the duration, and hence the prevalence, of symptomatic STDs.[29] These results were collaborated by a controlled clinical study in Malawi in which men with HIV infection and urethritis were shown to have eightfold higher HIV concentrations in semen as compared with men without urethritis. Two weeks after antibiotic therapy, the HIV level decreased significantly in both gonococcal and nongonococcal urethritis patients, although the decline was less dramatic for the latter.[30] Additional evidence from a clinical study among female SWs in Abidjan also showed that cervicovaginal shedding of HIV-1 was associated with ulcerative and nonulcerative STDs and decreased significantly following treatment of STDs.[31]

At question now is the treatment protocol most effective for case management of STDs, especially among women, in resource-poor settings. Ongoing research in Abidjan is comparing the effectiveness among SWs of the "traditional" approach of treating only when symptomatic with a more intensive approach of systematically examining women every month and treating according to a thorough diagnostic and treatment strategy.[32] Preliminary results from an on-going study in Uganda of mass antibiotic treatment of STDs indicated statistically significant declines in STD symptoms and prevalence in the intervention group, although it was too soon to determine the effect on HIV incidence.[33]

All available evidence suggested that combining STD treatment with targeted condom promotion has been highly effective in reducing the spread of STDs and HIV (Table 5). This mix of interventions brought about a 62% decrease in HIV incidence in a group of SWs in Kinshasa.[34] An intervention for SWs in Calcutta combined STD treatment at a small clinic located in a high-volume, red-light district with outreach activities to SWs that include condom distribution, training in condom negotiation skills, and STD symptom recognition. Over 3 years, condom use increased substantially, incidence syphilis rates declined, and HIV prevalence remained low.[35] In Mombasa, a 12-month program for truckers provided STD screening and treatment and promoted condom use and having fewer sexual partners. The results were significantly fewer sexual encounters with SWs and extramarital sexual contacts and a decline in STD incidence rates, although there was no change in condom use.[36]

Structural and Environmental Interventions

Structural interventions change laws, policies, and standard operating procedures in a society, and environmental interventions alter living conditions, resources, opportunities, and social pressures (Table 4).[37] These approaches to promoting healthier behavior are not new to public health; they have been used successfully in the United States, for example, to reduce motorcycle injuries and automobile accidents by, respectively, mandating helmet use and decreasing speed limits and seat-belt use. Although not many structural and environmental interventions in developing countries have been implemented or evaluated, they hold the promise of being effective in reducing HIV transmission.

The most prominent example of a structural intervention in HIV prevention in a developing country is the 100% condom policy in Thailand, which mandates and enforces condom use at all commercial sex establishments. Other countries have implemented smaller-scale structural interventions. For example, in Brazil, the removal of high taxes on imported condoms helped to lower the price of condoms and to increase demand.[38] In the Dominican Republic, a

Table 4. Examples of Structural and Environmental Interventions to Reduce HIV Transmission[a]

Structural	Environmental
Enact laws and policies requiring condom use in brothels	Employ the entire family at migrant work camps
Legislate requirements for family housing in migrant labor camps	Improve STD care and expand access
Reduce taxes on condoms	Expand availability of condoms in traditional and non-traditional settings
Require that hotels stock condoms in each room	Improve the social and economic status of women (thereby increasing their bargaining power in sex)
Enact laws outlawing wife inheritance	
Subsidize condoms for individuals who engage in high-risk behavior	Reduce poverty, which would reduce migration of men and need to work in sex industry
Repeal laws that criminalize the possession of drug injection equipment	

[a]SOURCE: Authors and Sweat and Denison.[37]

pilot program increased condom use by making condoms available in hotel rooms.[39] In December 1997, the Chinese government outlawed the sale of blood, which previously provided about half the nation's blood supply and was often contaminated, and now relies entirely on voluntary donations in an effort to make the blood supply safer.[40] Other structural interventions that have the potential to reduce HIV transmission include taxes on the consumption of commodities associated with risky behavior (e.g., alcoholic beverages sold at bars) and subsidies for condoms.

The most widely implemented environmental interventions that we have been able to identify are condom social marketing programs. These programs not only promote condom use, but they also strive to make condoms available for sale in more convenient locations and condom use to be more socially acceptable. Since 1987, one organization, Population Services International, has assisted 23 African countries to develop social marketing programs. Condom sales have increased exponentially in these countries: from less than 20,000 sold in 1987 to over 150 million sold in 1995.[41] In Uganda, the social marketing scheme resulted in an increase in the sales of Protector condoms from 1.3 million in 1992 to 10 million in 1996.[42] In many countries, these programs also have paved the way for more aggressive advertising and promotion of all brads of condoms and have encouraged market diversity and expansion of the condom sector in general.[43] Beyond an increase in condom sales, however, the impact of social marketing programs in developing countries on individual behavior is not known.

Some environmental interventions aim to expand the economic power of women as a means of improving their ability to negotiate safer sex with their partners and to expand their employment opportunities (beyond commercial sex). In one area of Zambia where women fish traders were often forced into sex in exchange for fish from fisherman, economic cooperatives were set up to bargain collectively for fish and provide credit to women, thereby reducing sexual exploitation.[44] In Bangladesh, the Grameen Bank provided access to credit for rural women, which resulted in increased control of their sexual behavior as evidenced by greater contraception use rates.[45]

Other potentially important environmental interventions include promoting policies that encourage spouses and families to move with migrant laborers and expanding education for women and girls. Policies that make STD treatment more widely available and more accessible also would help to reduce the spread of HIV. One way to do this is to expand the over-the-counter availability of STD treatment and improve the training of pharmacists in treating STDs. Research in Thailand suggests that men are more likely to self-treat their STDs than to seek care at a clinic.[46]

National-Level Response: Combining Interventions

As discussed earlier in the chapter, the epidemic in Thailand spread exponentially during the 1980s. Although the governmental response did not start until 1989, it was massive and was led by the Prime Minister. It began with a nationwide condom advertising campaign and was soon followed by the 100% condom use policy. In addition, STD services and over-the-counter antibiotics were widely available.

The enormous increase in condom use and the paralleled STD and HIV decline strongly suggest that this multifaceted government response to the epidemic helped to prevent many HIV infections in Thailand.[47] Between 1989 (the year the government response was initiated) and 1995, there was an 85% decrease in the number of male STD cases presented at governmental clinics. There was a corresponding increase in condom use in brothels from 14% in 1989 to 85% in 1991 to 91% in 1993.[48] At the same time, studies in large cohorts of 21-year-old enlisted men from northern Thailand at the time of conscription showed that HIV prevalence decreased from 10.4 and 12.5% in the 1991 and 1993 cohorts, respectively, to 6.7% in the 1995 cohort.[49] More recent data have demonstrated significant declines in STD and HIV incidence among the 1991 and 1993 cohorts during their 2-year period of military service* (D. Celentano, personal communication, December 17, 1996).

There are strong indications that HIV incidence also has declined in Uganda. In Nsambya (Kampala) and Jinja, HIV prevalence among pregnant women decreased 53% and 79%, respectively, in 15- to 19-year-olds between 1991 and 1996. At the same time, there has been a significant behavior change among youth, as suggested by a comparison of data from a nationwide Knowledge, Attitudes, Practices, and Behaviors (KAPB) survey in 1989 with the results of a 1995 cross-sectional, random cluster survey carried out in five urban and rural districts. The proportion of male and females aged 15 to 19 reporting that they have never had sex declined from 31% and 26%, respectively, in 1989 to 56% and 46% in 1995. Also, in the 1995 survey, 66% of men and 49% of women in urban areas reported the use of condoms during the last sexual intercourse of risk.[50]

These positive behavioral changes have been linked to the multiplicity of interventions initiated in Uganda. These include various individual and community-based interventions implemented during the past 10 years, many of which promoted monogamy and abstinence; the social marketing campaign; improved STD treatment; and the large number of people who have been counseled and tested for HIV. All benefited from the strong political support for HIV prevention provided by the Prime Minister. The importance of a multifaceted AIDs prevention program was confirmed by a recent study that identified the marked heterogeneity in risk factors for HIV, suggesting that a variety of approaches are needed to promote prevention in diverse circumstances.[51]

IMPLICATIONS FOR PREVENTION STRATEGIES

Four factors are particularly helpful in determining the appropriate mix of prevention interventions in a particular setting: (1) information on the epidemiology of HIV and the stage of the epidemic; (2) knowledge of what types of interventions are effective; (3) information about the cost-effectiveness of specific interventions; and (4) the level of resources available for HIV prevention. The mix of interventions will necessarily vary from country to country; no single combination of interventions is appropriate in all settings.

The epidemiology of HIV suggests two clear messages for prevention.[8] First, it is imperative to act early in the epidemic, when HIV spreads exponentially. Viral load is also highest during the first few months of infection, so that early in the epidemic a large proportion of those infected may be highly infectious. And, from a budgetary perspective, it is far less costly to prevent HIV than to treat people with AIDS. Second, it is crucial to target interventions initially to those with the highest-risk behavior. This will have the greatest impact in terms of the number of new HIV infections prevented, as individuals with large numbers of sexual and needle-sharing partners who do not use condoms or clean injecting equipment are those most likely to become infected and then spread HIV. Changing the behavior of these individuals, even if only a relatively few members of society, is essential to curbing the epidemic.

Knowing the stage of the epidemic and the characteristics of the population groups most

---

*Gonorrhea declined 10-fold, syphilis 9-fold, chancroid 16-fold, and HIV incidence declined 4-fold.

at risk in a particular country can help in the selection of the most appropriate HIV prevention interventions. In the context of a nascent epidemic, for example, targeting individuals with large numbers of sexual and needle-sharing partners may be enough, but where the epidemic is concentrated or generalized, expanded prevention activities are needed (more discussion later in this section).

As explained earlier in the chapter, two particular types of interventions—condom promotion and STD treatment, both alone and in combination—have been shown to be effective in reducing HIV transmission among high-risk population groups in developing countries. The effectiveness of voluntary counseling and testing has been mixed: VCT programs prevent transmission among discordant couples, but their effectiveness in other situations is inconclusive. Although there is only evidence from one study of a harm reduction program in a developing country,[26] it is likely that such programs also could be effective in reducing HIV transmission among IDUs, as they are in industrialized countries. Structural and environmental interventions, such as the 100% condom policy in Thailand and condom social marketing, also show promise for effective HIV prevention.

Since developing country governments work in an environment of scarce resources, it is particularly important to identify interventions that are cost-effective—those that will prevent the greatest number of infections for the lowest cost. Unfortunately, only a few studies have assessed the cost-effectiveness of HIV prevention interventions.* Furthermore, the results of cost-effectiveness studies are rarely transferable from one setting to another, since they depend on HIV prevalence and other factors that vary across settings. Consequently, decisions about which prevention interventions merit support must often be made in the absence of specific information on cost-effectiveness. As a general rule, however, it is likely that interventions focused on those most likely to contract and spread HIV are most cost-effective from the public perspective, as preventing infection in a person with risky behavior prevents many more infections among individuals with whom they mix.[8]†

Not all developing countries have the same level of resources, and this necessarily influences HIV prevention choices. The focus in the lowest-income countries, in general, should first be to reach those groups that are most likely to contract and spread HIV and expand to lower-risk groups as resources permit. Of course, the severity of the epidemic also must be taken into account, and in the context of a generalized epidemic it will be necessary to find additional resources to implement broad-based interventions. Middle-income countries may have enough additional resources to extend prevention efforts beyond those at highest risk, but first priority should always be to high-risk groups.[8]

We now illustrate how policy makers might use information about these four factors to select a combination of interventions for their country (Table 5). This discussion is meant to identify the highest-priority interventions and is not prescriptive or exhaustive, as the appropriate mix of interventions is necessarily country-specific. Overall, the prevention strategy requires an emphasis on prevention activities focused on those at highest risk of contracting and spreading HIV and then addressing as many other lower-risk population groups where the epidemic is more severe.

For a developing country with a nascent epidemic, the goal is to prevent any further spread of the epidemic among high-risk populations. Countries in this situation, such as

---

*Appendix B in Confronting AIDS: Public Priorities in a Global Epidemic (World Bank, 1997) provides a list of these studies.

†In some situations, however, it is difficult to reach those most likely to contract and spread HIV because of legal sanctions and social stigma. This can increase the cost of reaching these groups and can have a significant impact on the cost-effectiveness of intervention programs.

Table 5:   Research and Intervention Priorities for HIV Prevention by Stage of Epidemic

State of epidemic	Priority prevention research and interventions

Nascent epidemic	Research and information collection
	    Surveillance to monitor the levels of HIV and STDs among population groups at highest risk for HIV
	    Behavioral research to understand the behaviors of groups at highest risk for HIV and how to reach them
	    Sentinel surveillance to monitor the spread of the epidemic in the population at large, to the extent that resources permit
	Interventions
	    Individual-based and structural–environmental interventions to promote safe sexual practices and safe injecting behavior among those with many partners
	    STD treatment for groups at highest risk for HIV

Concentrated epidemic	Research and information collection
	    Surveillance to monitor the levels of HIV and STDs among population groups at highest risk for HIV
	    Surveillance to monitor the spread of HIV to population groups at lower risk for HIV (e.g., pregnant women and appropriate groups)
	    Behavioral research to understand the behaviors of those at highest risk and how to reach them
	Interventions
	    Individual-based and structural–environmental interventions to promote safe sexual practices and safe injecting behavior among those with many partners
	    STD treatment for groups at high risk and expanded to groups at lower risk to the extent that resources permit
	    Condom social marketing focused narrowly to those at highest risk and expanded to groups at lower risk to the extent that resources permit
	    School-based sex–HIV education to the extent that resources permit

Generalized epidemic	Research and information collection
	    Surveillance to monitor the epidemic in all population groups
	    Behavior research to understand the risk behaviors of groups at high and lower risk for HIV and how to reach them
	Interventions
	    Individual-based and structural–environmental interventions to promote safe injecting behavior among those with many partners, and among populations group at lower risk, to the extent that resources permit
	    High-quality STD treatment for all population groups
	    Broad-based social marketing of condoms
	    School-based sex/HIV education
	    Mass-media HIV education

[a]SOURCE: Authors' conclusions and recommendations in World Bank, 1997.[8]

Ecuador, Madagascar, and the Philippines, have the opportunity to prevent a more severe epidemic and thereby avert higher costs in human suffering and economic loss. The priority in these countries is twofold. First, epidemiological surveillance should monitor the prevalence and when possible the incidence of HIV and other STDs among groups at highest risk for contracting and spreading HIV. Behavioral research should examine risky behaviors among these populations, the contexts in which they occur, and the motivations of those who engage in them. It is equally important to implement individual-level interventions in these populations using this information that promote safe sexual practices and safe injecting behaviors (such as condom promotion and harm reduction programs). STD treatment for those at highest risk for HIV should be improved and expanded.

Policy makers in countries with a nascent epidemic also should consider focused structural and environmental interventions (such as the 100% condom use rule and targeted social marketing of condoms), which may result in behavior change among high-risk populations more quickly and at less expense than individually targeted programs. As resources permit, countries also may want to establish sentinel surveillance among pregnant women (and other populations such as military recruits) to monitor the spread of the epidemic in the population at large. A sensible approach is to start such surveillance in the areas expected to be hardest hit by the epidemic (usually the largest urban centers) and expand beyond these areas as resources permit.

A wide range of countries are currently confronting concentrated epidemics, including Brazil, Malaysia, and Ukraine. Surveillance and behavioral research among groups at highest risk for HIV continues to be important. These efforts will need to be expanded to include sentinel surveillance of pregnant woman and other suitable populations as a way to monitor the spread of the epidemic in the population at large. Individual-level interventions to promote safe sexual practices and safe injecting behavior among those most likely to contract and spread HIV, as well as STD treatment for these groups, should be sustained. Structural and environmental interventions, such as increasing the availability of condoms through social marketing, also should continue to target those at highest risk for HIV. To the extent that resources permit, some countries may be able to expand these interventions to groups at relatively lower risk, as well as implement additional ones such as school-based sex/HIV education.

In the context of a generalized epidemic, surveillance, behavioral research and prevention interventions focused on those at highest risk for HIV must continue. Containing the epidemic, however, will require prevention efforts to be expanded to people with relatively lower levels of risk for HIV. This could include expanded STD treatment, broad-based social marketing of condoms, and additional behavioral interventions such as school-based sex/HIV education. To the extent that resources permit, it is also important to provide mass media information on how to prevent HIV transmission. Expanding prevention activities to the population at-large will likely raise the costs of HIV prevention, but this will be necessary to contain the epidemic.

FUTURE DIRECTIONS FOR PREVENTION RESEARCH

Although developing countries have made impressive strides in documenting the spread of HIV and in preventing additional infections, the epidemic is still expanding in many places and increased effort is needed to contain it. Research on prevention plays a key role in identifying the most effective strategies to confront the epidemic. Priorities for future research include work in five key areas: behavioral research, evaluation of prevention interventions, cost assessment of prevention programs, research to improve prevention technologies, and training of researchers from developing countries.

More Information on the Characteristics and Behaviors of Those at Highest Risk

For many developing countries, we still do not know how many people engage in risky behaviors, how often they do so, and if and when they take precautions to reduce their risk. Our understanding of the risky practices themselves is also limited. Information about the rate of partner change and level of condom use in the general population is also unavailable. Studies by the World Health Organization Global Program on AIDS on behavioral risk factors and others, specifically on drug-injecting behavior, have expanded our knowledge, but coverage is still limited to a small part of the developing world.[8] Without this information it is impossible to predict how fast the epidemic will spread and how best to focus prevention interventions.

Evaluation of the Effectiveness of Prevention Interventions

Based on existing evaluations, we know that condom promotion and STD treatment are effective when targeted to high-risk groups and SWs in particular. Much less is known about the effectiveness of interventions targeted to other risk groups, such as IDUs, men who have sex with men, youth, and women who are not SWs. It is urgent that future prevention research address these gaps. While there have been several evaluations of VCT programs, the evidence is mixed and more rigorous evaluations would help us draw conclusions about what works. Analysis to assess the relative importance of testing versus counseling and issues related to the duration, timing, quality, and quantity of counseling also would be particularly useful. Finally, although it is rarely possible to conduct randomized controlled experiments in behavioral research, future prevention research should make more extensive use of quasi-experimental design and the statistical methods available to analyze these types of data.*

More evaluation also is needed of HIV-related structural or environmental interventions, as these programs hold tremendous potential to change behavior. For example, we do not know the impact of social marketing programs in developing countries. Are those who buy condoms those who are most at risk of transmitting HIV? What are the effects of these programs on condom use and HIV transmission rates? In addition, more extensive evaluation of national-level programs that combine structural, environmental, and individual-level interventions would be informative for policymakers.

Assessment of the Costs of Prevention and Mitigation Efforts

Very few studies of the cost-effectiveness of HIV prevention programs exist and most of these measure impact based on changes in intermediate behaviors believed to reduce risk (e.g., condom use). The only available assessment of the impact on secondary infections is based on model simulations.[8] Research that fills these gaps would make a strong contribution to decision making about how to allocate scarce resources for HIV prevention.

Research to Improve Prevention Technologies

Several new and developing technologies have the potential to change the scope and effectiveness of prevention interventions in significant ways. The most obvious example is research for an effective vaccine and efforts to support this effort should continue. The female condom and vaginal microbicides also hold promise as additional barrier methods for sexual transmission. These have the advantage over the traditional condom in that they can be used by women. Finally, research is needed to investigate what role, if any, the newly available drugs for HIV treatment can have in decreasing HIV transmission in the developing world. In particular, the analysis could assess how prevention goals can be addressed within the context of the recent UNAIDS initiative to provide wider access to HIV-related drugs in developing countries.[52]

---

*For a discussion of statistical methods available to evaluated non-randomized data, see Moffitt.[53]

Training More Researchers from Developing Countries

One reason that not enough prevention research is taking place in developing countries is that too few researchers from these countries have the appropriate training. A fundamental aspect of improving prevention research in developing countries therefore is to expand the training of researchers from developing countries. This includes training more social and behavioral scientists, epidemiologists, and economists, among other specialties, so that more of them are able to conduct much-needed prevention research.

REFERENCES

1. UNAIDS. *Report of the Global HIV/AIDS Epidemic*. Geneva: WHO; December 1997.
2. Quinn TC, Ruff A, Halsey N. Special consideration for developing countries. In: Pizzo PA, Wilfert CM, eds. *Pediatric AIDS: The Challenge of HIV Infection in Infants, Children and Adolescents*. Baltimore, MD: Williams and Wilkins; 1994:31–50.
3. May MM, Anderson RM. Transmission dynamics of HIV infection. *Nature* 1987; 326:137–142.
4. Royce RA, Sena A, Cates W, et al. Sexual transmission of HIV. *N Engl J Med* 1997; 336(15):1072–1078.
5. Hayes R, Mosha F, Nicoll A, et al. A community trial of the impact of improved sexually transmitted disease treatment on the HIV epidemic in rural Tanzania: Design. *AIDS* 1995; 9:919–926.
6. Laga M, Manoka A, Kivuvu M, et al. Non-ulcerative sexually transmitted diseases as risk factors for Hiv-1 transmission in women: results from a cohort study. *AIDS* 1993; 7:95–102.
7. Robinson NJ, Mulder DM, Auvert B, Hayes RJ. Proportion of HIV infections attributable to other sexually transmitted diseases in a rural Ugandan population: Simulation model estimates. *Int J Epidemiol* 1997; 26: 180–189.
8. World Bank. *Confronting AIDS: Public Priorities in a Global Epidemic*. New York: Oxford University Press; 1997.
9. Morris M, Podhisita C, Wawer M, Handcock MS. Bridge populations in the spread of HIV/AIDS. *AIDS* 1996; 10:1267–1271.
10. Anderson R. The spread of HIV and sexual mixing patterns. In: Mann J, Tarantola D, eds. *AIDS in the World II: Global Dimensions, Social Roots, and Responses*. The Global AIDS Policy Coalition. New York: Oxford University Press; 1996:71–86.
11. Vuylsteke B, Sunkutu R, Laga M. Epidemiology of HIV and sexually transmitted infections in women. In: Mann J, Tarantola D, eds. *AIDS in the World II: Global Dimensions, Social Roots, and Responses*. The Global AIDS Policy Coalition. New York: Oxford University Press; 1996:
12. Tyndall M, Malisa M, Plummer FA. Cefriaxone no longer predictably cures chancroid in Kenya. *J Infect Dis* 1993; 167:469–471.
13. Gangakhedkar RR, Bentley ME, Divekar AD, et al. Spread of HIV infection in married monogamous women in India. *JAMA* 1997; 278:2090–2092.
14. Murray C, Lopez AD. The global burden of disease. In: *Global Burden of Disease and Injury Series*, vol. 1 WHO, Harvard School of Public Health, World Bank. Cambridge, MA: Harvard University Press; 1996:
15. Mulder DW, Nunn AJ, Kamali A, et al. Two-year HIV-1 associated mortality in a Ugandan rural population. *Lancet* 1994; 343:1021–1023.
16. US Bureau of the Census. World population profile: 1998 with a special chapter focusing on HIV/AIDS in the developing world. US Department of Commerce, Washington, DC: US Government Printing Office; 1998.
17. UNAIDS. *HIV/AIDS: The Global Epidemic Fact Sheet*. Geneva: WHO; December 1996.
18. Mertens TE, Low-Beer D. HIV and AIDS: Where is the epidemic going? *Bull World Health Organ* 1996; 74(2):121–129.
19. Weniger BG, Limpakarnjanarat K, Ungchusak K, et al. The epidemiology of HIV infection and AIDS in Thailand. *AIDS* 1991; 5(suppl 2):S71–85.
20. Brown T, Sittitrai W, Vanichseni S, Thisyakorn U. The recent epidemiology of HIV and AIDS in Thailand. *AIDS* 1994; 8(suppl 2):S131–S141.
21. UNAIDS. *The Status and Trends of the Global HIV/AIDS Pandemic: Final Report*. Paper presented at Eleventh International Conference on AIDS, Vancouver, Canada; July 7–12, 1996.
22. Muller O, Ungchusak K, Leng HB, et al. HIV and AIDS in Southeast Asia. *Lancet* 1997; 350:288.

23. Monitoring the AIDS Epidemic (MAP). The status and trends of the HIV/AIDS/STD epidemics in Asia and the Pacific. Report for the Fourth International Conference on AIDS in Asia and the Pacific, Manila, Philippines; October 21–23, 1997.

24. Specter M. AIDS onrush sends Russia to the edge of an epidemic. *New York Times* November 1, 1997.

25. Moore M, Tukwasiibwe E, Marum E, et al. Impact of HIV counseling and testing in Uganda. XI International Conference on AIDS, Vancouver; July 1996. Abstract WS C 16-4.

26. Peak A, Rana S, Maharjan SH, et al. Declining risk for HIV among injecting drug users in Kathmandu, Nepal: The impact of a harm-reduction program. *AIDS* 1995; 9:1067–1070.

27. Klepp K, Ndeki S, Seha A, et al. AIDS education for primary school children in Tanzania: An evaluation study. *AIDS* 1994; 8:1157–1162.

28. Grosskurth H, Mosha F, Todd J, et al. Impact of improved treatment of STDs on HIV infection in rural Tanzania: Randomised controlled trial. *Lancet* 1995; 346:530–537.

29. Mayaud P, Mosha F, Todd J, et al. Improved treatment services significantly reduce the prevalence of sexually transmitted diseases in rural Tanzania: Results of a randomized controlled trial. *AIDS* 1997; 11:1873–1880.

30. Cohen MS, Hoffman IF, Royce RA, et al. Reduction of concentration of HIV-1 in semen after treatment of urethritis: Implications for prevention of sexual transmission of HIV-1. *Lancet* 1997; 349:1868–1873.

31. Ghys PD, Fransen K, Diallo MO, et al. The associations between cervicovaginal HIV shedding, sexually transmitted diseases and immunosuppression in female sex workers in Abidjan, Cote d'Ivoire. *AIDS* 1997; 11: F85–F93.

32. Ettiegne-Traore V, Ghys PD, Diallo MO, et al. HIV seroincidence and STD prevalence during an intervention study among female sex workers in Abidjan, Cote d'Ivoire: Preliminary Findings. XI International Conference on AIDS, Vancouver; July 1996. Abstract Mo C 442.

33. Wawer MJ, Sewankambo NK, Gray RH, et al. Community-based trial of mass STD treatment for HIV control, Rakai, Uganda: Preliminary Data on STD declines. XI International Conference on AIDS, Vancouver; July 1996. Abstract Mo D 443.

34. Laga M, Alary M, Nzila N, et al. Condom promotion, sexually transmitted diseases treatment, and declining incidence of HIV-1 infection in female Zairian sex workers. *Lancet* 1994; 344:246–248.

35. O'Reilly KO, Mertens T, Sethi G, et al. *Evaluation of the Sonagachi Project.* Geneva: World Health Organization; November 1995.

36. Jackson D, Rakwar, J, Richardson B, et al. Decreased incidence of sexually transmitted diseases among trucking company workers in Kenya: Results of a behaviour risk-reduction programme. *AIDS* 1997; 11:903–909.

37. Sweat MD, Denison JA. Reducing HIV incidence in developing countries with structural and environmental interventions. *AIDS* 1995; 9(suppl A):S251–S257.

38. Tawil O, Verster A, O'Reilly KR. Enabling approaches for HIV/AIDS prevention: can we modify the environment and minimize the risk? *AIDS* 1995; 9:1299–1306.

39. Guerrero E, De Moya EA, Rosario S. *Ongoing Impact of the Condom Use Promotion/Desensitization Program for preventing AIDS in the Dominican Republic.* Santo Domingo: Programa ETS/SIDA (PROCETS); 1988.

40. China outlaws selling of blood. *Washington Times*, December 30, 1997, p. A11.

41. Meekers D. Population Services International, Washington, DC. Personal communication, November 11, 1996.

42. *Contraceptive Social Marketing: 1996 Annual Sales Report.* Washington, DC: SOMARC/The Futures Group International; 1997.

43. *The Transition to the Commercial Sector: What happens to Socially Marketed Products after Graduating from USAID Support?* Special Study 1. Washington, DC: The Futures Group International; August 1997.

44. Msiska R. *An Intervention Study to Develop and Test the Benefits of an Enabling Approach in Reducing HIV Transmission in a Fish Trading Community in Zambia.* Lusaka: National AIDS Programme; 1994.

45. Schuler SR, Hashemi SM. Credit programs, women's empowerment and contraceptive use in rural Bangladesh. *Stud Fam Plann* 1994; 25:65–76.

46. Khamboonruang D, Seyrer C, Natpratam C, et al. Human immunodeficiency virus infection and self-treatment for sexually transmitted diseases among northern Thai men. *Sex Transm Dis* 1996; 23:264–269.

47. Robinson NJ, Hanenberg H. Condoms used during most commercial sex acts in Thailand. *AIDS* 1997; 11:1064–1065.

48. Hanenberg R, Rojanapithayakorn W, Kunasol P, Sokal D. Impact of Thailand's HIV-control programme as indicated by the decline of sexually transmitted diseases. *Lancet* 1994; 344:243–245.

49. Nelson KE, Ecentano D, Eiumtrakol S, et al. Changes in sexual behavior and a decline in HIV infection among young men in Thailand. *N Engl J Med* 1996; 335:297–303.

50. Asiimwe-Okiror G, Opio A, Musinguzi J, et al. Change in sexual behavior and decline in HIV infection among young pregnant women in urban Uganda. *AIDS* 1997; 11:1757–1763.

51. Quigley M, Munguti K. Grosskurth H, et al. Sexual behaviour patterns and other risk factors for HIV infection in rural Tanzania: A case–control study. *AIDS* 1997; 11:237–248.

52. UNAIDS. *UNAIDS HIV Drug Initiative: Providing Wider Access to HIV-Related Drugs in Developing Countries. Pilot Phase Background Document.* Geneva: WHO; October 1997.

53. Moffitt, R. The use of selection modeling to evaluate AIDS interventions with observational data. In: *Evaluating AIDS Prevention Programs.* Washington, DC: National Research Council; 1991:342–364.

54. Merson MH, Dayton JM, O'Reilly KR. Effectiveness of HIV prevention interventions in developing countries. *AIDS*, in press.

13

HIV Prevention in Industrialized Countries

KIM RIVERS and PETER AGGLETON

INTRODUCTION

Acquired immunodeficiency syndrome (AIDS) was first diagnosed in the United States in the early 1980s, and since that time every country in the world has reported cases. In the short term, the prospect of a preventive vaccine is not encouraging.[1] New therapeutic agents have offered some people with human immunodeficiency virus (HIV) a substantially improved quality of life and the possibility of a near-normal life span.[2] However, the consequences of HIV/AIDS continue to be very serious even in countries where there are resources to pay for new treatments. A combination of social and behavioral change therefore remains essential in reducing the risk of HIV infection.[2,3] Over the last 15 years, a great deal has been learned about the kinds of programs and interventions that are most effective in preventing HIV infection. In this chapter, we will describe and review some of the major HIV prevention initiatives that have taken place in Australia, Canada, New Zealand, and selected countries in Western Europe.

The Impact of HIV Infection in Industrialized Countries

Groups most affected by HIV and AIDS in industrialized countries include those already widely discriminated against and marginalized in society, such as gay men and injecting drug users. The consequences of HIV/AIDS have been felt not only by individuals, families, and communities, but by the health system, education and other public sectors, and the economy. People affected by AIDS routinely have experienced ignorance, stigmatization, and ostracization, which may lead to feelings of isolation and sometimes shame.[4,5] Not surprisingly, disclosure of HIV status constitutes another major source of stress for HIV-positive people.[6] Persons affected by HIV/AIDS report concerns about their continuing health, future welfare, longevity, and ability to earn a living.[4]

People with HIV additionally often face the stress of caring for other people who are ill.[4] Individuals, families, and networks of friends affected by HIV are not infrequently denied the support usually available to people who have another life-threatening diseases.[5] Women with HIV/AIDS in particular, who traditionally are expected to be carers and nurturers, may face the additional worry of caring for others.[6] In Australia, for example, some women with HIV/

KIM RIVERS and PETER AGGLETON • Thomas Coram Research Unit, Institute of Education, University of London, London, WC1H 0AA England.

Handbook of HIV Prevention, edited by Peterson and DiClemente.
Kluwer Academic/Plenum Publishers, New York, 2000.

AIDS have been faced with the choice of accessing services that are HIV-friendly but not necessarily woman-friendly, or services that are women-friendly but not necessarily HIV-friendly.[6] In some contexts, HIV-related services designed to meet the needs of women with children have been largely nonexistent.[6] Additionally, women of reproductive age who are infected with HIV face difficult choices about future childbearing.[7] Although perinatal zidovudine prophylaxis considerably reduces the risk of HIV transmission from mother to child, women still have to consider this risk alongside anxieties that they may not live long enough to raise their child.[7]

As well as these human costs, HIV/AIDS imposes a financial burden on society.[2] It has been estimated in Canada that every 1000 new HIV infection adds approximately $100 million to collective future direct medical costs and approximately $600 million to indirect costs.[8]

Epidemiological Data from Selected Industrialized Countries

An analysis of the patterns of HIV and AIDS within and between countries reveals that what appears to be a global epidemic is in fact a series of overlapping microepidemics, and there can be substantial variations in the course of the epidemic in different countries.[9] Across industrialized countries, then, there have been not one but several epidemics of HIV and AIDS. For example, in Ireland to the end of 1994, the incidence rate of AIDS was 10.2 per million population, while for the same period the rate for Italy was 73.9.[10] Trends also vary in relation to whether the incidence of AIDS is stabilizing, declining, or increasing. In some countries—Switzerland, Netherlands, and New Zealand, for example—the total number of AIDS cases reported per year has stabilized or is declining.[2,9] In other countries, such as Ireland and Portugal, the number of cases is increasing.[2] However, overall upward or downward trends in the number of new cases diagnosed nationally may disguise a more complex picture, whereby cases are rising among some groups and stabilizing or decreasing among others. In Canada, for example, there appears to be a plateau or decrease of cases of HIV infection among gay and bisexual men, but an increase in cases among injecting drug users and heterosexuals.[2]

While some groups of people have been disproportionately affected by AIDS, the groups most affected vary. In northwestern Europe, for example, gay men and their partners have been most affected, while in parts of southern Europe the majority of infections have been linked to injecting drug use.[11] So, for example, until December 1994, 66% of all cases of AIDS in Spain had been among injecting drug users, while for the same period in Great Britain 73.7% of cumulative cases of AIDS had been among gay and bisexual men.[10] The rates of infection for those groups most affected, however, vary widely between countries and even cities. HIV prevalence has been reported as less than 5% among injecting drug users in Glasgow, Scotland, while in some other European cities the prevalence of HIV among injecting drug users has been reported as being over 50%.[2] The incidence of HIV infection also varies within groups. For example, in some countries HIV incidence is declining among gay and bisexual men aged over 30 but not among younger gay men.[2] Conversely, in a number of settings older injecting drug users appear to be at greater risk of infection than those who are younger.[2]

While no developed country has experienced a heterosexual epidemic on the scale of those characteristic of many developing countries, heterosexual transmission is steadily increasing.[2] Moreover, there is potential for a further increase in HIV infection among heterosexually active adults, since national surveys in a number of industrialized countries suggest that many are reluctant to adopt safer sex practices.[2,12]

Variations in the nature of the epidemic across and within industrialized countries and between groups who are most affected reflect both diversity in behavioral patterns and differences in the responses of communities and national and regional systems of government. Local responses to HIV have been influenced by prevailing norms about drug use and sexual behavior, attitudes toward vulnerable groups, the role of the state in public health, and pre-existing systems of health care.[11] HIV prevention efforts have been characterized by both great successes and significant failures. It is important, therefore, to determine why and how certain responses and interventions have helped reduce and stabilize new cases of HIV infection, while in other contexts rates have increased.

STRATEGIES OF INTERVENTION

Responses to HIV and AIDS have varied widely between industrialized countries. Early in the epidemic many interventions for prevention were based on theoretical frameworks such as the theory of reasoned action, protection motivation theory, social learning, and the health belief model. These models placed the emphasis for HIV prevention on information-giving, discussion, and skills development to change individual behavior.

Many countries also undertook mass media campaigns to raise awareness about HIV and AIDS among the general public.[3,11] The often unspoken assumption of these approaches was that once people had acquired the necessary information and skills, they would change their behavior to protect themselves against HIV.[13,14] This simplistic analysis did not take adequate account of the social context in which behavior takes place. It also led to "victim blaming" whereby people infected with HIV were made to shoulder the responsibility for having become infected, marginalizing concern for the influence of the complex social and cultural factors affecting peoples' lives.

The middle years of the epidemic were characterized by a move away from such individualized models of intervention, largely because of the recognition that access to information does not necessarily lead to changes in behavior.[15] A discernable shift took place toward models focused more at the level of community.[11] Although programs and interventions that might be characterized as community-level are diverse, they share a common concern with changing norms by working with people assumed to share certain social experiences in common.[11,14]

Positive community responses have been cited as one of the most important factors in preventing HIV/AIDS.[16] Indeed, swift responses from within the communities most affected, such as gay men, have been characteristic of many successful responses to the epidemic.[2] Although such grassroots activity has played an important role in decreasing rates of HIV infection, success is largely dependent on preexisting levels of community organization[2] and the willingness of those providing health and other services to make links with affected groups. Some of the groups most vulnerable to HIV infection have been socially isolated, lacking in power, and least able to organize a united and concerted response to HIV/AIDS.

Although community-based interventions take greater account of the social context in which HIV risk-related behavior occurs than more individual-level approaches, both rely on communication to encourage individuals and groups to change their behavior. Elsewhere, it has been argued that efforts through communication to persuade individuals and groups to reduce risk behavior will have limited success in the absence of more generally supportive environments.[14,17] Tawil et al.,[13] for example, have distinguished between prevention approaches that aim to "persuade" people to change their behavior and those that "enable" changes to occur. The latter, they write, focus on the nonindividual, or social and environmental, determinants that facilitate or impede behavioral choice. Enabling approaches intend to remove barriers or constraints. Similarly, Baldo[18] has argued that social policies that might inhibit the growth of the epidemic must be in place to significantly reduce the risk of HIV infection. For example, policies that promote greater equality between men and women are important, since the power and economic disadvantage women commonly experience places them at increased vulnerability to HIV infection. Stryker et al.[1] also have highlighted the cultural constraints that often restrict the frank and open discussion of sex and drug use. Legal restraints, as well as political, religious, and other considerations, may also pose a barrier to the implementation of appropriate HIV prevention programs.

Individualized, community-level, and structural interventions are rarely independent of each other.[17] Often a combination of approaches is built into HIV prevention programs so that both persuasive and enabling techniques are combined. Tawil et al.[13] have suggested that it is important to consider how enabling approaches can work with rather than replace persuasive initiatives. The impact of any single approach will inevitably be limited and the most successful interventions are those that combine a number of different ways of working so as to achieve the common goal of the prevention of HIV infection.[14]

The need to evaluate HIV prevention strategies has been widely acknowledged,[19] and it is crucial to know whether or not what we do in relation to HIV prevention has the desired effect. Important questions recently have been raised about the evaluation methods that are the most appropriate.[20] Early in the epidemic systematic evaluation to determine whether or not programs had been effective was unusual. Recently, there has been a noticeable move toward what has been called evidence-based HIV prevention interventions, which means that program planners must take more care to offer concrete evidence of effectiveness.[20]

The success of HIV prevention can be evaluated using observation, objectives-based evaluation, experimental evaluation, and comparative designs.[17] Recently, it has been suggested that experimental methods and randomized controlled trials offer a gold standard in terms of providing evidence of whether or not a program is effective.[21] However, in addition to being costly, the evidence generated through randomized controlled trials and other experimental methods may not be easily generalizable.[20] It also may be difficult to apply these designs to the evaluation of programs aimed at large population groups or national strategies.[19] In relation to the evaluation of mass media campaigns, it may be difficult to attribute outcomes to specific interventions, since it may not be possible to distinguish campaign effects from those due to other interventions and activities.[11]

HIV-RELATED HEALTH PROMOTION IN SELECTED INDUSTRIALIZED COUNTRIES

Wellings and Field[11] identify two strategic options that need to be balanced in HIV and AIDS education: addressing the entire population universally, or working with specific groups. In the industrialized world, where while the entire population is potentially at-risk, specific groups have been disproportionately affected; thus, both approaches have been used. Usually, those interventions designed to reach the general population have used the mass media as a vehicle for providing education about HIV and AIDS, while particular groups have been selectively targeted at individual and community level.

The General Population and Mass Media Approaches

National mass media campaigns have been the most important measures targeted at the population as a whole in an effort to provide information and raise awareness about HIV/

AIDS.[11,22] Wellings and Field,[11] for example, have written that the AIDS epidemic has seen "the use of the mass media in health promotion on a scale unprecedented in the sphere of public health" (p. vii). While public awareness about HIV and AIDS may be raised by the use of mass media, the effects on behavior may be negligible.[11] Nevertheless, mass media activity continues to be important, since these campaigns can create an environment that is conducive to other types of interventions.[11] Additionally, media campaigns may help to create agenda that render grassroots and other initiatives more credible and acceptable.[11] In the Netherlands, Kok et al.[23] have concluded that the most important contribution made by media campaigns has been one of getting people's attention and involvement and providing an umbrella for other local and risk-group-oriented interventions. Public recognition of HIV as an issue worthy of attention may therefore be "an important precondition for mobilization against AIDS and the emergence and stabilization of community-based work."[11,p.5]

The mass media also can be important in changing social norms. For example, open discussion related to sex, sexuality, and drug use have become more common in industrialized countries since the beginning of the epidemic. While there have been controversies and obstacles in producing clear messages about HIV/AIDS, a great deal of progress has been made in a short time and many barriers have been eroded.[11] For example, a ban on the advertising of condom use in Belgium was lifted in the face of the epidemic in 1987, and the more general " normalization" of condoms "across Europe reflects the success of efforts to change the social context in which AIDS public education has been carried out."[11,p.115]

An evaluation of the impact of mass media campaigns in France during the early 1990s reached similar conclusions. Nearly all respondents remembered seeing television advertisements about condoms, while 71% reported remembering seeing advertisements about HIV/ AIDS. Over 48% of those sampled felt that they had been influenced by the campaigns and over 25% declared that they had become more concerned about personal risk of HIV infection. While there is little evidence that mass media campaigns in france led directly to behavioral change, the mass media exerted an influence on social norms and increased people's perceptions of normative pressure to use practice safer sex. Moatti et al.[24] suggest than that media campaigns "contributed to change [in condoms] social image" (p. 245). Additionally and importantly, people who reported being influenced by the campaigns were less like to express discrimination toward people infected with HIV.[24] Such normative effects may only be sustained, however, if regular media messages continue to be presented.

The importance of regular and consistent HIV/AIDS information is emphasized by Wellings and Field[11] in their evaluation of the effects of campaigns that have concentrated on condom use. Examining data on condom use in Europe, they claim that remarkable achievements were made between 1986 and 1989. However, cross-cultural comparisons demonstrate that the most sustained increases in condom use took place in countries where campaigns have been maintained over time, for example, in Switzerland where the well-known Stop AIDS campaign has consistently promoted condom use as its main message. Here, the use of condoms with nonregular partners among people aged 17–30 years increased from 8% in 1987 to 56% in 1994, and from 22% in 1989 to 42% in 1994 among those aged 31–45.[25] Conversely, in Great Britain, where there have been variable and inconsistent campaigns for condom use, reported increases in condom use have been less marked and more variable both between groups and over time.[11]

In the early 1980s, national mass media messages played an important role in efforts to counter the negative, sensationalized, and inaccurate reporting widespread in much unpaid-for press coverage. Since 1987, French media campaigns had the dual aim of preventing HIV infection and countering discrimination through messages designed to promote empathy, understanding, and solidarity with people living with HIV/AIDS.[11] In Norway, the Care Campaign of the late 1980s also was designed to prevent discrimination against people affected by HIV/AIDS.[22] However, surveys after the campaign indicated that large numbers of people continued to approve of discriminatory measures, including the compulsory HIV testing of foreigners and laws to prohibit people with HIV from having sexual relations. Indeed, 21% of those surveyed in 1991 advocated the isolation of people with AIDS.[22] These attitudes were most prevalent, however, among those who had the poorest knowledge of the ways in which HIV is transmitted, which may suggest that at the time of the evaluation certain sectors of the population had not yet been exposed to adequate information about HIV/AIDS.

Elsewhere, some of the messages about HIV/AIDS in the mass media have been contradictory and may have reinforced negative stereotypes and misinformation. Wellings and Field[11] have noted that in Sweden, for example, mass media images of sex workers gave the impression that they were predatory and a reservoir of infection. In Spain, a 1987 campaign mentioned a number of highly theoretical risks through which no cases of transmission had actually been reported, including sharing a toothbrush. Not surprisingly, research in the early 1990s showed that one third of Spanish people surveyed believed HIV could be transmitted through saliva.[26] Clearly the content of the messages about HIV/AIDS is crucial if misinformation and discrimination are to be reduced.

Early prevention campaigns often relied on fear to motivate behavior change. Characteristic of this approach was the Don't Die of Ignorance campaign, which ran between 1986 and 1987 in Great Britain. This campaign featured coffins, icebergs, and erupting volcanoes. While Wellings and Field[11] do not completely discount the value of fear-inducing approaches, they note that they are likely to produce limited results and only then in very particular circumstances, for example, where the threat is perceived by the audience as real and preventive action is available and understood.

People may react more positively to messages based on humor rather than fear.[27,28] The Danish Think Twice campaign included a series of humorous TV advertisements.[11] Evaluation research showed that recall was highest for these humorous advertisements when compared with fear-inducing messages reaching Denmark from overseas, which interestingly were thought by some respondents to be "un-Danish."[11] Danish respondents also reported that fear-inducing messages were difficult to take seriously, unintentionally funny, propagandalike, and likely to lead to blame and discrimination. This evaluation underlines the importance of context as well as content.

HIV-Related Risk Reduction with Gay Men

In industrialized countries, the majority of cases of HIV infection have occurred within a few particular groups, including gay and bisexual men, who still represent more than 50% of cases of AIDS in western Europe, Australia, Canada, and New Zealand. This has raised a number of issues for prevention, including the importance of promoting awareness among those at highest risk, while not generating panic or reinforcing widespread stigmatization.[29]

Pollack et al.[29] offer an overview of programs aimed at gay men in western Europe during the early 1980s. They note that almost everywhere the active involvement of voluntary and grassroots gay organizations preceded national and governmental initiatives. In Australia, too, gay communities responded to the epidemic before government funding was available and organized a wide range of preventive education activities including pamphlets, posters, newspaper advertisements, seminars, and conferences.[30] The effects of these early community activities were reported decreases in the incidence of gonorrhoea among gay men from early 1980s onward, at a time long before national HIV preventive education had occurred.[30]

By 1985, surveys across Europe showed that there was a high level of knowledge about HIV/AIDS among gay and bisexual men.[29] Behavior changes were observed soon after, with research in Great Britain and France demonstrating that the number of reported sexual partners among gay and bisexual men dropped substantially in the mid- to late-1980s.[29] Surveys also showed a substantial decrease in anal sex and an increase in condom use in contexts where anal sex continued to take place.[29] In Denmark, for example, reported condom use at last intercourse increased from 3% among gay men in the early 1980s to 82% in 1987.[31] The major changes observed among gay men across Europe in the first 10 years of the epidemic were modifications in their sexual repertoire from anogenital to orogenital practices and mutual masturbation, a reduction of numbers of sexual partners, more widespread condom use, and the adoption of different safer sex strategies with steady and nonregular partners.[29] Factors associated with the adoption of safer sex included the amount of information to which gay men have been exposed, attitudes and beliefs about transmission, perceived personal risk, social proximity to AIDS, relationship type, and self-identity.[29] In Australia, gay community attachment also was found to be an important predictor of safer sex practice.[30] In Canada, a range of factors, including "Personal characteristics of age and education, and lifestyle variables including relationship status, number of sexual partners and substance use all were shown to be correlated with ... behaviour."[32,p.166]

In Switzerland, Dubois-Auber et al.[33] measured attitude and behavior changes among gay men between 1987 and 1990, to evaluate the effectiveness of AIDS prevention activities. Interventions, including posters, advertisements, articles in the press, telephone helplines, discussions, workshops, and self-help groups, were delivered to gay men through the Swiss AIDS Foundation and grassroots organizations from 1986 onward. Reported behaviors changed very little between 1987 and 1990, with the majority of gay men reporting practicing safer sex.[33] Interviewees reported, however, that it was difficult to maintain safe sex on every occasion and that exceptions were made. Inconsistent condom use was linked to holidays, emotional health, and fear of jeopardizing relationships.[33] Conversely, sustained condom use was associated with having a friend or acquaintance with HIV/AIDS and being reminded of the need to continue to practice safer sex by close friends. The authors concluded that the most important reason for continuing interventions with men who have sex with men in the 1990s should be the maintenance of safer behavior,[33] a conclusion that has been widely echoed elsewhere.[34]

It may be that some men who practice unprotected anal sex may not be abandoning safer sex but making informed choices about HIV-related risks. Research in Australia and other countries not demonstrates that a number of gay men practice "negotiated safety" or an agreement between seroconcordant HIV-negative partners to dispense with condom use within the primary relationship while continuing to practice safer sex with other nonregular partners.[33] While not entirely free of risk, negotiated safety appears to be a successful way or preventing HIV infection for a significant number of men (i.e., between those in regular relationships and their nonregular partners). The concept of negotiated safety also allows researchers and practitioners to distinguish between relapses into unsafe sex and the sustained adoption of unprotected anal intercourse with regular seroconcordant partners. Kippax et al.[35] suggest that the strategy may become more widely and successfully used if "well-funded education campaigns that deal with the issues of honesty, testing, trust and talk between men are implemented" (p. 197).

Bochow et al.[36] have compared the recent sexual behavior and HIV risk reduction of gay and bisexual men in eight European countries. In common with other studies, the survey showed that the majority of gay men had substantially modified their behavior since becoming aware of HIV/AIDS. However, the greatest success in effecting change had taken place in environments where there had been close collaboration between government and medical institutions, and between the gay community and nongovernmental AIDS organizations. In the Netherlands, where there has been a strong involvement of gay men in HIV prevention from the onset of the epidemic, gay men have been able to directly influence policy and intervention development.[37] Australia has also seen a partnership model of response to the epidemic.[6] In this country, where the response to HIV/AIDS has been considered exceptional by many, the active participation of affected communities has been consistently encouraged, with bipartisan support from the major political parties.[38]

Across a range of industrialized countries around 80% of gay men now report that they have taken preventive measures to avoid HIV infection and another 11% report that they have always practiced a form of safer sex.[39] Research indicates, however, that continuing efforts are needed to reinforce safer sex practices, particularly in regular partnerships where unprotected sex may connote intimacy and commitment and among members of particularly vulnerable subgroups of homosexually active men, such as some younger gay men and men who are unsure of their sexual identity.

HIV-Related Risk Reduction with Injecting Drug Users

Like gay men, people who inject drugs were affected by HIV early in the epidemic. Indeed, in some industrialized countries injecting drug users have been and continue to be the most affected group. However, perhaps even more than for other groups, there have been wide variations in the nature of the epidemic of HIV/AIDS among injecting drug users. These variations can be observed both between and within countries. In Spain, for example, injecting drug use accounted for 66% of the cumulative cases of AIDS up until the end of 1994, while in Sweden only 10% of cases were among injecting drug users.[10] Within counties rates also have varied widely, with some areas being more affected than others. In Scotland in the mid-1980s, for example, around 50% of injecting drug users in Edinburgh were infected with HIV, while in Glasgow only 5% or so were infected.[40] Some of these variations can be accounted for by looking at the behavior patterns of injecting drug users in different contexts, but others are related to national and regional responses to injecting drug use and HIV/AIDS.

From the late 1980s onward, a number of prevention activities have been implemented to reduce the incidence of HIV infection among injecting drug users.[41] Programs have included information campaigns, HIV testing and counseling, AIDS prevention through community outreach, promoting safer injecting and sexual behavior, methadone substitution programs, and needle and syringe exchange schemes.[41]

Drug use is stigmatized and in many contexts it is illegal. This has made prevention efforts with injecting drug users, who may fear persecution and prosecution, more difficult. However, there has been some remarkable success in reducing HIV-related risk behavior among injecting drug users, especially where concern with HIV infection has taken precedence over concerns about the illegality of drug use.[40] Stimson[40] has described responses to the epidemic among injecting drug users, the government, and others in Great Britain. The prevalence of HIV infection among injecting drug users is stable in some cities and declining in others.[40] Prior to the onset of the epidemic of HIV/AIDS, the sharing of syringes and needles was usual behavior for many people injecting drugs; studies in the early to mid-1980s, for example, show that between 59 and 83% of injecting drug users shared equipment, providing an environment conducive to the rapid transmission of HIV infection.[40] However, swift action on the part of the British government, voluntary groups, some sections of the medical community, and injecting drug users themselves had an enormous impact. In 1986, pilot syringe exchange schemes were set up in England and Scotland.[40] Major changes in philosophy and practices in drug services also took place, as the ideas of harm minimization, accessibility, flexibility, and multiple and intermediate goals were developed.[40] From 15 pilot projects providing clean syringes in 1987, these prevention efforts have grown and now about two thirds of all drugs agencies are involved in some type of syringe distribution.[40] In parallel, there has been a growing use of literature, including posters, leaflets, and comics, to advise injecting drug users about safer injecting behavior. These strategies have led to significant changes in behavior among injecting drug users. Rates of syringe sharing in 1995 were one quarter to one third of the levels found in Great Britain before 1988.[40] Those who continue to share equipment tend to do so within a more discrete, groups, sharing only with sexual partners and close friends, which indicates a greater awareness of HIV/AIDS and attempts at risk reduction, albeit not risk elimination. Stimson[40] concludes that "injecting drug users have done more to change their behavior in the face of AIDS than many in the general population. Along with other marginalized and stigmatized groups, they showed that people can respond favorably to the threat of HIV infection" (pp. 712–713).

Loxley et al.[41] have suggested that age and social context may be important in relation to injecting behavior. In research conducted in Australia, the authors found that relative to older injecting drug users, younger users were more likely to be women, inject in larger groups of people, have fewer HIV tests, be more mobile, and less likely to be in drug treatment. Although this research did not demonstrate higher sharing of needles among younger people, the social context of younger injecting drug users' lives and difficulties of access should be taken account of in designing harm reduction strategies.

Research in Glasgow, as well as other cities worldwide, has shown that factors associated with reduction in HIV-related risk behavior among injecting users include talking about drug-using with friends and talking with sexual partners and families about AIDS.[42] Risk reduction therefore should be conceptualized as a social process rather than as isolated individual behavior, and prevention programs should be based on models that help groups to positively influence the behavior of individuals within groups.[42]

In some European countries, up to 40% of people in prison have injected drugs. Furthermore, people may continue to inject drugs and share needles while in prison.[43] Approximately 8% of prisoners in England and Wales, and possibly more in Scotland, have injected drugs in the period immediately preceding imprisonment and there have been confirmed cases of HIV infection through injecting drug use while in prison.[40] Although education about HIV/AIDS has taken place in prisons,[43] enabling factors, such as provision of clean injecting equipment and condoms for male prisoners, have proved more problematic, except in a few countries such as Switzerland where syringe and needle exchange programs have been introduced.

HIV-Related Risk Reduction with Sex Workers

From early in the epidemic sex workers have been recognized as a key group to involve in prevention.[11] However, in many countries, sex workers have been difficult to reach with HIV-preventive messages as the illegality of their activities means that they are not always visible.[3] Sex work is also highly stigmatized in many societies. In early reports about AIDS, the mass media often presented sex workers as conduits of infection,[44] and even in the Netherlands, often considered the most open and liberal of societies, many people continue to hold negative attitudes toward sex workers.[45]

Sex workers are often highly mobile, making grassroots organization and HIV-prevention programs difficult to implement. Additionally, while many sex workers do use condoms, the largely illicit and sometimes illegal nature of sex work in many countries renders sex workers vulnerable. In contexts where soliciting for clients is illegal, carrying large numbers of condoms may lead to arrest and fines.[45] Similarly, the hidden nature of sex work may render sex workers more vulnerable to rape and sexual coercion.[44,46]

Sex workers, like other groups, are far from homogeneous. They include women and men, including those who identify as gay or bisexual and those who do not[47]; young people, who may be relatively powerless and particularly vulnerable to exploitation[44]; and injecting drug users.[45] There also are large differences in the socioeconomic position of sex workers, and some research demonstrates that those sex workers who are able to charge more per transaction are less at risk of sexually transmitted diseases (STDs) and HIV infection than those who cannot.[44]

Despite difficulties, sex workers in some industrialized countries, including Germany, Italy, New Zealand, and Great Britain, have organized for the prevention of HIV infection.[44] Rates of HIV infection among sex workers who do not inject drugs in these countries have remained consistently low.[45] Peer education programs have proved particularly effective in Europe, aided by the fact that sex workers often work in pairs and/or small groups.[3]

Research has shown that sex workers of both sexes who consistently use condoms with clients are less likely to do so with their own regular partners.[46,48] Future interventions involving sex workers therefore may include strategies that focus on safer sex within regular partnerships, initiatives for sex workers who inject drugs, and programs that seek to work with those who have newly begun sex work. Additionally, environments in which the promotion of safer sex is given precedence over concerns about the illegality of sex work may enable sex workers to better protect their health. It is particularly important to provide a safer working environment.[44] Not surprisingly, given that few HIV-prevention initiatives have taken place with men generally, few prevention initiatives have taken place with the clients of sex workers, and this should be addressed through future programming.

HIV-Related Risk Reduction with Women

In most industrialized countries, the number of women infected with HIV was initially low but has increased over the years. Between 1985 and 1994, cases of AIDS among women in Europe doubled from 20% to 40%.[49] In Italy, the incidence of AIDS among women increased from 2.1 per 100,000 in 1987 to 17.2 per 100,000 in 1994.[50] In Great Britain, girls and women now outnumber men by 2 to 1 among people diagnosed with AIDS aged 13–29 years and reporting heterosexual contact.[51] There are a number of factors that render women vulnerable to HIV infection. First, the research suggests that women are physiologically more vulnerable than men to HIV infection and STDs.[52] Second, and most importantly, exposure of women to HIV is exacerbated by cultural and economic factors. Inequalities in social and economic power, as well as entrenched stereotypes and differences in role expectations between the sexes, mean that women often have less say in decisions about when and how intercourse takes place, including whether or not a condom will be used.[53]

Gallois et al.[54] have argued that women do not constitute a risk group for HIV infection in the usual sense of the term because women do not usually infect each other, but rather acquire HIV mainly through their relationships with men. Research in a variety of contexts shows that women's sexual behavior may differ from that of men. For example, women have fewer sexual partners than men and markedly ore women than men report having only one lifetime sexual partner.[55] In addition, women report a preference for sexual relations based on mutual fidelity, intimacy, and open communication.[55] Long and Ankrah[55] recently have argued that sexual responsibility among men is central to the health of both men and women. Women's empowerment cannot be achieved by women alone, but requires the support of men for its successful realization.[56] Despite increasing recognition of the importance of more equal gender roles in preventing HIV infection[57] and dominant ideologies of masculinity, which value the display of sexual prowess and encourage men to have multiple partners, few HIV-related prevention interventions so far have been targeted specifically at men.[58]

Exner et al.[59] have reviewed a number of interventions aimed at "at-risk" women in Canada. When examining interventions for at-risk women, the authors concluded not surprisingly that brief informational sessions were of limited effectiveness. Community-based interventions involving multiple and sustained contacts, however, showed more promising results. Out reach work, which included individual counseling and provided access to condoms, appeared to be effective in reaching women not easily accessed through more traditional techniques. Most importantly, the authors emphasize the importance of environmental conditions that impede behavior change among women, as well as an enhanced understanding of realistic and acceptable long-term sexual behavior for women.[59]

HIV-Related Risk Reduction with Young People

Young people have been identified as being at particular risk of HIV infection. Estimates from the Joint United Nations Programme on HIV/AIDS suggest that globally up to 60% of new HIV infections occur among those aged 15–24 years.[60] Although less than 1% of cumulative AIDS cases reported up until the end of September 1994 in Europe were among those aged 13–19 years, nearly 30% of the total were reported among young adults aged 20–29 years.[51] A considerable number of these young adults became infected with HIV during their youth and adolescence. Furthermore, studies demonstrate that in many industrialized countries the age of first sexual intercourse is decreasing.[61] In Australia, for example, Dunne et al.[62] have reported that 10% of young people surveyed reported having sex by the age of 13. In Canada, research has suggested that 31% of boys and 21% of girls in the ninth grade already have had sex.[63]

Work with young people offers an important opportunity to decrease the number of new HIV infections, since sexual and drug use habits may not be firmly established and behavior modification strategies may be more effective than with older people.[3,64] However, there has been a great deal of uncertainty about how to approach HIV prevention with young people. First, the literature on young people has tended to characterize them in narrow and stereotypical ways.[65] Young people are routinely seen as unknowledgeable and prone to risk-taking.[65] Second, accounts of young people often fail to differentiate between their needs in relation to class, culture, ethnicity, gender, and sexuality.[65] For example, Kippax and Crawford[66] observe that studies focusing on young people often ignore gay and bisexual young people. Third, there has been widespread concern among adults that talking openly to young people may encourage premature sexual relationships.[17] As a consequence, many sex education programs have focused unduly on abstinence, even though several studies suggest that well-designed programs of sex education, combining messages about safer sex as well as abstinence, may delay sexual debut, as well as increase preventive behaviors among those young people who are already sexually active.[67,68]

Many studies have looked at the view's held by young people, including their level of knowledge about HIV/AIDS.[69] Systematic evaluations of programs aimed at reducing HIV-related risk behavior among young people are much less common.[69] HIV-related health promotion has taken place with young people in a number of ways. In industrialized countries, schools have been seen as important environments in which work with young people on HIV/AIDS is undertaken.[65] Out-of-school approaches often have taken place in the setting of youth groups led by youth workers.

There has been much discussion of the merits of peer-led education, which involves the recruitment and training of groups of young people who will disseminate information and messages to other young people about HIV/AIDS.[65] Svenson and Hanson[70] found that peer education at Lund University in Sweden enjoyed a high degree of success. Students reached by the project reported significantly higher consistent condom use with new partners than those who were not. In one year, consistent condom use with new partners was reported as increasing from 46.8 to 60%.

In Switzerland, Blanchard et al.[71] report that the media-based Stop AIDS campaign, combined with specific interventions for young people in school, youth centers, and other settings, led to an increase in regular condom use among 16- to 19-year-olds from 22% and 10% for males and females, respectively, in 1987, to 42% and 32% in 1992. In France in 1989, Daures et al.[72] evaluated an individualized program for 15- to 18-year-olds on sexual health including STDs and found that the 3-year follow-up STDs among the experimental group were 4.3% compared with 11.5% among control groups. Similarly, girls involved in the program were 2.3 times less likely than controls to have intercourse without using contraception.

Grunseit[73] has described a number of characteristics shared by successful sex and HIV/AIDS education programs. First, programs appear to have a great impact if they are undertaken prior to the onset of sexual activity. Second, successful programs often have clearly focused aims but are delivered at a number of levels using different media and means of communication. Third, skills rehearsal has proved pivotal to the success of programs in improving young people's confidence of sexual negotiation and communication. Additional issues that may be crucial include appropriate and effective training for adult trainers, multiple rather than single interventions, and a variety of participatory and interactive activities rather than those that are didactic.[73] Elsewhere, Aggleton and Rivers[17] have identified a number of principles that underpin successful work with young people. These include listening to the expressed needs of young people and acknowledging the realities that they face, recognizing diversity among young people and providing opportunities to address issues of gender and sexuality, undertaking more interventions with young men as well as young women, and examining the positive aspects of sexual health including pleasure as well as negative aspects such as STDs.

Enabling as well as persuasion is essential to the longer-term success of work with young people, since their sexual behavior does not take place in a vacuum but in a broader social and cultural context. For example, Grunseit[73] has suggested that the negotiation of safer sex challenges culturally constructed notions of femininity and masculinity. Therefore, seeking to change female sexual behavior without taking into account its relationship to male behavior is unlikely to be successful. Most important, in addition to programs that aim to persuade young people to change their behavior, structural changes that enable young people to do so and are supportive of such behavior are critical.[17,18] Structural issues of relevance to the sexual health of young people include good access to condoms and appropriate sexual health services.

People Living with HIV Disease

An important component of HIV-related health promotion is the provision of services for people with HIV disease. It also is important to ensure that people affected by HIV are included in the planning and provision of prevention initiatives and services. Some commentators have noted that the patterning of the epidemic in some countries has led to the development of services that may be appropriate for certain people affected by HIV but are less so for others.[6,74] In Australia, because of the nature of the epidemic in that country, many services have been oriented toward gay men but may not serve the needs of some women living with HIV.[6] Similarly, in Britain the impact of AIDS on gay men led to the development of services for them but failed initially to serve other groups.[74] Conversely, in some southern European countries where levels of homophobia may be higher and the epidemic is reported as being largely among injecting drug users, access of homosexually active men to services may be especially problematic.

Coates et al.[2] have noted that HIV prevention efforts usually have not targeted potentially infected individuals to encourage testing and preventive behavior. This has been in part so as not to entrench discrimination. However, such action may be a useful way of decreasing new cases of HIV infection, particularly in contexts where knowledge of HIV status is high. In Australia, where there has been a great deal of success in HIV prevention, 90% of gay en are reported to know their HIV status.[2] Clearly, a great deal more can be done to encourage the proper involvement of people with HIV in prevention efforts: as advisers and active participants in programming and as the deliverers of key prevention messages.

Stryker et al.[1] have commented that HIV/AIDS thrives "in a medium of poverty, joblessness, homelessness, discrimination and despair" (p. 1146). Vulnerable population groups require improved access to health and social services, testing and counseling, drug services, affordable condoms, and appropriate care and support. Research in France has shown that HIV-positive patients who were defined as destitute (having no permanent residence, without regular income or employment, and without regular health coverage) were three times more likely than nondestitute people who were HIV-positive to develop tuberculosis.[75] Services to reach the most vulnerable, including primary and secondary prevention, are therefore crucial.

STRUCTURAL AND ENABLING FACTORS

Altering the environment may help to significantly reduce HIV transmission, even in the absence of widespread behavioral changes. Tawil et al.[13] point out that comprehensive treatment of STDs, for example, can result in a decreased incidence of HIV. While clearly a medical intervention, the comprehensive treatment of STDs require appropriate structural interventions to ensure that adequate levels of funding are available, that service delivery is enhanced and that all people with STDs, including young people and others who for whatever reason are unable to easily access treatment, are encouraged to do so. Restrictive legislation may act as a major barrier to the adoption of preventive measures.[13] In acknowledgment of this, some countries have changed laws relating to sexual behavior and drug use. For example, in New Zealand homosexual acts and the possession of syringes and needles were decriminalized in 1986 and 1987, respectively.[9] Needle and syringe exchange programs were established in retail pharmacies and community outreach groups in 1988.[9] The prevalence of HIV among injecting drug users in this country has remained low, attributable to both the effectiveness of educational campaigns and needle and the introduction of needle and syringe exchange schemes.[9] Where persuasive techniques have been combined with the provision of clean syringes, such as in Lund (Sweden), Sydney (Australia), and Toronto (Canada), low levels of HIV prevalence among injecting drug users can be maintained.[2]

Stimson[40] has described in detail the important changes in philosophy, policy, practice that took place in British governmental departments and drug agencies during the mid- to late-1980s and resulted in remarkable changes in HIV-related risk behavior among injecting drug users. Similarly, while the prescription of methadone may have helped some people reduce their risk of HIV infection in countries such as Great Britain and the Netherlands, in other countries, such as France and Greece, methadone prescription have remained limited or prohibited.[76]

There also have been considerable structural and environmental changes in relation to the advertisement and sale of condoms. For example, in Ireland restrictions on the sale of condoms were amended in 1992 and 1993.[11] However, in many industrialized countries fierce debate continues around the distribution of condoms and clean injecting equipment to particular population groups including young people and prisoners.[13]

Research across Europe demonstrates the importance of governmental and medical institutions entering into collaboration with the gay community and nongovernmental AIDS service organizations.[36] The largest and most sustained changes in HIV-risk related behavior have occurred in environments where this has taken place, including Denmark, the Netherlands, and Switzerland. Similarly, in Australia the government pursued a policy of active cooperation and consultation with gay communities, who had been organizing prevention programs since 1983 with little initial assistance.[30] This type of liaison and involvement requires not only a social climate in which gay men are able to have a level of visibility, but political will on the part of governments. So long as homophobia and prejudice, sometimes reinforced by legislation, remains widespread, the involvement of stigmatized and marginalized groups such as gay men in the protection of their own health will be limited.

SUMMARY AND FUTURE DIRECTIONS

There is no one epidemic of HIV in industrialized countries but a number of overlapping epidemics that vary within and between countries. As a result, the groups most affected can vary widely between countries and even cities. Across the developed world those most affected have included people who belong to groups who are discriminated against, marginalized, powerless, and subject to social inequalities. Members of such groups have faced not only an epidemic of HIV infection but increased prejudice and stigmatization. Yet these same groups have nonetheless and often against the odds made remarkable strides in changing their behavior to decrease the risk of HIV infection. Concurrently, except in a few countries, there have not been major changes in behavior among adult heterosexuals, reflected in the rate of increasing HIV infection among women. While it is not possible to describe all the initiatives that have been successful in bringing about a reduction in HIV infections in the industrialized world, it is becoming clear which prevention strategies and approaches work best in which contexts and under particular circumstances.

There is now clear evidence that the mass media may help to create an environment conducive to HIV prevention. In particular it can foster awareness that HIV is an issue worthy of debate, concern, and public funding. In numerous European countries, in Canada, New Zealand, and Australia, an agenda thus has been set that renders other activities, including those at grassroots level, more widely acceptable. Additionally, messages about HIV disseminated through the mass media may facilitate more open discussion of drug use and sexuality in circumstances, which before was not possible. The widespread promotion of condoms, for example, which is commonplace now in most industrialized countries of Western Europe, was unimaginable prior to the onset of the HIV epidemic and the attention given to it through the mass media.

In several counties in the industrialized world, gay men have made substantial changes to their sexual behavior that have led to a stabilizing and decreasing incidence of HIV. Success has been most pronounced when gay organizations have been able to collaborate with governmental and medical institutions. This, however, requires an environment in which gay men are able to be open about their sexuality, as well as able to cooperate with gay opinion leaders and voluntary groups. The long-term maintenance of safer sexual behaviors is now a key issue in many countries, and the factors that explain why some gay men may not practice safer sex with all partners need to be better understood.

In some countries, injecting drug users have been able to make significant changes in their behavior resulting in the stabilization and decline of new cases of HIV infection. Changes in governmental and medical philosophy, policy, and practices in relation to injecting drug use have been instrumental in providing an appropriate environment for change. Policies that have given precedence to the prevention of HIV infection over concerns about the illegality of drug use have been crucial in helping those injecting drug users who are not able or wiling to stop injecting drugs to reduce risk behavior. However, while many injecting drug users have changed their behavior in relation to drug use, sexual behavior remains a key factor influencing HIV-related risks.

Sex workers are a diverse group and have diverse needs. While in some countries sex workers have been able to organize politically for HIV prevention, in other contexts the hidden and often illegal nature of sex work often means that this is not possible. Additionally, while many sex workers in industrialized countries use condoms with clients, safer sex practices may be less likely with regular partners. New programs and interventions are therefore needed to enable sex workers to protect their sexual health across a range of contexts and relationships.

Levels of HIV infection are increasing among women in industrialized countries. However, prevention interventions with women only rarely acknowledge the pervasive social and economic inequalities that underpin HIV risk-related behavior. Structural changes to bring about great equality between the sexes are important not only in terms of social justice, but also to help women and men protect their sexual health. Importantly, work with heterosexual men is still marginal to most HIV prevention activities; yet, if women are to be empowered to change sexual behavior, the support and involvement of men are crucial.

Concerns about discussing sexuality and drug use openly with young people have determined the nature of many initiatives for HIV prevention, and there has been insufficient recognition that young people are diverse in attitudes and behavior. Programs that aim to help young people talk openly about sex and drugs have been hindered because of worries among adults that young people may be encouraged to engage in premature sexual activity and drug use. However, there are now clear indications of the prevention strategies that are most likely to help young people protect their sexual health, and there is clear evidence that well-designed sex education programs do not encourage an increase in risk-related behaviors.

People who are directly affected by HIV disease have a valuable contribution to make to the development of policy, practice, and implementation of HIV prevention programs. Partnerships with affected individuals and communities are therefore important. As improvements in the quality of life of people with HIV occur, it is vital to involve them more fully and appropriately in local, national, and international prevention efforts.

In addition to HIV-related health promotion that attempts to persuade people to change their sexual and drug-related behavior, it is crucial that structural changes take place to ensure that people are enabled to make the desired changes in behavior. These can include changes in the law, public health policy, and the context and circumstances in which sex and injecting drug use occur, including those linked to sex work. Policies and structures to help young people change their behavior and opportunities for young people to be included in program planning are especially crucial in this respect. Inequalities, stereotyping, and discrimination facilitate the epidemic of HIV. Women, whose social and economic power may be less than that of men, may experience significant constraints when it comes to negotiating safer sex. Acknowledging these inequalities is central to the success of future HIV-related health promotion work.

Beyond the issues already discussed is the need for continuing research. This includes descriptive and analytic studies of the meanings attached to unsafe sex and unsafe injecting behaviors in different relationship contexts, continuing enquiry into intervention effectiveness, studies of the key constructs and strategies of successful programs for prevention, and studies of ways of involving people with HIV more fully in prevention activities.

Recent advances in treatment effectiveness raise important questions about changing public perceptions of the epidemic and its effects. It is important to know more about how these changes impact on attitudes to prevention and prevention behaviors. It is also important to identify and challenge the new forms of discrimination and stigmatization that may arise in circumstances where HIV and AIDS become long-term, if expensive to manage, health conditions.

Finally, we need to know more about how best to ensure that HIV prevention receives the funding and political support it needs amid a plethora of other concerns. There is evidence from some European countries that resources for prevention are falling as treatment costs rise, and some politicians and policy makers are reluctant to make continuing investments in prevention research and programs. Such responses are shortsighted and will in time lead to a worsening of the epidemic. The challenge for behavioral and prevention science lies in prioritizing the issues, problems, and activities that will have the greatest impact on the epidemic in these changing times.

ACKNOWLEDGMENTS.   We would like to thank the following for their advice, suggestions, and support while preparing this chapter: Susan Kippax (Sydney, Australia), Jo Kittelsen (Oslo, Norway), Anne-Lise Middelthon (Oslo, Norway), Ted Myers (Toronto, Canada), Theo Sandfort (Utrecht, Netherlands), Bengt Sundbaum (Stockholm, Sweden), Gary Svenson (Lund, Sweden), and Anne Vassall (Montréal, Canada).

REFERENCES

1. Stryker J, Coates TJ, DeCarlo P, et al. Prevention of HIV infection. *JAMA* 1995; 273(14):1143–1148.
2. Coates TJ, Aggleton P, Gutzwiller F, et al. HIV prevention in developed countries. *Lancet* 1996; 348:1143–1148.
3. Coleman LM, Ford NJ. An extensive literature review of the evaluation of HIV prevention programmes. *Health Educ Res* 1996; 11(3):327–338.
4. Colletta ND. *Understanding Cross-cultural Child Development and Designing Programs for Children.* Richmond, VA: Christian Children's Fund; 1992.
5. Auer C. Women, children and HIV/AIDS. In: Long LD, Ankrah EM, eds. *Women's Experiences with HIV/AIDS: An International Perspective.* New York: Columbia University Press; 1996:236–263.
6. Crawford J, Lawless S, Kippax S. Positive women and heterosexuality: problems of disclosure of serostatus to sexual partners. In: Aggleton P, Davies P, Hart G, eds. *AIDS Activism and Alliances.* London, England: Taylor & Francis; 1997:1–14.
7. Bedimo AL, Bessinger R, Kissinger P. Reproductive choices among HIV-positive women. *Soc Sci Med* 1998; 46(2):171–179.

8. Strathdee SA, Hogg RS, Hanvelt R. *Evaluating HIV/AIDS Prevention Programs in Canada: Where Do We Go From Here?* Ottawa, Canada: Canadian Policy Networks Inc; 1996.

9. Sharples KJ, Dickson NP, Paul C, et al. HIV/AIDS in New Zealand: An epidemic in decline? *AIDS* 1996; 10:1273–1278.

10. European Centre for Epidemiological Monitoring of AIDS. *AIDS surveillance in Europe.* Quarterly report. December 1994.

11. Wellings K, Field B. *Stopping AIDS: AIDS/HIV Public Education and the Mass Media in Europe.* Harlow, England: Longman; 1996.

12. Buzy JM, Gayle HD. The epidemiology of HIV and AIDS in women. In: Long LD, Ankrah EM, eds. *Women's Experiences with HIV/AIDS: An International Perspective.* New York: Columbia University Press; 1996:181–204.

13. Tawil O, Verster A, O'Reilly KR. Enabling approaches for HIV/AIDS prevention: Can we modify the environment and minimize the risk? *AIDS* 1995; 9:1299–1306.

14. Aggleton P. *Success in HIV Prevention.* Horsham, England: AVERT; 1997.

15. Aggleton P. Global priorities for HIV/AIDS intervention research. *Int J STD AIDS* 1996; 7(suppl 2):13–16.

16. Canadian AIDS Society and the National Health Promotion Demonstration Project. *Paradigms Lost: Examining the Impact of a Shift from Health Promotion to Population Health on HIV/AIDS Policy and Programs in Canada.* Ottawa, Canada: Canadian AIDS Society and the National Health Promotion Demonstration Project; 1997.

17. Aggleton P, Rivers K. Behavioral interventions for adolescents. In: Gibney L, DiClemente R, Vermund S, eds. *Preventing HIV infection in developing countries.* New York: Plenum Press; 1999:in press.

18. Baldo M. *Youth and AIDS: adapting to an evolving epidemic.* Paper presented at the 6th Congress on Adolescent Health/Youth Health. Vancouver, Canada; 1995.

19. Dubois-Arber F, Paccaud F. Assessing AIDS/HIV prevention: What do we know in Europe? *Soc Prev Med* 1994; 39(suppl 1):S3–S11.

20. Aggleton P. Behavior change communication. *AIDS Educ Prev* 1997; 9(2):111–123.

21. Oakley A, Fullerton D, Holland J, et al. Sexual health education interventions for young people: A methodological overview. *Br Med J* 1995; 310:158–162.

22. Norwegian Board of Health. *An Evaluation of AIDS Prevention in Norway: A Summary Report.* Oslo, Norway: Norwegian Board of Health; 1995.

23. Kok G, Kolker L, de Vroome E, et al. "Safe sex" and "compassion": Public campaigns on AIDS in the Netherlands. In: Sandford T, ed. *The Dutch Response to HIV.* London, England: UCL Press; 1988:19–39.

24. Moatti JP, Dab W, Loundou H, et al. Impact on the general public of media campaigns against AIDS: A French evaluation. *Health Policy* 1992; 21:233–247.

25. Dubois-Arber F, Jeannin A, Meystre-Agustoni G, et al. *Evaluation of the AIDS Prevention Strategy in Switzerland: Fifth Synthesis Report 1993–1995,* abridged version. Lausanne, Switzerland: University Institute of Social and Preventive Medicine; 1996.

26. Ministerio de Sanidad y Consumo. *Estudio cuantitivo. Segundo barometro sanitario epigrafe.* Conocimiento y actitudes sociales ante al SIDA. Madrid, Spain; 1993.

27. Servant AM. *Love object ... condoms with humor.* Paper presented at VIIIth International Conference on AIDS, Amsterdam, Netherlands; 1992.

28. Dubé LG, Reaidi G, Descombes C. *Comparing affective and cognitive responses to informational vs emotional messages on AIDS prevention: a field study among Canadian young adults.* Paper presented at IXth International Conference on AIDS, Berlin, Germany; 1993.

29. Pollack M, Dur W, Vincineau M, et al. Evaluating AIDS prevention for men having sex with men: The west European experience. *Soc Prev Med* 1994; 39(suppl 1):S47–S60.

30. Kippax S, Connell RW, Dowsett GW, et al. *Sustaining Safe Sex: Gay Communities Respond to AIDS.* London, England: Falmer Press; 1993.

31. Bottzauw J, Hermansen K, Tauris P. Alterations in the sexual habits of a group of homosexual persons after information about AIDS. *Ungeskr Laeger* 1989; 151:1920–1922.

32. Myers T, Kurtz RG, Tundiver F, et al. Predictors of change, poor outcome and premature drop-out in a randomized control study of AIDS education: The Talking Sex Project. In: Paccaud F, Vader JP, Gutzwiller F, eds. *Assessing AIDS Prevention.* Basel, Switzerland: Birkhauser Verlag; 1992:65–78.

33. Dubois-Arber F, Masur J-B, Husser D, et al. Evaluation of AIDS prevention among homosexual and bisexual men in Switzerland. *Soc Sci Med* 1993; 37(12):1539–1544.

34. Van De Ven P, Campell D, Kippax S, et al. Factors associated with unprotected anal intercourse in gay men's casual partnership in Sydney, Australia. *AIDS Care* 1997; 9(6):637–649.

35. Kippax S, Noble J, Prestage G, et al. Sexual negotiation in the AIDS era: Negotiated safety revisited. *AIDS* 1997; 11:191–197.

36. Bochow M, Chiarotti F, Davies P, et al. Sexual behavior of gay and bisexual men in eight European countries. *AIDS Care* 1996; 6(5):533–548.

37. Hospers H, Blom C. HIV prevention activities for gay men in the Netherlands 1983–93. In: Sandfort T, ed. *The Dutch Response to HIV*. London, England: UCL Press; 1988:40–60.

38. Edwards M. AIDS policy communities in Australia. In: Aggleton P, Davies P, Hart G, eds. *AIDS: Activism and Alliances*. London, England: Taylor & Francis; 1997:41–57.

39. Schiltz M-A, Adam P. Reputedly effective risk reduction strategies and gay men. In: Aggleton P, Davies P, Hart G, eds. *AIDS: Safety, Sexuality and Risk*. London, England: Taylor and Francis; 1995:1–19.

40. Stimson G. AIDS and injecting drug use in the United Kingdom, 1987–1993: The policy response and the prevention of the epidemic. *Soc Sci Med* 1995; 41(5):699–716.

41. Loxley WM, Bevan JS, Carruthers SJ. Age and injecting drug use revisited: The Australian study of HIV and injecting drug use. *AIDS Care* 1997; 9(6):661–670.

42. Des Jarlais DC, Friedman SR, Friedmann P, et al. HIV/AIDS-related behavior change among injecting drug users in different national settings. *AIDS* 1995; 9:611–617.

43. Rezza G, Rota MCh, Buning E, et al. Assessing HIV prevention among injecting drug users in European Community countries: A review. *Soc Prev Med* 1994; 39(suppl 1):S14–S46.

44. Alexander P. Making a living: Women who go out. In: Long LD, Ankrah EM, eds. *Women's Experiences*. New York: Columbia University Press; 1996:

45. Vanwesenbeeck I, de Graaf R. Sex work and HIV in the Netherlands: Policy, research and prevention. In: Sandford T, ed. *The Dutch Response to HIV*. London, England: UCL Press; 1998:86–106.

46. Aggleton P. *Men Who Sell Sex*. London, UCL Press; 1998.

47. Boulton M, Fitzpatrick R. Bisexual men in Britain. In: Aggleton P, eds. *Bisexualities and AIDS: International Perspectives*. London, England: Taylor and Francis Ltd; 1996:3–22.

48. Hart G, Boulton M. Sexual behaviour in gay men: towards a sociology of risk. In: Aggleton P, Davies P, Hart G, eds. *AIDS: Safety, Sexuality and Risk*. London, England: Taylor & Francis; 1995:55–67.

49. European Centre for Epidemiological Monitoring of AIDS. *AIDS Surveillance in Europe*. Quarterly report. March 1995.

50. Conti S, Lepri AC, Farchi G, et al. AIDS: A major health problem among young Italian women. *AIDS* 1996; 10:407–411.

51. Elford J. HIV and AIDS in adolescence: Epidemiology. In: Sherr L, ed. *AIDS and Adolescents*. Amsterdam, the Netherlands: Harwood Academic Publishers; 1997:25–50.

52. European Study Group on Heterosexual Transmission of HIV. Comparison of female to male and male to female transmission of HIV in 563 stable couples. *Br Med J* 1992; 304:809–813.

53. Davies AG, Dominy NJ, Peters AD, et al. Gender differences in HIV risk behaviour of injecting drug users in Edinburgh. *AIDS Care* 1996; 8(5):517–527.

54. Gallois C, Statham D, Smith S. *Women and HIV/AIDS Education in Australia*. Canberra, Australia: Commonwealth Department of Health, Housing and Community Services; 1992.

55. Giffin K. Beyond empowerment: Heterosexualities and the prevention of AIDS. *Soc Sci Med* 1998; 46(2): 151–161.

56. Long LD, Ankrah EM, eds. *Women Experiences with HIV/AIDS: An International Perspective*. New York: Columbia University Press; 1996.

57. Gupta GR, Weiss E, Mane P. Talking about sex: A prerequisite for AIDS prevention. In: Long LD, Ankrah EM, eds. *Women Experiences with HIV/AIDS: An International Perspective*. New York: Columbia University Press; 1996:

58. Rivers K, Aggleton P. Men and the HIV Epidemic. New York: United Nations Development Programme, 1999.

59. Exner TM, Seal DW, Ehrhardt AA. A review of HIV interventions for at-risk women. *AIDS Behav* 1997; 1(2): 93–124.

60. Panos. AIDS and young people. In: *AIDS Briefing 4*. London: Panos; 1996:

61. Rosenthal D. Australian adolescents' behaviors and beliefs about HIV/AIDS and other STDs. In: Sherr L, ed. *AIDS and Adolescents*. Amsterdam, the Netherlands: Harwood Academic Publishers; 1994:91–106.

62. Dunne M, Donald M, Lucke J, et al. Age-related increase in sexual behaviours and decrease in regular condom use among adolescents in Australia. *Int J STDs AIDS* 1994; 5:41–47.

63. King AJC, Beazley RP, Warren WK, et al. *Canada Youth and AIDS Study*. Kingston, Canada: Social Program Evaluation Group; 1988.

64. Mann J, Tarantola DJM, Netter TW, eds. *AIDS in the World*. Cambridge, MA: Harvard University Press; 1992.

65. Aggleton P, Warwick I. Young people, sexuality and AIDS education. In: Sherr L, ed. *AIDS and Adolescents*. Amsterdam, the Netherlands: Harwood Academic Publishers; 1997:79–90.

66. Kippax S, Crawford J. Fact and fictions of adolescent risk. In: Sherr L, ed. *AIDS and Adolescents*. Amsterdam, the Netherlands: Harwood Academic Publishers; 1998:63–78.

67. Baldo M, Aggleton P, Slutkin G. *Does sex education lead to earlier or increased sexual activity in youth?* Poster presented at IXth International Conference on AIDS. Berlin, Germany; 1993.

68. Grunseit A, Kippax S, Aggleton P, et al. Sexuality and young people's sexual behavior: A review of studies. *J Adoles Res* 1997; 12(4):421–453.

69. Sherr L. Adolescents and AIDS in our midst. In: Sherr L, ed. *AIDS and Adolescents*. Amsterdam, the Netherlands: Harwood Academic Publishers; 1997:5–24.

70. Svenson GR, Hanson BS. Are peer and social influences important component to include in HIV–STD prevention models? *Eur J Public Health* 1996; 6:203–211.

71. Blanchard M, Narring F, Michaud PA, et al. *The effect of the Swiss Stop-AIDS campaigns 1987–1992: increase in condom use without promotion of sexual promiscuity*. Poster presentation, IXth International Conference on AIDS. Berlin, Germany; 1993.

72. Daures JP, Chaix-Durand G, Maurin M, et al. Etude préliminaire sur la prévention des interruptions volontaires de grossesse (TVG) et des maladies sexuellement transmissibles (MST) chez l'adolescent par une information en classes de troisieme. *Contraception-Fertilité Sex* 1989; 17:1021–1026.

73. Grunseit A. *Impact of HIV and Sexual Health Education on the Sexual Behaviour of Young People: A Review Update*. Geneva, Switzerland: UNAIDS; 1997.

74. Feldman R, Crowley C. HIV services for women in east London: The match between provision and needs. In: Aggleton P, Davies P, Hart G, eds. *AIDS: Activism and Alliances*. London, England: Taylor & Francis; 1997: 122–141.

75. Chauvin P, Mortier E, Carrat F, et al. A new outpatient care facility for HIV-infected destitute populations in Paris, France. *AIDS Care* 1997; 9(4):451–459.

76. van Ameijden E, van den Hoek A. AIDS among injecting drug users in the Netherlands: The epidemic and the response. In: Sandfort T, ed. *The Dutch Response to HIV*. London, England: UCL Press; 1998:61–85.

Implications of HIV Intervention Research

Technology Transfer
Achieving the Promise of HIV Prevention

RONALD O. VALDISERRI

Early national plans to prevent and control the spread of acquired immunodeficiency syndrome (AIDS), called for "the implementation of community risk reduction and health education programs to effect behavior change regarding high-risk sexual practices and the use of intravenous drugs."[1(p.454)] As a means of furthering prevention efforts, the US Public Health Service plan recommended the dissemination of "research findings" and "accurate information" to other scientists, educational authorities, and organizations serving individuals at high risk for AIDS. When the first Presidential Commission on the Human Immunodeficiency Virus Epidemic issued its report in 1988, it too called for the implementation of "risk reduction interventions" by state and local health departments as well as community based service organizations.[2] State and local health departments were widely recognized as necessary components in the national response to preventing the spread of human immunodeficiency virus (HIV) because of their traditional and constitutionally defined role in protecting the public's health. Community-based service organizations were considered to be essential partners in national HIV prevention efforts because of their unique access to high-risk populations, such as gay men,[3] who were often suspicious and mistrustful of government-sponsored health care systems and services, no matter how well meaning.

CHALLENGES TO PREVENTION CAPACITY

Developing behaviorally based interventions in these two settings (i.e., clinic-based health department settings and community-based organizational settings) posed unique problems. Exceptions notwithstanding, in the earliest years of the epidemic, most health departments were better prepared to deliver the more traditional sexually transmitted disease (STDs) control measures of case identification and contact tracing than they were to provide interactive, client-centered prevention counseling.[4] And community-based organizations (CBOs), despite their credibility with high-risk populations such as gay men and injecting drug users, were often found lacking in their capacity to develop scientifically sound interventions and to evaluate intervention effectiveness.[5,6]

These challenges to prevention capacity have not disappeared over time. In 1993, when the National Commission on AIDS published a report on "Behavioral and Social Sciences and

RONALD O. VALDISERRI • National Center for HIV, STD, and TB Prevention, Centers for Disease Control and Prevention, Atlanta, Georgia 30333.

Handbook of HIV Prevention, edited by Peterson and DiClemente.
Kluwer Academic / Plenum Publishers, New York, 2000.

the HIV/AIDS Epidemic," it recommended that "technology transfer and feedback between behavioral and social science research and prevention efforts must be improved, increased, and accelerated."[7(p.28)] A similar theme was reiterated 2 years later in September 1995, when the Congressional Office of Technology Assessment (OTA) published its report, "The Effectiveness of AIDS Prevention Efforts," and found that "there is a gap between what is known about effective intervention and what is actually delivered as prevention."[8(p.3)]

Shortcomings in program implementation do not mitigate the fact that definite progress has been made in the field of HIV prevention. Exhaustive reviews of the published literature have consistently demonstrated that effective HIV prevention programs can result in long-term behavior change[9] and that "when delivered with sufficient resources, intensity, and cultural competency"[10(p.142)] HIV prevention efforts can yield highly favorable results. Today, it would seem that the salient question regarding HIV prevention is no longer "Does HIV prevention work," but rather, "How can we make HIV prevention work as it should?" Stated another way, important scientific advances in HIV prevention by themselves cannot ensure that our subsequent HIV prevention efforts will become more highly targeted, more scientifically sound, or even more effective. It is only when these scientific advances are appropriately operationalized that they achieve their true promise in terms of HIV prevention.

Therefore, this chapter will focus on the critical issue of ensuring that HIV prevention programs and activities incorporate the most current scientific thinking and practices on HIV prevention. Barriers to incorporating new and emerging HIV prevention technologies will be identified to better inform our discussion. Then, using examples from publicly funded HIV prevention activities in health department and nongovernmental organization (NGO) settings, we will review a sample of actual technology transfer products. A brief summary of future challenges will conclude the chapter.

THE UPTAKE OF NEW PREVENTION TECHNOLOGY

When considering deficiencies in the uptake of new prevention technologies and how best to rectify them, it is important to keep in mind that a number of factors mediate the incorporation of emerging behavioral and biomedical research findings into HIV prevention programs. Among the most obvious is the level and quality of available research. If research findings are lacking or equivocal, persons who are responsible for funding, designing, or implementing HIV prevention activities may not have sufficient information to make the most informed choices. Consequently, existing prevention programs may not be as effective as they might be, had they access to conclusive research findings providing detailed information on specific interventions tailored toward their populations of interest. For example, when Wingood and DiClemente[11] reviewed the published literature on HIV risk reduction interventions for sexually active women, from 1981 through May 1995, they found "relatively few behavioral interventions that have been designed specifically for women" (p. 213) and concluded that there is an urgent need to develop and test risk reduction interventions specific to women, especially interventions that address the realities of gender roles. The OTA report, mentioned earlier, noted a paucity of intervention research for African-American and Latino populations as well as a scarcity of inquiries into interventions needed to maintain safer behaviors over long periods of time.[8]

Yet, important as sound research is, its existence is only one of the ingredients necessary for the transfer of emerging behavioral and biomedical technologies into ongoing HIV prevention efforts. Other important variables influence the extent to which findings move from the pages of scientific journals into clinic and community-based practice settings. After his study of technology transfer initiatives undertaken by various federal agencies in the area of substance abuse prevention, Backer[12] identified four fundamental conditions that must be met in order for technology transfer to result in individual or system wide change:

> individuals and organizations must be aware that the new knowledge exists and have access to it.... there must be credible evidence that behavior change will lead to improved practice without either excessive costs or undesirable side effects.... the money, materials, and personnel needed to implement the new technology must be available.... active interventions are required to overcome resistances, fears, and anxieties about change among the people who will need to implement the innovation. (p. 3–4)

Access to the New Technology

In an analysis of community capacity to implement and maintain HIV risk reduction programs, Freundenberg and colleagues[13] noted substantial disparities between optimal HIV prevention interventions and reported community practices. In their opinion, one of the major reasons for this discrepancy was the fact that "very few community organizations have access—or a desire—to engage with those who could provide a theoretical framework for their efforts" (p. 300). This is especially problematic when one considers Leviton's[14] admonition that basing HIV prevention interventions on a sound theoretical foundation is an important defense against the repetition of past mistakes and a safeguard against supporting ineffective programs that are predicated on implicit, untested, and often inaccurate belief systems.

Ensuring access to emerging HIV prevention technologies means not only providing scientific information in terms that nonscientists can understand but also providing materials that are accessible to persons who may not speak English as a first language. In 1993, when the United States Conference of Mayors (USCM) conducted a national assessment of the HIV prevention needs of gay and bisexual men or color, they found that there were very few HIV prevention materials (for either clients or program managers) printed in Asian and Pacific Islander languages.[15] Furthermore, scientific findings are not the only form of technical information that may be required in order to conduct effective HIV prevention programs. The same USCM report also called for technical assistance in grant writing as a strategy to ensure that fledgling community organizations could compete effectively for HIV prevention funding.

Credibility of the New Technology

Even after promoting access, the technological innovation may not be adopted if it is not deemed to be credible. Consider the following. Even among persons who are in drug treatment, relapse is a well-known and widely accepted aspect of addiction to opiates. Therefore, early on, HIV prevention specialists thought it important to provide education to drug users who were in treatment about the dangers of needle sharing and steps they could take to disinfect injection equipment. However, these efforts were often thwarted by well-meaning, drug treatment clinical staff who, after devoting their careers to extinguishing injection behaviors, were extremely wary of the notion of making injection practices "safer" and were fearful that delivering such messages to their clients might precipitate relapse.[3]

Another poignant example of a credibility threat interfering with the uptake of new technology derives from the shameful legacy of the Tuskegee Syphilis Study and the subsequent distrust that many African Americans have of the public health establishment. Thomas and Quinn,[16] writing on the implications of the Tuskegee Syphilis Study on HIV education and risk reduction programs in the African-American community, delivered the following warning:

> [Public health authorities] must be willing to listen respectfully to community fears, share the facts of the Tuskegee study when it arises as a justification of those fears, and admit to the limitations of science when they do not have all the answers. This approach may help public health authorities to regain the credibility and the public trust they need to successfully implement HIV risk reduction strategies in the Black community. (p. 1503)

Cost of the New Technology

Many would likely identify financial constraints as among the most easily recognized of barriers to the adoption of new prevention technologies. In 1992, when the National Commission on AIDS reported on the multifaced challenges of AIDS in communities of color, they specifically identified low levels of funding as a reason why HIV prevention efforts in communities of color were often inadequate.[17] In support of this assertion, a case study of 28 black and Latino community organizations in the Washington Heights/Inwood section of New York City revealed that lack of resources was a frequently cited reason why these organizations (many of which described themselves as already "overwhelmed" with existing activities, even prior to the AIDS epidemic) were often unable to implement or expand HIV prevention activities.[18] In the spring of 1995, when 25 CBOs from San Francisco were randomly selected to answer questions about their access to HIV prevention research, 54% cited lack of resources as a significant barrier to incorporating social and behavioral research into their existing activities.[19]

However, it would be a mistake to assume that inadequate financial resources is the only resource constraint to operationalizing new prevention technologies. Human resources are equally important, especially if the new intervention requires specialized skills to implement and oversee. Consider the following advice, provided by a US Public Health Service Task Force,[20] writing on the necessity of strengthening public health capacity in the United States.

> For public health and health care professionals, publication of research findings is only the first step in making new information accessible. Professionals need to understand and accept a study's implications for their practice and may need to acquire new knowledge or develop new skills to apply advances effectively. (p. 13)

Unfortunately, as many community-based prevention service providers know from first-hand experience, staff training expenses generally fare poorly when competing against unmet needs for client services and other organizational priorities. Nor is this phenomenon limited to NGOs. Based on information collected from eight states, the Public Health Foundation[21] estimated that in 1993, per capita public health expenditures for training and education ranked the lowest, among a listing of ten essential public health functions.

Resistance to the New Technology

As discussed earlier, specific concerns about the credibility of a particular prevention technology may impede its uptake. For example, contrary to extant evaluation data, some opponents of comprehensive HIV education in schools may still continue to object to its implementation, fearing that school-based condom skills training will result in an increase in sexual frequency or hasten the sexual debut of adolescents. However, in addition to specific concerns about the credibility of a particular prevention intervention, there may be broader, more global impediments to the adoption of a new prevention technology; impediments that are not specific to a particular innovation, but rather relate to the discomfort that comes from changing from an accustomed mode of doing business to a new, less familiar, one. Backer et al.[12] refer to these barriers as "resistances, fears, and anxieties about change among the people who will need to implement the innovation" (p. 4).

Resistance to change is a common occurrence in all manner of organizations, whether those organizations manufacture products, distribute goods, deliver health care, or provide HIV prevention services. So pervasive is the occurrence of organizational resistance to change that those who specialize in the field of organizational development often speak of the importance of "managing" change.[22] Cummings and Worley,[23] in describing a model of effective change management, emphasize the necessity of sustaining momentum, once the change is initiated, through a variety of strategies, including the positive reinforcement of new behaviors.

Think about a hypothetical primary care clinic that provides HIV counseling and testing services to its clients, many of whom are women of color at increased risk for HIV infection through sexual contact with injecting drug users. A new director who comes to the clinic performs an assessment of services and discovers that current counseling efforts are largely didactic, nonspecific, and not tailored to the specific needs and circumstances of the clients served. The new director quickly mounts several corrective actions targeting the counselors, including required readings from the peer-reviewed literature on counseling theory and a series of in-service presentations on client-centered HIV counseling techniques.[24] Satisfied that the new form of counseling has been successfully implemented, the director's attention turns to other matters. However, the next time an assessment of counseling services is conducted several months later, it is discovered that three of the four counselors have reverted to delivering standardized, nonspecific, HIV prevention messages during their counseling sessions rather than tailoring the messages to the clients' needs and circumstances. A follow-up focus group session of the counselors reveals that all had received verbal warnings from their supervisor (the program manager) about the increased length of time they had been spending counseling clients. Further, their job plans (which had not been updated for several years) continued to emphasize speed and efficiency of counseling rather than client-centered counseling acumen as a key performance element. Therefore, rather than jeopardize their salary increase (which was determined in large part by their performance evaluation), all but one of the counselors had reverted to the older, quicker (and less effective) form of "generic" counseling. In this hypothetical illustration, the historical emphasis on speed of counseling was a major disincentive to the adoption of client-centered counseling and would likely continue to interfere with its adoption until the job plans were changed.

Public Attitudes about the New Technology

To this listing, we can add another critical variable mediating the uptake of new technologies, one that is especially relevant to discussions of HIV prevention technologies: public attitudes about the intervention.[25] As an example of this phenomenon, let us consider in greater detail how social reactions to sexuality, especially homosexuality, can influence the uptake of HIV prevention technology.

As historically has been the case with other STDs,[26] persons with HIV infection may become victims of stigmatization and moralizing. Nor is this merely historical artifact. In a recent review of STDs in the United States, the Institute of Medicine affirmed that, sadly, "the portrayal of STDs as symbols of immoral behavior continues today."[27(p.89)] Furthermore, because gay and bisexual men account for a substantial portion of the HIV epidemic in the United States, the powerful stigma of homosexuality is added to the already substantial stigma of STD. It is precisely these stigmatizing attitudes that may interfere with the uptake of new HIV prevention technologies.

To wit, scientifically credible research has demonstrated that opinion leaders recruited through gay bars and clubs are effective agents in influencing the adoption of safer sexual practices in a community level intervention.[28] Regardless of the credibility that this intervention has with behavioral scientists and the target population, however, others may be skeptical of the notion of health outreach in a bar or nightclub setting. If these others are in policy- or grant-making positions, their skepticism could inhibit meaningful support for these activities.

Issues surrounding interventions that seek to enhance the adoption of safer sexual practices among gay men by eroticizing those practices have been even more controversial. In 1985, the Gay Men's Health Crisis (GMHC) in New York pioneered a safer sex workshop for gay men in which men could "discuss and share their feelings about changing patterns of their sex lives."[29(p.1)] Other GMHC efforts to encourage safer sex norms among sexually active gay men included a series of erotic "safer sex comics" produced in 1986 and 1987, for distribution in gay bars and bathhouses. When viewed by some members of Congress, these efforts were described as "hard-core, pornographic, lustful, and ugly."[30] Although the provocative comics were not funded with federal dollars, legislative language soon followed that directed the CDC and the recipients of CDC funds to adhere to the following when producing AIDS educational materials: "... none of the funds made available to the Centers for Disease Control shall be used to provide AIDS education, information, or prevention materials and activities that promote or encourage, directly or indirectly, homosexual sexual activities."[31(p.289)]

These restrictions (which have been modified since 1987, but are still in place at the time of this writing) were a direct outgrowth of the notion that eroticization of safer sex for gay men was a means of "promoting" homosexuality.

The importance of popularizing risk reduction as a means of facilitating its uptake among the gay community was well-understood by behavioral scientists. Although the gay community is not a homogeneous entity, many gay men at risk for HIV consider eroticization an appropriate and important intervention to further the acceptance of safer sexual practices, especially given its emphasis on self-empowerment. However, as this example shows, general public attitudes can have great influence on the uptake of HIV prevention technology, even when that technology is deemed valid by scientists and members of the target population. In fact, when a group of State AIDS Program Managers were surveyed in 1993 to learn more about the obstacles to planning HIV prevention programs, the managers reported that "they were especially concerned about public or political acceptance of, or opposition to, controversial and important HIV prevention activities."[32(p.210)]

TECHNOLOGY TRANSFER VERSUS TECHNOLOGY UPTAKE

The gap between what is known and what is practiced is not unique to the HIV/AIDS realm. As most readers doubtless recognize, the term "technology transfer" is neither derived from nor specific to HIV prevention. In fact, the concept of technology transfer transcends a single contextual paradigm and can be found among the terminologies of various disciplines. For example, in the context of international community development, technology transfer is seen as a mechanism by which developing countries can implement new technologies that improve the quality of life while preserving the environment for future generations.[33] In other disciplines, the use of the term "technology transfer" can describe activities as diverse as assessing the speed of the transfer of new statistical methods into peer reviewed medical journals,[34] determining the length of time it takes primary care providers to adopt new drugs into clinical practice,[35] and facilitating the uptake of new laboratory procedures for the diagnosis of infectious diseases.[36]

Hope[33] describes technology transfer as a "two-way relationship of sending and receiving technology primarily between and among firms, industries, and governments"; technology he defines as the "skills, knowledge, and procedures used in the provision of goods and services" (p. 196). His definition, though written in the context of international community development, is particularly relevant to our discussion of HIV prevention technology transfer. One of the critical aspects of technology transfer has been given light in Hope's definition: the mirror-image duality of his activity. In reality, technology transfer is not just about the *transfer* of technology, it is also about the *uptake*: being able to "receive" the new technology is every bit as critical as having it "sent" in the first place.

An example from basic biology illustrates this point. There are two ways in which essential materials move into a living cell from the extracellular environment: passive transport, which does not require the cell to expend energy (materials always move from an area of higher to lower concentration), and active transport, which does require cells to expend energy, since materials are moving against a concentration gradient (i.e., from an area of lower to higher concentration).

Why the biology lesson? Simply stated, because the way in which we conceptualize a process influences both how we define problems within that process and also what types of solutions we identify to address those problems. Specifically, if we think about HIV prevention technology transfer as a "passive' transfer model, our approaches will focus primarily on developing transferable technology products, assuming that once these products become available, they will be taken up spontaneously by individual and organizational providers of HIV prevention services. Whereas, if we think about HIV prevention technology transfer as an "active" transfer model, we will be acutely concerned about individual and organizational capacity to operationalize new technology, in addition to considering the availability of transferable technology products. In this discussion of HIV prevention technology transfer, we will embrace an active transfer model, recognizing that the policies, strategies, and systems that may be required to facilitate the uptake of transferable technology products are as essential as the development of the products themselves. In many areas of the country, for example, one of the major impediments to the uptake of HIV prevention technology is the lack of adequate infrastructure to carry out prevention activities.[15,37] We also must acknowledge that activities seeking to translate technology from scientific jargon into language and formats that prevention providers can understand may be distinctly different from activities aimed at increasing organizational capacity to adopt and sustain the use of new HIV prevention technology.

A TYPOLOGY OF HIV PREVENTION TECHNOLOGIES

Borrowing from Hope's[33] definition, we will define HIV prevention technology as the skills, knowledge, and procedures needed to provide effective HIV prevention services. Implicit in this definition is the understanding that HIV prevention technology is a heterogeneous grouping. There is no question that there are many potential ways of characterizing the variety of technologies that might fall under this heading.

One might choose to classify HIV prevention technologies on the basis of their scientific origin. For instance, a community-level intervention endorsing safer sexual behaviors within a large urban housing project where many women who are sex partners of injecting drug users reside would be classed as behavioral science prevention technology. In this same taxonomy, the use of antiretroviral drugs to reduce the chances of vertical HIV transmission from pregnant, HIV-infected women to their unborn children would be classed as biomedical science prevention technology.

Another taxonomy of HIV prevention technology might distinguish among technologies in terms of the level of intervention they informed. Such a schema could have the following designations: individual level, couples level, group level, community level, and general public. Still another taxonomy might typify HIV prevention technology in terms of where HIV prevention services are delivered, for example, clinic/health care delivery setting, CBO setting, street or other public venue, or at home (e.g., electronically through television or via home based services). However, for our discussion we will categorize HIV prevention technology depending on which aspect of the HIV prevention program cycle the technology is meant to influence.

HIV Prevention Programs

An HIV prevention program can be defined as a set of coordinated and interrelated activities undertaken to prevent the transmission or acquisition of HIV. Figure 1 shows the optimal sequence of events in such a program's life cycle: planning, setting priorities, obtaining resources, implementing prevention activities, and evaluating program outcomes. Plainly, this definition does not specify what manner of HIV prevention intervention(s) will be undertaken, what population(s) will be targeted to receive those intervention(s), or what kind of organization(s) will be providing the HIV prevention services. Furthermore, the life cycle depicted in Fig. 1 is not specific to HIV prevention, but could be easily used to describe a variety of health or social service activities.

Nevertheless, the generic nature of this typology serves our discussion well, for it

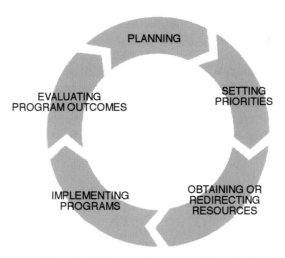

Figure 1. HIV prevention program life cycle.

underscores the diversity of needs related to HIV prevention technology. It helps us to avoid the common pitfall of emphasizing one aspect of HIV prevention technology need while ignoring others that, though less readily apparent, may be equally critical for successful prevention outcomes. Also, using a holistic model such as this one provides those involved in improving the transfer and uptake of HIV prevention technology with a basis for developing specific tools and processes to diagnose the exact nature of a technology deficit and to develop customized solutions to address deficits.

The remainder of this section will identify and discuss a variety of illustrative HIV prevention technology transfer products. Borrowing again from Hope's[33] definition, we will think of HIV prevention technology transfer products as those materials or methods that seek to improve or increase the skills, knowledge, and procedures that are required to provide effective HIV prevention services. Examples from both governmental and nongovernmental sectors will be given for each of the five stages of the HIV prevention program cycle.

Technologies Related to HIV Prevention Planning

An important dimension of program planning relates to the ability to assess in an accurate and timely manner unmet service needs. Yet, technical deficits have been cited as one of the major barriers to conducting needs assessments for HIV prevention programs, especially given the methodological complexity that can attend the measurement of need.[38] To help address this problem, the USCM developed a technical assistance report on the subject of needs assessment for HIV/AIDS prevention that offered "general guidance and practical suggestion to CBO and local health departments for designing and conducting needs assessments in their communities."[39(p.1)] The document provided readers with an operational definition of needs assessment, profiled three common methods of information collection, and suggested approaches to evaluating needs assessment processes.[39] Especially helpful was a step-by-step flowchart walking readers through the design of a model needs assessment.

In 1994, when the CDC directed health departments receiving federal funds to enhance the targeting, scientific bases, and cultural relevance of their HIV prevention programs, a chronic need to improve HIV prevention planning became suddenly and dramatically amplified.[25] HIV prevention community planning, as the process has come to be known, placed a number of new demands on health departments and community partners and highlighted the need to develop materials and methods in support of this undertaking. Two such products are described: "Do's and Don'ts for an Inclusive HIV Prevention Community Planning Process"[40] and a "Self-Assessment Tool for Community Planning Groups."[41] The former gave users specific, easy-to-understand pointers on how to maintain an open recruitment process, achieve true participation in decision making about HIV prevention priorities, and how to avoid and manage conflicts of interest.[40] The guide was formatted to be used either in group trainings or as an individual self-help tool. A particularly useful feature of this technology transfer product was its clever use of "scenarios to avoid" and "a better scenario"—brief story narratives providing readers with realistic examples of negative and positive planning experiences.

The "Self-Assessment Tool for Community Planning Groups"[41] was developed in 1995, at the end of the first year of HIV prevention community planning. This product consisted of a series of "diagnostic" questions about various aspects of the community planning process, among them: "ground rules" and written policies describing meeting-related processes, sources of qualitative and quantitative data used for decision making, and the use of epidemiological data to assess ongoing trends in the HIV epidemic. The instrument, which was developed based on the results of first-year evaluation findings, was promoted as a means of orienting new members to the major tasks of community planning, providing a means of periodically assessing community planning groups' progress, and better pinpointing specific technical assistance needs.

Technologies Related to Setting HIV Prevention Priorities

Holtgrave[42] outlined a number of formal decision analytic models that might be used to identify HIV prevention priorities, including decision tree analysis; multiattribute utility theory; economic evaluation techniques of cost, cost benefit, cost-effectiveness, and cost-utility analysis; linear programming; or scenario analysis. In his review of various decision analysis models, he identified ten steps that are found in common with most of the models studied; these were the steps he suggested would be most useful to persons who were involved in setting HIV prevention priorities through the community planning process.[42]

In actual practice, it appears that community planning groups find the job of setting HIV prevention funding priorities to be daunting. When Schietinger and colleagues[43] evaluated HIV prevention community planning at the end of its first year, they concluded that the prioritization process was often contentious and poorly understood by many of the 80 community planning group members they surveyed from nine sites across the country. Subsequently, several products have been developed to help improve the priority setting aspects of HIV prevention community planning, including "Overview of HIV/AIDS Prevention Interventions"[44] and "HIV Prevention Priorities: How Community Planning Groups Decide."[45]

Prioritization, by definition, involves rating or ranking from among a series of activities or items. If multiple groups are involved in the same priority-setting exercise (as is the case with HIV prevention community planning), it is critical that they share a common understanding of the universe of activities from among which they are selecting. Outlining a comprehensive list of HIV prevention interventions is particularly important in an evolving, multi-disciplinary field such as HIV/AIDS prevention, where essential interventions can range in diversity from clinic-based HIV counseling and testing, through community-level mobilization activities, to hotlines and clearinghouses. Therefore, providing HIV prevention community planning groups with a workable taxonomy of HIV/AIDS prevention interventions helped to encourage the adoption of a common vocabulary within the priority-setting process.[44]

Readers were informed that the taxonomy would help them make meaningful distinctions and choices among possible interventions.[44] Planners of HIV prevention activities were further advised to consider five broad parameters when reviewing the strengths and weaknesses of potential interventions: (1) What is the intervention's objective? Is it meant to increase information levels, develop skills, or change social norms? (2) At what level will the intervention be targeted: individual, group, community, or general public? (3) How often will the intervention be delivered? (4) In what type of institutional or community setting will this intervention be delivered? (5) What is the manner or method by which the intervention is provided (e.g., one-on-one, group process, via media, via community mobilization, etc.)

Ongoing evaluations of priority setting activities within the context of HIV prevention community planning have substantiated recurrent needs for certain kinds of data (especially information about intervention effectiveness), tension between evidence-based and value-based decision making, and the need for models demonstrating how diverse data can be reviewed, rated, and utilized in the context of a group decision making process.[45] An important contribution to priority-setting technology was created in 1996, by the Academy for Educational Development and the National Alliance of State and Territorial AIDS Directors. Their document, "How Community Planning Groups Decide," provided in-depth profiles of HIV prevention priority-setting approaches in six states—diverse in terms of geography, HIV epidemiology, and the configuration of their respective community planning processes.[45] Clear, concise writing helps the reader understand the advantages and disadvantages of various priority-setting approaches. Further, each profile is accompanied by the name and telephone number of an expert consultant who can provide additional information to interested readers. Another section of the document contains key findings and issues about priority setting culled from information provided by 44 state AIDS directors, with an eye toward ensuring a successful prioritization process that can be endorsed by the entire group.

Technologies Related to Obtaining HIV Prevention Resources

"A poorly written proposal for an extraordinary program will cause funders to question the capability of the applicant."[45(p.1)] This statement, taken directly from one of the technology transfer products described in this section, underscores the fact that granting agencies (whether public or private) consider issues in addition to need when they allocate prevention resources through a competitive process. They also consider the quality of the proposal itself as a surrogate for the applicant's capacity to meet critical program objectives.

With federal support, the USCM first produced a technical guidance on preparing funding proposals in 1989; this was updated in September 1992.[46] In addition to practical tips listed as "do's" (e.g., describe how the project meets a unique need and that it will not duplicate existing services) and "don'ts" (e.g., avoid using letters of support that are form letters), this technology transfer product provided important insights into how granters evaluate proposals; what funders look for. Examples of program goals, objectives, and strategies were profiled for an intended audience composed largely of CBOs. Readers were counseled to be extremely specific when justifying program needs to potential funders, with the admonishment that "developing a project without utilizing a needs assessment is much like taking a long trip without knowing your destination."[46(p.4)] In addition to identifying unmet needs, persons seeking funding for HIV prevention activities were advised to specify current barriers to service delivery and to indicate how their organizations were uniquely qualified to meet prevention gaps, in terms of both organizational capacity and the organization's present relationship with the target population.

In 1995, the Support Center for Nonprofit Management and the National Minority AIDS Council[47] created an "action handbook" for a specific subset of the NGO audience: boards of directors. Recognizing the critical developmental role of boards of directors, this product detailed specific strategies to be undertaken for boards to productively increase their involvement in fundraising. The suggested strategies are straightforward (e.g., form a fundraising committee, recruit new board members who have an interest in fundraising, talk to other non-AIDS agencies to learn how they raise money for their organizations) and do not require specialized expertise in financial management to understand or operationalize.

Technologies Related to Implementing HIV Prevention Activities

Of all the technology needs related to HIV prevention, arguably this is the one that is most frequently identified. Because we know that HIV prevention programs can have a favorable impact on reducing HIV transmission when they are delivered with scientific fidelity, sufficient intensity, and cultural competency,[10] there is an understandable urgency to ensuring that technological advances in the behavioral and biomedical realms are translated so that their HIV prevention benefits are realized.

Recommendations to improve the implementation of HIV prevention activities and the quality of HIV prevention services rendered have been made throughout the epidemic (see first section, this chapter, "Challenges to Prevention Capacity"). Analyses from both the first and second decades of the HIV/AIDS epidemic have been remarkably similar in their call for bettering the implementation of HIV prevention programs. Reviewing community-based experience from the first decade of the epidemic, Freudenberg and Zimmerman[48] found that organizations attempting to provide HIV prevention services often "had difficult in setting realistic goals, implementing the intervention, and integrating the new program with existing services."[48(p.189)] More recently, when a nonfederal panel of experts was convened to develop an objective assessment of behavioral intervention methods to reduce the risk of HIV infection. They[49] found:

> Prevention interventions are effective for reducing behavioral risk for HIV/AIDS and must be widely disseminated. Their application in practice settings may require careful training of personal, close monitoring of the fidelity of procedures, and ongoing monitoring of effectiveness. Results of this evaluation must be reported, and where effectiveness in field settings is reduced, program modifications must be undertaken immediately. (p. 27)

Among the multiple barriers to using published scientific research for the purposes of implementing scientifically sound HIV prevention programs are turgid, academic language, inadequate information on the content and process of actual interventions, and multiple issues related to the "transferability" of controlled scientific research from one setting and population to another setting and perhaps a somewhat different population.[50]

The technology transfer products described in this section have in common the goal of improving the quality of HIV prevention efforts by improving the quality of HIV interventions. The Center for AIDS Prevention Studies (CAPS) at the University of California, San Francisco, and the Harvard AIDS Institute jointly publish a series of bilingual (English and Spanish) fact sheets on various aspects of HIV prevention science that economically synthesize relevant scientific theory and research into pithy, easy to understand summaries. One offering[51] gives readers brief summaries of successful and unsuccessful attempts to adapt prevention interventions in different settings and populations. Examples include a description of the successful adaptation of a peer-based sex education program for American junior high school students to address Balinese youth at increased risk for HIV and an unsuccessful effort to adapt an intervention originally designed for gay men to serve women in inner-city housing projects. Both examples are highly instructive.

The AIDS Community Demonstration Projects (1989–1994) tested HIV prevention community level interventions in five US cities: Dallas, Denver, Long Beach, New York City, and Seattle.[52] Using a common study protocol based on behavior change theories, these five projects focused on groups considered difficult to reach and specifically sought to increase the prevalence of consistent condom use among sexually active persons and to increase the proper use of bleach to clean injection equipment among active drug users. A stated goal of this research, which is described in greater detail elsewhere,[52] was to transfer effective interventions from a study protocol into community practice settings. Corby and colleagues[53] support a critical dimension of this transfer in their detailed outline of how to develop effective role model stories.

According to Corby et al.,[53]

> a role model story relates the experience of a member of a priority population in changing a risky behavior so that other members of the same populations can identify with the story and begin to change their perceptions, beliefs, and/or attitudes in a direction that will facilitate their own behavior change. (p. 137)

Readers are guided through the steps involved in developing credible role model stories: defining target populations, recruiting credible role models, interviewing role models, transcribing the interview, constructing a role model story, and publishing a role model story. Details of this process are extraordinarily complete and address important though often neglected topics such as how to make the story culturally, ethnically, and gender specific; how to assess the literacy level of the story; and what type of artwork should be used to illustrate the story—even what type and color of paper should be used. The chapter is rounded out with directions on pretesting the story and suggestions on materials distribution.

Technologies Related to Evaluating Program Outcomes

In a 3-year review (1989–1992) of the program management aspects of California's HIV prevention efforts, evaluators noted that organizations receiving contract funds from California had difficulty evaluating their programs.[54] Contractors, consisting of CBOs, AIDS service organizations, county health departments, and community clinics and hospitals, reported that their greatest needs for technical assistance were in the realm of evaluating prevention programs.[54] These findings are consistent with experiences in other jurisdictions and call attention to another important dimension of technology transfer: evaluating HIV prevention program outcomes.

The National Council for La Raza's Center for Health Promotion published an introductory guide to evaluating HIV/STD programs in 1991.[55] A major emphasis of this document was to stress the benefits of evaluation, not just to highlight its accountability functions. Users were informed that evaluation can: (1) help to run an effective program; (2) show that HIV/STD funding is a good investment; (3) identify and fix problems quickly; and (4) identify and share program models that can be replicated to save lives. Evaluation systems were described in terms of four basic components: a record-keeping system, process(es) for content and format review of prevention materials, mechanism(s) for postassessment of presentations or training sessions, and ways to perform a periodic analysis of project activities. Finally, readers were provided with 14 sequenced steps to follow when implementing a basic evaluation system.

Somewhat more detailed was the 1993 offering of the National Community AIDS Partnership.[56] The authors specifically noted that their work was not meant to be perceived as a "how-to" document. Nevertheless, this particular guide contains a wealth of useful information, including articulate and intelligible descriptions of techniques for collecting and analyzing evaluation data; straightforward summary narratives outlining the distinctions between experimental, quasi-experimental, and nonexperimental evaluation research designs; and options for evaluating four basic HIV prevention approaches (i.e., interactive small-group sessions, one-on-one sessions in nonclinical settings, telephone hotline and referral services, and media-based prevention campaigns).

The third and final example of an evaluation technology transfer product is what has been euphemistically referred to as the "evaluation cookbook." Its formal title is somewhat less terse: "Planning and Evaluating HIV/AIDS Prevention Programs in State and Local Health Departments: A Companion to Program Announcement #300."[57] This product was specifically developed for health departments as the primary audience in order to address in adequate detail the planning and evaluation requirements outlined in the CDC's official program guidance to health department recipients of federal HIV prevention funds. It became unofficially known as the "evaluation cookbook" because of its expansion of terse program guidance language into detailed, step-by-step instructions for program managers and others on how to conduct the referenced evaluation activities.

For example, the program guidance informs grantees that they are responsible for "documenting and describing the success of referral systems, including the numbers of persons referred and the number actually receiving services, by site, and how well the system functions in identifying sources of services and in assisting persons in obtaining and receiving them,"[58(p.40681)] but does not provide particulars as to how this will be accomplished. The evaluation cookbook devotes an entire chapter to this requirement, defining key terms, providing examples of what does and does not meet basic criteria for a referral, and suggesting several options that can be used to document clients' follow-through with referrals. To round out the offering, a case study is presented of one organization's experience with collecting referral data on HIV-seropositive injecting drug users referred into drug treatment.

FACILITATING THE UPTAKE OF HIV PREVENTION TECHNOLOGIES

Earlier in this chapter, a distinction was made between the passive transfer of HIV prevention technology products versus the actions required to encourage the uptake and operationalization of these products. Experience to date suggests that, deficits notwithstanding, our knowledge and practices related to the development of technology transfer products are further advanced than our knowledge and practices related to uptake and operationalization of new HIV prevention technologies. Parcel and colleagues,[59] writing on the diffusion of health promotion interventions, sounded a similar note: "Most of the research in this area has focused on the adoption of health behavior innovations by individuals, and we know very little about how organizations are influenced to adopt innovative health promotion programs."[59(p.239)]

Advancing our understanding of how organizations, including the individual providers within those organizations, are influenced to adopt and maintain innovations in HIV prevention is clearly an area in need of further study. This research agenda requires that we further elucidate provider, organizational, and environmental barriers to the uptake and operationalization of new HIV prevention technologies and that specific strategies to ameliorate or remove these barriers be evaluated in a scientifically rigorous fashion.

However, research alone cannot solve all of the impediments discussed in this chapter. Equally critical is the need to invest in the development of sustainable systems and processes that have as their primary goal the active transfer of new HIV prevention technologies into rapid and widespread use in both community and clinic-based settings. To believe that technology transfer can be accomplished without paying serious attention to the underlying gaps and inadequacies in the infrastructure responsible for supporting the transfer and uptake of new prevention technologies is misguided.

Those in a position to craft policy also have a role to play in supporting HIV prevention technology transfer, regardless of whether their purview extends across an entire state or only within the bounds of a CBO. Individuals in leadership positions, whether governmental or nongovernmental, elected or hired, must encourage the formulation of funding and staff development policies that recognize and support the ongoing role of technology transfer in effective HIV prevention efforts. Sound research and substantial infrastructure count for little in the face of policies that discourage or prevent (either directly or inadvertently) the implementation of new advances in HIV prevention.

Because of its bidirectional nature (i.e., sending and receiving), HIV prevention technology transfer cannot exist in a milieu that does not strongly endorse, in theory and practice, equitable partnerships between the providers and receivers of technology transfer products and services. Further, these partnerships must not be left to develop after the research described above is completed; instead, they should be prominent throughout the entire process, from research development, to delivery, through evaluation of the technology transfer initiative. Asking HIV prevention researchers to work proactively with communities and providers to frame technology transfer needs and issues at the start of the research process can maximize outcomes and minimize many of the important barriers to uptake.

By taking these steps, we can assure that scientific findings move beyond the pages of research journals and technical reports to the level of providers and program managers, where they will achieve their promise in terms of reduced HIV transmission.

REFERENCES

1. Public Health Service Executive Task Force on AIDS. Public Health Service plan for the prevention and control of Acquired Immune Deficiency Syndrome (AIDS). *Public Health Rep* 1985; 100:453–455.
2. Presidential Commission on the Human Immunodeficiency Virus Epidemic. *Report of the Presidential Commission on the Human Immunodeficiency Virus Epidemic.* Washington, DC: US Government Printing Office: 1988 0-214-701:QL3:
3. Valdiserri RO. Planning and implementing AIDS-prevention programs: A case study approach. In: Valdiserri RO, ed. *Preventing AIDS: The Design of Effective Programs.* Rutgers University Press; 1989:129–208.
4. Valdiserri RO. HIV counseling and testing: Its evolving role in HIV prevention. *AIDS Educ Prev* 1997; 9S:2–13.
5. Thomas SB, Morgan CH. Evaluation of community-based AIDS education and risk reduction projects in ethnic and racial minority communities: A survey of projects funded by the US Public Health Service. *Eval Prog Plann* 1991; 14:247–255.
6. Thompson PI, Jones TS. Monitoring and documenting community-based organization outreach activities for populations at risk for HIV. *Hygie* 1990; 9:34–38.
7. National Commission on AIDS. *Behavioral and Social Sciences and the HIV/AIDS Epidemic.* Washington, DC: National Commission on AIDS 1993:1–52.
8. Gluck M, Rosenthal E. *The Effectiveness of AIDS Prevention Efforts.* Washington, DC: Office of Technology Assessment, Congress of the United States; September 1995; OTA-BP-H-172.
9. Choi KH, Coates TJ. Prevention of HIV infection. *AIDS* 1994; 8:1371–1389.
10. Holtgrave DR, Qualls ML, Curran JW, et al. An overview of the effectiveness and efficiency of HIV prevention programs. *Public Health Rep* 1995; 110:134–146.
11. Wingood GM, DiClemente RJ. HIV sexual risk reduction interventions for women: A review. *Am J Prev Med* 1996; 12:209–217.
12. Backer TE, David SL, Soucy G. The challenge of technology transfer. In: Backer TE, Davis SL, Soucy G, eds. *Reviewing the Behavioral Science Knowledge Base on Technology Transfer.* NIDA Research Monograph 155. Rockville, MD: National Institutes on Drug Abuse; 1995:1–19.
13. Freudenberg N, Eng E, Flay B, et al. Strengthening individual and community capacity to prevent disease and promote health: in search of relevant theories and principles. *Health Educ Q* 1995; 22:290–306.
14. Leviton L. Theoretical foundations of AIDS-prevention programs. In: Valdiserri RO, ed. *Preventing AIDS: The Design of Effective Programs.* New Brunswick NJ: Rutgers University Press; 1989:42–90.
15. United States Conference of Mayors. *Assessing the HIV Prevention Needs of Gay and Bisexual Men of Color.* Washington, DC: United States Conference of Mayors; 1993.
16. Thomas SB, Quinn SC. The Tuskegee Syphilis Study, 1932 to 1972: Implications for HIV education and AIDS risk reduction education programs in the Black community. *Am J Public Health* 1991; 81:1498–1504.
17. National Commission on AIDS. *The Challenges of HIV/AIDS in Communities of Color.* Washington, DC: National Commission on AIDS; 1992.
18. Freudenberg N, Lee J, Silver D. How black and Latino community organizations respond to the AIDS epidemic: A case study in one New York City neighborhood. *AIDS Educ Prev* 1989; 1:12–21.
19. DeGroff A. Is prevention research reaching front line prevention programs: A descriptive study from San Francisco. In: *Abstracts from the XI International Conference on AIDS.* vol 2, Th.C. 4773. Vancouver, BC; 1996:372.
20. Public Health Service Task Force. A plan to strengthen public health in the United States. *Public Health Rep* 1991; 106:5–15.
21. Public Health Foundation. Measuring state expenditures for core public health functions. *Am J Prev Med* 1995; 11(S2):58–73.

22. French WL, Bell CH. *Organization Development: Behavioral Science Interventions for Organization Improvement*. Englewood Cliffs, NJ: Prentice Hall; 1995.
23. Cummings TG, Worley CG. *Organization Development and Change*. Minneapolis: West Publishing Company; 1993.
24. Centers for Disease Control and Prevention. Technical guidance on HIV counseling. *MMWR Morb Mortal Weekly Rep* 1993; 42:8–17.
25. Valdiserri RO. Managing system-wide change in HIV prevention programs. *Public Adm Rev* 1996; 56:545–553.
26. Brandt AM. *No Magic Bullet: A Social History of Venereal Disease in the United States since 1880*. New York: Oxford University Press; 1985.
27. Institute of Medicine. *The Hidden Epidemic: Confronting Sexually Transmitted Diseases*. Washington, DC: National Academy Press; 1997.
28. Kelly JA, St. Lawrence JS, Stevenson LY, et al. Community AIDS/HIV risk reduction: the effects of endorsements by popular people in three cities. *Am J Public Health* 1992; 82:1483–1489.
29. Palacios-Jiminez L, Shernoff M. *Facilitator's Guide to Eroticizing Safer Sex: A Psychoeducational Workshop Approach to Safer Sex Education*. New York: Gay Men's Health Crisis, Inc.; 1986.
30. Booth W. Another muzzle for AIDS education? *Science* 1987; 238:1036.
31. Congress of the United States of America. Departments of Labor, Health, and Human Services and Education and Related Agencies Appropriation Bill, 1988. Washington, DC: 1987; Section 514.
32. West GR, Valdiserri RO. Understanding and overcoming obstacles to planning HIV prevention programs. *AIDS Public Policy* 1994; 9:207–213.
33. Hope KR. Promoting sustainable community development in developing countries: The role of technology transfer. *Community Dev J* 1996; 31:193–200.
34. Altman DG, Goodman SN. Transfer of technology from statistical journals to the biomedical literature. *JAMA* 1994; 272:129–132.
35. Markson LE, Cosler LE, Turner BJ. Implications of generalists' slow adoption of Zidovudine in clinical practice. *Arch Intern Med* 1994; 154:1497–1504.
36. Centers for Disease Control. A strategic plan for the elimination of tuberculosis in the United States. *MMWR Morb Mortal Wkly Rep* 1989; 38(S-3):1–25.
37. Valdiserri RO, West GR, Moore M, et al. Structuring HIV prevention service delivery systems on the basis of social science theory. *J Community Health* 1992; 17:259–269.
38. Valdiserri RO, West GR. Barriers to the assessment of unmet need in planning HIV/AIDS prevention programs. *Public Adm Rev* 1994; 54:25–30.
39. United States Conference of Mayors. *Needs Assessment for HIV/AIDS Prevention and Service Programs*. HIV/AIDS Technical Assistance Reports. Washington, DC: United States Conference of Mayors; 1993.
40. McKay EG. *Do's and Dont's for an Inclusive HIV Prevention Community Planning Process: A Self-Help Guide*. Washington, DC: National Council of LaRaza; 1994.
41. Academy for Educational Development. *Self-Assessment Tool for Community Planning Groups*. Washington, DC: Academy for Education Development; 1995.
42. Holtgrave D. Setting priorities and community planning for HIV-prevention programs. *AIDS Public Policy* 1994; 9:145–151.
43. Schietinger H, Coburn J, Levi J. Community planning for HIV prevention: Findings from the first year. *AIDS Public Policy* 1994; 10:140–147.
44. Academy for Educational Development. *Overview of HIV/AIDS Prevention Interventions*. Washington, DC: Academy for Educational Development; 1995.
45. Academy for Educational Development, National Alliance of State and Territorial AIDS Directors. *HIV Prevention Priorities: How Community Planning Groups Decide*. Washington, DC: Academy for Educational Development; 1996.
46. United States Conference of Mayors. *Proposal Writing for HIV/AIDS Prevention Grants*. HIV/AIDS Technical Assistance Reports. Washington, DC: United States Conference of Mayors; 1992.
47. Support Center for Nonprofit Management, National Minority AIDS Council. *Action Handbook for Boards*. Washington, DC: National Minority AIDS Council; 1995.
48. Freudenberg N, Zimmerman, MA. The role of community organizations in public health practice: The lessons from AIDs prevention. In: Freudenberg N, Zimmerman MA, eds. *AIDS Prevention in the Community: Lessons from the First Decade*. Washington, DC: American Public Health Association Press; 1995:183–197.
49. National Institutes of Health. *Consensus Development Statement on Interventions to Prevent HIV Risk Behaviors*. National Institutes of Health: Bethesda, MD: February 11–13, 1997:19; No. 104.
50. Collins C, Franks P. *Improving Use of Behavioral Research in the CDC's HIV Prevention Community Planning Process*. Center for AIDS Prevention Studies Policy Monograph; July 1996.

51. Center for AIDS Prevention Studies, University of California, San Francisco and Harvard AIDS Institute. *Can Prevention Programs Be Adapted?* Center for AIDs Prevention Studies and Harvard AIDS Institute Publication No. 23E, October 1996.

52. Centers for Disease Control and Prevention. Community-level prevention of HIV infection among high-risk populations: The AIDS Community Demonstration Projects. *MMWR Morbid Mortal Wkly Rep* 1996; 45(RR-6): 1–24.

53. Corby NH, Enguidanos SM, Padilla S. Preparing culturally relevant HIV prevention materials: Role model stories. In Corby NH, Wolitski RJ, eds. *Community HIV Prevention: The Long Beach AIDS Community Demonstration Project.* Long Beach: California State University Press; 1997:135–157.

54. Marx R, Franks PE, Kahn JG, et al. HIV education and prevention in California: Problems and progress. *AIDS Public Policy* 1997; 12:31–45.

55. National Council of La Raza Center for Health Promotion. *Evaluating HIV/STD Education and Prevention Programs: An Introduction.* Washington, DC: National Council of La Raza AIDS Center; 1991.

56. National Community AIDS Partnership. *Evaluating HIV/AIDS Prevention Programs in Community Based Settings.* Washington DC: National Community AIDS Partnership; 1993.

57. *Planning and Evaluating HIV/AIDS Prevention Programs in State and Local Health Departments.* A Companion to Program Announcement #300. Atlanta, GA: Centers for Disease Control and Prevention; 1993.

58. Centers for Disease Control. Cooperative agreements for HIV; prevention projects program announcement and availability of funds for fiscal year 1993. *Fed Reg* 1992; 57:40675–40682.

59. Parcel GS, Perry CL, Taylor WC. Beyond demonstration: Diffusion of health promotion innovations. In: Bracht N, ed. *Health Promotion at the Community Level.* Newbury Park, CA: Sage; 1990:229–252.

15

The Economics of HIV Primary Prevention

DAVID R. HOLTGRAVE and STEVEN D. PINKERTON

Every hour, an average of approximately five people in the United States become infected with human immunodeficiency virus (HIV).[1] If the US government decided to open a trust fund and place in it enough money to pay for the future care and treatment of newly HIV-infected persons, it would have to deposit between $750,000 and $1,000,000 every hour (or between $6.57 billion and $8.76 billion per year), assuming current projections of medical care costs and HIV incidence.[2]

Clearly, effective HIV primary prevention programs have the potential for tremendous savings in terms of human lives and fiscal resources. Unfortunately, resources to fund these prevention programs are limited. For example, in 1997, the Centers for Disease Control and Prevention (CDC) made available approximately $18,000,000 to directly fund community-based organizations (CBOs) to provide important HIV prevention services. These monies funded 94 organizations; however, over five times that many CBOs applied for these funds. Hence, there are a great many unmet HIV prevention needs, and the available, limited resources must be used wisely to maximize their prevention potential.

Fiscal policy makers, public health program managers, and HIV prevention community planners who must judiciously prioritize programs and allocate fiscal resources often ask three types of key questions:

1. How much do specific types of HIV prevention interventions cost to deliver?
2. Are HIV primary prevention programs cost-effective compared to health programs in other disease areas?
3. Which HIV prevention programs are most cost-effective compared to each other?

Here, we provide an overview of recent studies designed to answer one or more of these key questions and discuss in detail the implications of the available study results for fiscal decision makers. Additionally, we make several recommendations for behavioral intervention researchers so as to facilitate further economic evaluation studies of primary prevention interventions; we also identify a number of needed areas of further methodological and applied research.

DAVID R. HOLTGRAVE • Division of HIV/AIDS Prevention, Intervention Research and Support, National Center for HIV, STD, and TB Prevention, Centers for Disease Control and Prevention, Atlanta, Georgia 30333. *STEVEN D. PINKERTON* • Center for AIDS Intervention Research, Medical College of Wisconsin, Milwaukee, Wisconsin 53202.

Handbook of HIV Prevention, edited by Peterson and DiClemente. Kluwer Academic/Plenum Publishers, New York, 2000.

OVERVIEW OF RESEARCH LITERATURE

The literature review is divided into two subsections: pre-1995 and post-1995.

Pre-1995

Holtgrave et al.[3] reviewed all economic evaluation studies of HIV-related prevention and treatment programs published in 1995 or earlier. They found a total of 93 such studies, of which 78% examined domestic programs. Of the domestic studies, 16 were focused on care and treatment, 29 on screening programs, and 28 on programs that may in some way involve changes in HIV-related risk behaviors.

The review identified several studies that found that HIV prevention efforts can be cost-effective and perhaps even cost-saving to society.[3] (Simply put, "cost-saving" interventions avert more medical care and treatment costs than the prevention intervention costs to deliver, "cost-effective" HIV prevention interventions cost more than they save yet still compare favorably to other life-saving interventions; we return to this topic below.) These efficient programs include counseling, testing, referral, and partner notification services for clients at high behavioral risk of infection; needle and syringe exchange programs; outreach services for persons who inject drugs; and information, education, and counseling activities for persons who inject drugs. (Several other behavioral modification interventions have since been identified as cost-effective, as discussed below.)

However, not all HIV prevention programs are cost-effective. Among the less efficient programs that have been studied are antibody screening programs in low seroprevalence populations, such as marriage license applicants and the general population.[3] On a methodological note, the review found that the wide diversity of economic evaluation methods employed across studies makes comparison of the results of one study to another highly problematic; we return to this important topic below.

The review also found that, at the time, no economic evaluations had been done on some of the most promising interventions for the primary prevention of sexual transmission of HIV, namely, small-group and community-level interventions.[3-6] Studies have found small-group and community-level behavioral interventions to be effective in reducing HIV-related sexual risk behaviors among at-risk women, gay and bisexual men, and adolescents, among other populations.[7-14] Further, the economic evaluation literature review found that no studies had examined the cost-effectiveness of interventions to reduce perinatal transmission of HIV through voluntary counseling and testing of pregnant women and administration of anti-retroviral therapy to HIV-infected women before and during childbirth as well as to the infant postnatally. Such an intervention was found in a clinical trial to reduce perinatal transmission of HIV from approximately 25% to 8%.[8]

Post-1995

However, there have been important developments since this review[3] was published. Table 1 lists several recent studies that have attempted to fill key literature gaps regarding the cost-effectiveness of the highly effective interventions noted in the previous paragraph. The table also includes a recent peer-reviewed economic evaluation study of a critical HIV prevention intervention strategy for injection drug users now receiving a great deal of attention and debate in the US Congress and several stage legislatures, namely, needle and syringe exchange programs. Further, there has been recent movement in this literature toward stan-

Table 1.   Selected Economic Evaluation Studies of HIV Primary Prevention Interventions

Investigator [source]	Intervention	Population	Base case results	
			Cost-per-client	Cost-effectiveness
Sexual transmission				
Holtgrave[15]	Group, 5-session behavioral risk reduction	At-risk women	$269	$2024 per QALY[a]
Holtgrave[16]	Group, 12-session, behavioral risk reduction	Gay men	$470	Cost saving[b]
Pinkerton[17]	Group, 1-session, behavioral skills training	Gay men	$40[c]	Cost saving
Pinkerton[18]	Community-level, peer opinion leader, behavioral risk reduction	Gay men	$38	Cost saving
Perinatal transmission				
Gorsky[19]	Counseling and testing, and AZT therapy if HIV+	Pregnant women	$20[d]	Cost saving
Mauskopf[20]	Counseling and testing, and AZT therapy if HIV+	Pregnant women	$60[d]	Cost saving
Injection-associated transmission				
Kaplan[21]	Needle and syringe exchange	Injection drug users	$25[e]	Cost saving

[a]"QALY" indicates "quality-adjusted life years" saved by the intervention.
[b]"Cost saving" indicates that the present value of the HIV-related medical costs saved by the intervention are greater than the cost of the intervention itself.
[c]This $40 cost is the incremental cost of the skills training intervention relative to a group lecture intervention.
[d]This gross cost for the intervention is per pregnant woman counseled and tested regardless of test result.
[e]The $25 cost is per client, per month for 168 syringes at $0.15 each.

dardization of methodologies for cost-effectiveness analysis; this greatly improves the possibilities for cross-study comparisons.

Table 1 displays the intervention type, population served, and base case results (both gross cost of the service per client and the cost-effectiveness finding) for each of seven studies. All these analyses included extensive sensitivity analysis to gauge the robustness of the base case results to changes in model parameters (the original sources should be consulted for the complete analyses).

Four studies have shown that small-group and community-level behavioral interventions are not only effective at reducing sexual behavioral risk, but are also cost-saving or cost-effective.[15–18] ("Cost-saving" interventions are those for which the medical costs averted by preventing HIV infection outweigh the programmatic cost of the intervention; "cost-effective" interventions are those that generally have a cost-per-quality-adjusted-life-year-saved less than roughly $50,000.) This is true even if the intervention is especially intensive (as many as 12 sessions per client were required by one intervention) and the overall cost of the intervention is measured in the tens of thousands of dollars. Hence, interventions for preventing the sexual transmission of HIV may at first blush seem expensive, but may very well be worth the expenditure because they avert future medical costs of care and treatment. These studies find via sensitivity analyses, however, that the cost-effectiveness ratios appear less favorable if assumptions of very low local HIV seroprevalence are made in the analyses; therefore, the cost-effectiveness of intensive behavioral interventions may be questioned for populations or geographic areas with extremely low HIV seroprevalence.

Illustrative Study

All four of these studies were retrospective. They were extensions of previously conducted, empirical, prospective studies of the behavioral effects of small-group or community-level interventions. Here we describe one study in some detail to illustrate the analytic steps taken by the authors.

Holtgrave and Kelly[16] retrospectively conducted a cost-utility analysis of a small-group intervention for gay men. A randomized controlled trial was previously conducted to assess this intervention (relative to a wait-list control) with 104 gay men.[10,16] Eighty-seven percent of the participants identified their race/ethnicity as white, and 45% had completed college or higher. Their average age was 31 years, and all had engaged in HIV-related high risk behaviors in the previous year.

The 12 intervention sessions were offered weekly, and each lasted about 1.5 hours. Groups of about 17 persons each discussed several important topics, including (1) basic information about HIV disease, transmission, and protection; (2) self-management and identification of situations likely to result in high risk behaviors; (3) safer sex assertiveness role-playing; (4) skills building to enhance relationships and social support; and (5) self-reinforcement of successful strategies to engage in safer sexual behaviors. Recalling behaviors from the past 4 months, the intervention group improved from 23% condom use at baseline to 65% at 4-month follow-up and 77% at 8-month follow-up. The group randomized to the wait-list control condition actually decreased condom use from 24% at baseline to 19% at 4-month follow-up. For ethical reasons, the wait-list control condition was provided the intervention after the 4-month follow-up rather than the 8-month follow-up as originally planned.

Holtgrave and Kelly[16] retrospectively determined the cost of providing the intervention on a per-client basis. They identified the categories of resources consumed by the intervention (e.g., an hour of group facilitator time; an hour of transportation time for a client; materials cost per client per session). For each resource category, they estimated the number of units of the resource consumed and the dollar value of each unit of each resource category. This information provided the basic data with which to estimate the cost per client for the intervention. The best estimate was $470 per client for the entire 12-session intervention (or $23,507 for all study participants immediately receiving the intervention).

Next, the authors used the observed behavioral results from the randomized trial as input to a mathematical model of HIV transmission. The purpose of this step was to make a careful estimate of the number of HIV infections averted by the intervention in the group of participants over the follow-up time period. The Bernoullian model they used posits that the cumulative probability of HIV infection over a given time period is a function of (1) the client's number of sexual partners, (2) the number of sexual acts per partner, (3) the infectivity of each sexual act, (4) the level of condom use, (5) the effectiveness of condom use at reducing infectivity, and (6) the HIV seroprevalence level among the network of one's sexual partners. These terms combine via a standard cumulative probability equation. Some terms, such as infectivity values, were obtained from the epidemiological literature. Holtgrave and Kelly[16] employed this equation to estimate the number of HIV seronegative study participants who were protected from HIV infection and a variant of this equation to approximate the number of HIV seronegative sexual partners of already HIV-seropositive study participants who were saved from HIV infection. Under base case estimates for parameter values, it was estimated that the intervention averted 0.75 HIV infections among study participants (and some partners) over the short follow-up period.

Holtgrave and Kelly[16] used a published estimated of the present value of the lifetime cost of medical treatment for HIV disease; this value was $56,000 when discounted at a 5% rate (this cost-of-illness estimate was published before the advent of protease inhibitors). Multiplying $56,000 by 0.75 (the number of infections averted by the intervention) yields the medical costs saved by this intervention; the result is a figure much higher than the $23,507 cost of the intervention. Hence, under base case assumptions, the intervention was determined to be cost-saving to society.

The authors also reported a large number of sensitivity analyses to gauge the robustness of their base case results to uncertainty in some model parameters. They found the results to be quite robust to uncertainty in parameter values. The intervention would not appear to be cost-effective only if it were to be delivered in areas of very low HIV seroprevalence or if the condom effectiveness parameter or number of sexual partner parameter were set to unrealistically low values. However, within realistic ranges of key parameter values, the results of the analysis were very robust; in each case the intervention was either cost-saving or cost-effective. Hence, the sensitivity analyses were very reassuring in this case.

The other studies of small-group and community level intervention summarized in Table 1 also followed similar analytic strategies. The original studies contain complete analytic details.[15–21]

Perinatal Studies

As summarized in Table 1, two studies[19,20] have found that voluntary counseling and testing for pregnant women [along with azidothymidine (AZT) therapy if the client tests HIV seropositive] can be a cost-saving strategy for the prevention of HIV transmission to infants. These results are somewhat sensitive to local HIV seroprevalence. They also are sensitive to assumptions made about the cost of HIV counseling, because relatively few pregnant women (out of the population of all pregnant women) will test HIV-seropositive. These studies raise the question of how intensive the routine counseling should be that accompanies HIV testing among pregnant women. If the counseling is as intensive (and costly) as that conducted in much higher seroprevalence environments [such as sexually transmitted disease (STD) treatment clinics], then the results appear slightly less favorable.

Needle and Syringe Exchange Study

Kaplan[21] recently published a peer-reviewed analysis of needle and syringe exchange programs for persons who inject drugs. For a typical drug user who injects 168 times per month, a supply of sterile syringes would cost about $25 per month.[21] However, empirically based mathematical models suggest that the preventive power of the sterile syringes would reduce the probability of HIV infection significantly; in fact, the HIV infections prevented would avert sufficient medical cost for HIV care and treatment to outweigh the cost of sterile syringe purchase, distribution, exchange, and disposal.[21] Kaplan's article complements and expands on the results of previously published reports about this intervention.[3] The cost–effectiveness of this intervention compares favorably to other life-saving interventions in other disease areas.[22]

The Advent of New Treatments

Even though the studies in Table 1 were conducted recently, they were all completed before protease inhibitors became part of comprehensive HIV treatment. Recent studies have estimated that the lifetime cost of treating a case of HIV disease has more than doubled with the availability of these new, effective yet expensive therapies.[2,23] Pinkerton and Holtgrave[23] have estimated the cost of illness for HIV disease per case under scenarios of low, intermediate, and high levels of access to treatment. Under intermediate assumptions, they estimated the per-case cost of treating HIV disease and acquired immunodeficiency syndrome (AIDS) to be between $217,000 and $275,000 (undiscounted; discounted at a 5% rate, this range becomes $125,000 to $157,000).[2,23]

Hence, effective primary prevention programs generally are now an even better investment of funds. Indeed, if the studies in Table 1 were all redone with the new, much higher cost-of-illness estimate, the cost-effectiveness of the prevention programs generally would be even more positive and would justify the use of the prevention interventions with even lower seroprevalence populations or areas.

Postexposure Prophylaxis

The advent of new therapies and their promising efficacy has led to an intensive debate over whether or not they should be taken immediately after a possible exposure to HIV. For instance, if a person had unprotected sex with a partner who might (or is known to) be HIV-infected, he or she may wish to take a course of double- or triple-combination therapy in an attempt to block the virus from taking hold in the body. A typical course of treatment might be 1 month in length. This intervention might be used in cases ranging from sexual assault, to accidental condom breakage during consensual sex, to intentional unprotected sex.

This strategy has theoretical plausibility, but the empirical evidence for the effectiveness of such an intervention is limited to a single case–control study of postexposure prophylaxis for occupationally exposed health care workers. The relevance of this particular study for the use of antiretroviral drugs as a "morning after" (or "month after") therapy to prevent infection after potential sexual exposure is unclear.

A myriad of factors must be considered in choosing whether or not to employ post-exposure prophylaxis in any given case; one, and only one, factor is cost-effectiveness. Pinkerton et al.[24] have estimated the cost-effectiveness of a month-long course of postexposure treatment. They found that the cost-effectiveness depends heavily on the joint probability that the client's partner is HIV-infected and the per-contact probability of transmission for the particular type of sexual behavior being considered. The cost-effectiveness ratio varies very widely depending on the value of these two parameters. Pinkerton et al.[23] concluded that when considering only cost-effectiveness, postexposure prophylaxis would be indicated only for partners of persons known to be HIV-infected, clients reporting unprotected receptive anal intercourse, and cases in which the client's partner was not known to be HIV-infected but for whom the probability of infection was very high. Again, in any real-world situation, cost-effectiveness would be only one of many factors considered (e.g., in the case of sexual assault, postexposure prophylaxis might not be cost-effectiveness but might be used for ethical reasons or to attempt to allay the very justifiable fears of the survivor of the assault).

INCREASING APPLICATIONS OF ECONOMIC EVALUATION

Although there have been important advances in the economic evaluation of HIV prevention literature, further work remains to be done. Clearly it is important for decision makers to have economic information on all types of HIV prevention interventions. This calls, in part, for continued retrospective work on interventions with known behavioral effects. To assist in the conduct of HIV prevention economic evaluation studies, Pinkerton and Holtgrave[25] have published a methodological guide that provides step by step information on the conduct of such analyses. The guide is intended mainly for use by behavioral researchers wishing to do cost-effectiveness studies of sexual risk reduction interventions.

Comparability is critical for such studies to be useful by decision makers. Holtgrave and Pinkerton have argued for standardization in the methods used to conduct economic evaluation studies,[2,25] in the cost-of-illness and quality of life parameter estimates,[2,23] and in the collection of behavioral data to support such analyses.[26] In particular, they have calculated estimates of two main parameters needed for such studies: the cost of illness saved and the number of quality adjusted life years (QALYs) saved each time an HIV infection is averted. Researchers using these figures then need to calculate the cost of the intervention as delivered and estimate (or measure) the number of HIV infections prevented by the intervention of interest. This serves to simultaneously reduce the burden on the individual researcher and to increase cross-study comparability.

Prospective intervention studies beginning in the future might well include a prospective economic evaluation component. Even if such a component is not included in the study, the behavioral intervention researchers can enable ex-post cost-effectiveness analyses by collecting a minimum set of behavioral variables needed for retrospective economic evaluations (such as those summarized by the first four studies in Table 1). Pinkerton and colleagues[26] have described such a minimum data set based on the requirements of the Bernoullian model of HIV transmission. In particular, behavioral intervention studies focused on sexual behavior change should include for each client and each type of relevant sexual behavior: (1) the number of sexual partners, (2) the number of sexual acts per partner, and (3) the number of these acts protected by condom use (or other relevant protection, such as a dental dam). Information about the HIV serostatus of study participants and their sex partners might be estimated from local HIV seroprevalence studies; however, it would be very useful if the HIV serostatus of study participants could be assessed directly and participants at least asked about their knowledge of their partners' HIV serostatus. With the advent of oral fluid HIV testing, assessment of study participants' HIV serostatus has become much more practical. Collection of such minimal sexual behavior data will greatly facilitate economic evaluation analyses and will further improve cross-study comparability.

OTHER RESEARCH NEEDS

Besides those research needs noted in the previous section, there are still other important gaps in this economic evaluation research literature. One is the need to investigate the cost-effectiveness of HIV primary prevention interventions for adolescents at high risk of infection, among other specific populations. Another is the need to research the cost-effectiveness of social marketing and mass media programs.[27] Third, it will be important to do additional validations of the epidemiological models of HIV transmission employed in retrospective economic evaluation studies. Fourth, it is imperative that attention be paid to cost-effectiveness analyses addressing the optimal configuration of various HIV intervention components in a comprehensive HIV prevention program. Ultimately, cost-effectiveness analyses should be usable to support decision makers faced with the allocation of resources to configure a comprehensive HIV program in a given locale. Research in this area can now partially meet this goal but studies expressly addressing *comprehensive* programs are most urgently needed.

IMPLICATIONS FOR DECISION MAKERS

In the introduction, three major types of policy questions were described. In this section, we describe the implications of the economic evaluation literature for answering each type of policy question.

Affordability

The HIV prevention economic evaluation literature now contains estimates of the cost per client of a wide variety of HIV prevention programs: HIV counseling and testing, small-group behavioral interventions, community-level interventions, interventions to prevent peri-natal transmission, needle and syringe exchange, outreach to injection drug users, and other interventions. Fiscal decision makers interested in learning how much specific types of HIV primary prevention programs cost are likely to find at least one relevant estimate in the literature.[3,15–21] This will help them determine if they can afford the intervention in question.

Of course, cost estimates from the literature must be generalized to local circumstances (just as efficacy estimates must be generalized from the literature to local circumstances). This external validity question is important. Local decision makers may feel that their economic circumstances do not well match the conditions under which the cost analysis studies were conducted. Even if this is true, however, the cost analytic framework can be of use. For instance, the cost analyses available (for instance from the studies displayed in Table 1) specify in detail the resource categories (e.g., staff time, flip chart papers, condoms) used by the intervention, the number of units of each resource category consumed, and the dollar value of each resource unit. Local decision makers may find the resource category listings and number of units of each category needed for the intervention very helpful for local planning purposes even if the local cost to buy a unit of a resource category is different from the original study. If a decision maker wants to know what it would take to implement a particular type of HIV prevention intervention, the cost analysis framework will provide useful information to them regardless of differences in the local purchasing power of a dollar, or slight differences in target population characteristics.

The cost analytic information also serves another key function for decision makers. Historically, persons responsible for expressing in financial terms the unmet HIV prevention needs in an area have had difficulty in doing so. Now, HIV prevention community planning as implemented in the United States has provided much more support for the conduct of prevention needs assessments.[28] This information is beginning to provide estimates of the number of persons in given locales in need of particular types of HIV prevention services. Combining such estimates of service needs with cost analytic information about the cost of such services yields an overall estimate of the cost of unmet HIV prevention needs in a community. Hence, the emerging availability of cost estimates of HIV prevention services will serve to strengthen our ability to make specific estimates of the cost of unmet HIV prevention service needs.

Investing in HIV Prevention versus Other Disease Areas

Without question, the economic evaluation literature indicates that investment in HIV prevention programs is a very wise expenditure for society. Several types of HIV prevention interventions actually save society money when they are implemented. (The exceptions are certain types of intensive programs delivered in very low seroprevalence areas and programs of quite limited effectiveness at reducing risk behaviors.) These bargains are much too good to pass up; the programs save lives and fiscal resources. To fail to invest in these programs is to waste fiscal resources and subject people to unnecessary suffering and even death. This is undoubtedly clear from the economic evaluation literature.

Even when the precise effectiveness of an intervention is not known, a variant of cost-effectiveness analysis can be of great help. Threshold analysis can be useful for determining whether an HIV prevention intervention (perhaps a new or untested intervention) is likely to be cost-saving to society.[29,30] The analysis would seek, for example, to determine the number of HIV infections that would have to be averted by an intervention in order for it to be considered cost-saving. Recent cost-of-illness estimates indicate that the discounted, present value of a lifetime of caring for a person with HIV disease is approximately $125,000 to $157,000, at a 5% discount rate.[2,23] Therefore, if a new HIV prevention intervention costs, say, $1,000,000 to implement, then it would only need to prevent approximately six to eight infections in order to be considered cost-saving. Decision makers can determine whether this minimum goal of six to eight prevented infections is a reasonable and feasible minimum standard for the intervention.

This technique was employed to assess whether the Wisconsin Division of Health's investment in HIV counseling and testing might be considered cost-effective.[30] Although the exact number of HIV infections prevented by the program was not known, a threshold analysis was possible. It was known that the state spent $565,499 on this intervention (for the year 1994). Of course, this amount spent may not equal the true societal cost of the services (just as a hospital charge to a patient may not equal the true underlying cost of the treatment). Combining budget and cost analytic information with estimates of the cost of HIV illness, Holtgrave and colleagues[30] estimated that the counseling and testing program in Wisconsin only had to avert between 1 and 18 infections (depending on model assumptions) in order for the expenditures to be considered cost-effective. All parties involved agreed that although the exact number of HIV infection averted by the program was not known, it was very likely to exceed such a modest threshold for efficiency. Hence, in this case, threshold analysis was quite useful in informing policymakers though a comprehensive cost-effectiveness analysis was not possible.

Which HIV Prevention Intervention Is Most Cost-Effective?

This is the most challenging of the three types of policy questions. Answering it requires estimation of the cost-effectiveness of a broad array of HIV prevention efforts in a rather precise fashion and in a way that is highly relevant for decision making in a given locale. The growing economic evaluation literature is nearly able to meet these criteria, but requires further maturation before, say, HIV prevention community planning groups will be able to use the economic evaluation to create a rank-ordered table of the cost-effectiveness of all interventions in their community. For this to happen, at least two important developments will need to occur: (1) further cost-effectiveness studies of different types of interventions (such as social marketing programs and interventions for at-risk youth) will need to be completed, and (2) computerized software will need to become available to make it easy for local decision makers to supply local parameters of interest (such as a state or city's HIV seroprevalence level) and thereby customize studies in the literature for local purposes.

Although this goal has not yet been met, local decision makers can take advantage of the cost-effectiveness literature to create rank-ordered menus of a limited set of HIV prevention efforts for their locale. Further, decision makers such as HIV prevention community planning groups can approach the issue of relative cost-effectiveness in a qualitative rather than a quantitative manner. This can be achieved in two ways. First, community planning groups can use general, qualitative lessons learned from the cost-effectiveness literature. For instance, one lesson is that the cost-effectiveness of interventions generally decreases as HIV seroprevalence decreases; hence, community planning groups may wish to qualitatively question very intensive interventions for the general population.[31]

Second, community planning groups can simply ask themselves the following question for each HIV prevention intervention they consider: "Why do we want to do this intervention?" Answers to this question can include evidence from the following categories: (1) empirical effectiveness data, (2) client experience, (3) service provider experience, (4) theoretical rationale, (5) affordability, and (6) making the best use of available resources. In other words, if a local decision maker wishes to field a particular intervention, he or she might ask, "Can we afford this intervention in terms of available human and fiscal resources?" and "Is there some better way to spend this pool of resources—that is, could be we a better job of preventing HIV infection by spending the resources in some other way?" Qualitative deliberation of these questions provides an excellent beginning to tackling issues of cost-effectiveness in a given locale.

CONCLUSION

Local policy makers will greatly benefit from further maturation of the HIV prevention economic evaluation literature. However, the field already has provided a number of important and useful studies for guiding public health resource allocation. The studies are most useful at addressing the question, "Is HIV prevention a good investment of resources vis-à-vis expenditures on programs in other disease areas?" Clearly, the answer is yes. Indeed, intensive and seemingly expensive programs may still be well worth the expenditure. Further, even imperfect, partially effective programs may be well worth the resources invested. The economic evaluation literature tells us that investment in HIV prevention must continue. The remaining question is how to fine-tune the allocation of these resources across different interventions at the local level so as to maximize their prevention potential. HIV prevention is a good investment for society.

ACKNOWLEDGMENT.   Preparation of this manuscript was supported by grants R01-MH55440 and P30-MH52776 from the National Institute of Mental Health.

REFERENCES

1. Centers for Disease Control and Prevention. *HIV/AIDS Surveillance Report*. Atlanta, GA: Centers for Disease Control and Prevention; 1996. Year end edition.
2. Holtgrave DR, Pinkerton SD. Updates of cost of illness and quality of life estimates for use in economic evaluations of HIV prevention programs. *J Acquir Immune Defic Syndr Hum Retrovirol*, 1997; 16:54–62.
3. Holtgrave DR, Qualls NL, Graham JD. Economic evaluation of HIV prevention. *Annu Rev Public Health* 1996; 17:467–488.
4. Choi KH, Coates TJ. Prevention of HIV infection. *AIDS* 1994; 8:1371–1389.
5. Holtgrave DR, Qualls NL, Curran JW, et al. An overview of the effectiveness and efficiency of HIV prevention programs. *Public Health Rep* 1995; 110:134–146.

6. Kelly JA, Murphy DA, Sikkema KJ, et al. Psychological interventions to prevent HIV infection are urgently needed: New priorities for behavioral research in the second decade of AIDS. *Am Psychol* 1993; 48:1023–1034.

7. Kelly JA, Murphy DA, Washington CD, et al. The effect of HIV/AIDS intervention groups for high-risk women in urban clinics. *Am J Public Health* 1994; 84:1918–1922.

8. Hobfoll SE, Jackson AP, Lavin J, et al. Reducing inner-city women's AIDS risk activities: A study of single, pregnant women. *Health Psychol* 1994; 13:397–403.

9. Valdiserri RO, Lyter DW, Leviton LC, et al. AIDS prevention in homosexual and bisexual men: Results of a randomized trial evaluating two risk reduction interventions. *AIDS* 1989; 3:21–26.

10. Kelly JA, St. Lawrence JS, Hood HV, et al. Behavioral intervention to reduce AIDS risk activities. *J. Consult Clin Psychol* 1989; 57:60–67.

11. Kelly JA, St. Lawrence JS, Stevenson LY, et al. Community AIDS/HIV risk reduction: The effect of endorsement by popular people in three cities. *Am J Public Health* 1992; 82:1483–1489.

12. Jemmott JB, Jemmott LS, Fong GT. Reductions in HIV risk-associated sexual behaviors among black male adolescents. *Am J Public Health* 1992; 82:372–377.

13. Rotheram-Borus MJ, Koopman C, Haignere C, et al. Reducing HIV sexual risk behaviors among runaway adolescents. *JAMA* 1991; 266:1237–1241.

14. Connor EM, Sperling RS, Gelber R, et al. Reduction of maternal–infant transmission of human immunodeficiency virus type 1 with zidovudine treatment. *N Engl J Med* 1994; 331:1173–1180.

15. Holtgrave DR, Kelly JA. Preventing HIV/AIDS among high-risk urban women: The cost-effectiveness of a behavioral group intervention. *Am J Public Health* 1996; 86:1442–1445.

16. Holtgrave DR, Kelly JA. The cost-effectiveness of an HIV prevention intervention for gay men. *AIDS Behav* 1997; 1:173–180.

17. Pinkerton SD, Holtgrave DR, Valdiserri RO. Cost-effectiveness of HIV prevention skills training for men who have sex with men. *AIDS* 1997; 11:347–357.

18. Pinkerton SD, Holtgrave DR, DiFranceisco WJ, et al. Cost-effectiveness of a community-level HIV risk reduction intervention. *Am J Public Health* 1998; 88:1239–1242.

19. Gorsky RD, Farnham PG, Straus WL, et al. Preventing perinatal transmission of HIV—Costs and effectiveness of a recommended intervention. *Public Health Rep* 1996; 111:335–341.

20. Mauskopf JA, Paul JE, Wichman DS, et al. Economic impact of treatment of HIV-positive pregnant women and their newborns with zidovudine. *JAMA* 1996; 276:132–138.

21. Kaplan EH. Economic analysis of needle exchange. *AIDS* 1996; 9:1113–1119.

22. Tolley G, Kenkel D, Fabian R. *Valuing Health for Policy.* Chicago: The University of Chicago Press; 1994.

23. Pinkerton SD, Holtgrave DR. Lifetime costs of HIV/AIDS. *J Acquir Immune Defic Syndrome Hum Retrovirol*, 1997; 14:380–381.

24. Pinkerton SD, Holtgrave DR, Bloom FR. Postexposure treatment of HIV. *N Engl J Med* 1997; 337:500–501.

25. Pinkerton SD, Holtgrave DR. A method for evaluating the economic efficiency of HIV behavioral risk reduction intervention. *AIDS Behav* 1998; 2:189–201.

26. Pinkerton SD, Holtgrave DR, Leviton LC, et al. Toward a standard sexual behavior data set for HIV prevention evaluation. *Am J Health Behav* 1998; 22:259–266.

27. Holtgrave DR. Public health communication strategies for HIV prevention: Past and emerging roles. *AIDS* 1997; 11(suppl A):S183–S190.

28. Valdiserri RO, Aultman TV, Curran JW. Community planning: A national strategy to improve HIV prevention programs. *J Community Health* 1995; 20:87–100.

29. Holtgrave DR, Qualls NL. Threshold analysis and programs for prevention of HIV infection. *Med Decis Making* 1995; 15:311–317.

30. Holtgrave DR, DiFranceisco W, Reiser W, et al. Setting standards for the Wisconsin HIV counseling and testing program: An application of threshold analysis. *J Public Health Manage Practice* 1997; 3:42–49.

31. Pinkerton SD, Abramson PR. Model-based allocation of HIV-prevention resources. *AIDS Public Policy J* 1996; 11:153–155.

SELECTED, ADDITIONAL BIBLIOGRAPHY

Gold MR, Siegel JE, Russell LB, Weinstein MC, eds. *Cost-effectiveness in Health and Medicine.* New York: Oxford University Press; 1996.

Haddix AC, Teutsch SM, Shaffer PA, Dunet DO, eds. *Prevention Effectiveness: A Guide to Decision Analysis and Economic Evaluation.* New York: Oxford University press; 1996.

Holtgrave DR, ed. *Handbook of Economic Evaluation of HIV Prevention Programs.* Plenum Press; 1998.

Kaplan EH, Brandeau ML, eds. *Modeling the AIDS Epidemic: Planning, Policy and Prediction.* New York: Raven Press; 1994.

Kahn JG. Are NEPs cost-effective in preventing HIV infection? In: Lurie P, Reingold AL, ed. *The Public Health Impact of Needle Exchange Programs in the United States and Abroad.* San Francisco: Institute for Health Policy Studies, University of California at San Francisco; 1993:475–509.

16

Ethical Issues of Behavioral Interventions for HIV Prevention

SANA LOUE

BACKGROUND

The Nuremberg Code and the Helsinki Declaration

The world was shocked by the accounts of the experiments conducted by Nazi physicians on concentration camp prisoners. These experiments included the exposure of prisoners to cold water and to extremely low air pressure,[1] the injection of dye into persons' eyes in an attempt to change their eye color, and the inoculation of prisoners with typhus bacilli.[2] These events provided the impetus for the formulation of the Nuremberg Code, which enumerated ten principles to be universally applied to research involving human participants:

1. The voluntary consent of the prospective participant is essential.
2. The experiment must be expected to produce results beneficial, for society that cannot be obtained by any other means.
3. The study should be based on the results of animal experimentation and a knowledge of the natural history of the disease in question so that the anticipated results justify conducting the experiment.
4. All unnecessary physical or mental suffering or injury should be avoided during the course of the experiment.
5. No experiment should be conducted where it is believed that death or disabling injury will occur, except where the research physicians also serve as subjects.
6. The degree of risk should not exceed the humanitarian importance of the problem to be solved.
7. The participant should be protected against death or injury through the use of adequate facilities and preparations.
8. The experiment should be conducted only by scientifically qualified persons.
9. The participant has the right to end his or her participation in the experiment if he or she has reached a point where continuation seems to be impossible.
10. The scientist in charge must be prepared to terminate the experiment if he or she has probable cause to believe that continuation would be likely to result in the injury, disability, or death of the research participant.[3]

SANA LOUE • Department of Epidemiology and Biostatistics, Case Western Reserve University, MetroHealth Medical Center, Cleveland, Ohio 44109.

Handbook of HIV Prevention, edited by Peterson and DiClemente.
Kluwer Academic/Plenum Publishers, New York, 2000.

The Helsinki Declaration was formulated to address the shortcomings of the Nuremberg Code, including its failure to distinguish between therapeutic clinical research and clinical research on healthy subjects and its failure to provide for a mechanism for the review of researcher conduct.[4] Adopted by the World Medical Association in 1964, the Helsinki Declaration provides for the obtaining of informed consent from a surrogate in cases where the prospective research participant is legally or physically unable to give consent and distinguishes between clinical research combined with professional care and nontherapeutic research. Later revisions in 1975, 1983, and 1989 provided increased emphasis on obtaining individual informed consent to participate in experimentation.[4–6]

Four first-order principles have emerged from the Nuremberg Code: respect for persons or autonomy, beneficence, nonmaleficence, and justice. A principlistic approach to the resolution of ethical dilemmas demands that action or inaction be consistent with these principles. The operationalization of these principles is reflected in the United States in the regulations governing research involving human participants that has been promulgated by the Department of Health and Human Services and the Food and Drug Administration. It should be noted, however, that neither the Nuremberg Code nor the Helsinki Declaration provides guidance on how to simultaneously maximize compliance with each of these principles. US regulations are similarly silent on this issue and also fail to provide significant guidance on how these principles can be applied in significantly different social and cultural settings.

Various alternative approaches to the resolution of ethical dilemmas have been developed that address some of the difficulties of the principlistic approach. These alternative approaches are reflected in varying degrees in the provisions of the *International Guidelines for Ethical Review of Epidemiological Studies*[7] and the *International Guidelines for Biomedical Research Involving Human Subjects*,[8] which also incorporate the four basic principles of autonomy, beneficence, nonmaleficence, and justice. These documents are promulgated by the Council for International Organizations of Medical Sciences (CIOMS). It is critical that researchers engaged in cross-cultural human immunodeficiency virus (HIV) research understand these various approaches and their use or acceptability in and to the communities with which they are working. Insistence on a "cookie-cutter" US-based approach without consideration of the cultural and social context could invite charges of ethical imperialism.[9–12]

Uganda, for instance, has accepted the four principles enumerated by the Nuremberg Code and the Helsinki Declaration but relies on a modified form of casuistry as the primary strategy for analyzing and resolving ethical issues.[13] Uganda's decision to embark on this course, rather than utilizing a strictly principlistic approach, is a direct result of the country's past experience with a central government that relied heavily on torture and tyranny and its present experiences with a high rate of HIV infection, limited economic resources, and widespread poverty and illiteracy.[13]

Unlike principlism, which requires the deductivistic application of formulated principles to particular fact situations, casuistry requires that dilemmas be resolved through nuanced interpretations of individual cases. Casuistry, then, also known as a "case-based" approach, resembles common law traditions in that it is a process or evolution by which the principles are discovered in the cases themselves.[14] Consequently, the principles cannot be enunciated apart from their factual contexts. Just as with legal cases, the principles derived from an examination of cases remain subject to further revision and elucidation through new cases.[15–16]

Like principlism, casuistry is subject to criticism for its lack of comprehensiveness with respect to various issues. First, casuistry does not delineate how a case description is to be judged with respect to its adequacy and sufficiency. Second, casuistry provides no guidance on how to choose which cases should be deeply scrutinized. Third, a casuistic approach may unintentionally omit alternative perspectives of particular individuals.[15] (This particular criticism also can be leveled against principlism, which quite often places emphasis on the opinions of professionals to the exclusion of other participants in the process.) Fourth, criteria for constructing linkage between cases, required for the application of precedents, remains relatively undefined. Fifth, at least one writer has contended that casuistical analyses will provoke conflicting interpretations and consequently is an inappropriate strategy for the development of moral consensus.[15–17] And, finally, casuistry has been criticized for its failure to consider the economic and power relations that shape the social consensus.[18]

Other approaches often relied on to address ethical dilemmas include communitarianism, utilitarianism, and the ethics of care, also known as feminist ethics. Communitarianism is based on the concept of community as a "network of social relationships among people bound together by shared understandings, a sense of mutual obligation, emotional bonds, and common interests that encompass the whole of life."[19(p.139)] Communitywide agreements provide the basis for moral rules; communal intervention is required to address socially disruptive outcomes. Analysis of an ethical dilemma requires an assessment of which communal values and relationships are present or absent, which actions will express communal values, and which actions will have a positive impact on the community.[20]

Utlitarianism is premised on the production of the maximal balance of positive value over disvalue. This is accomplished by balancing the interests of all persons who are affected in a particular situation. In this sense, utilitarianism can be seen as an attempt to maximize beneficence. The positive value is subject to measurement by a variety of standards, including happiness or pleasure[21]; friendship, health, and knowledge[22]; or personal autonomy, understanding, and deep relations.[23]

Feminist ethics seek to expand what is seen as a professionally driven male perspective on the nature of ethics.[24] It is founded on two basic assumptions: that the subordination of women is morally wrong and that women's experience must be treated as respectfully as that of men.[25] The field of feminist ethics encompasses feminist ethical work in two dimensions: attention to contemporary issues, such as abortion, heterosexuality, and rape, and attention to traditional ethical theory and its male bias.[25] This work calls into question the appropriateness of relying on traditional ethical theory and its underlying assumptions to address a broad range of issues. The concept of rights in the context of abortion, for instance, postures the mother and fetus as adversaries.[25] Contract theory's premise that each contracting party is equal, independent, and mutually disinterested is inconsistent with the experiences of many women.[26,27] Accordingly, feminist ethics demands a "rethinking [of] the deepest issues in ethical theory … in light of a moral sensibility perceived as distinctively feminine."[25(p.82)] Clearly, how "feminine" is to be defined is an issue to be acknowledged.

The existence of a "distinctively feminine" moral sensibility appears to be supported by research in the area of developmental psychology. Gilligan[28] found that in contrast to males' construction of moral dilemmas as conflicts of rights, females construed these dilemmas as conflicts of responsibilities, often requiring resolution in a manner that would repair damaged relationships. Unlike males, whose morality of justice was premised on values of fairness and equality, females emphasized a morality of care premised on inclusion and protection from harm (an "ethics of care").

Feminist ethics do not, however, imply that there are issues unique to women. For instance, the availability of abortion and the types of birth control available have implications for both men and women. It is recognized, though, that women may have a gender-specific interest in specific issues.

CONFRONTING THE ISSUES

Respect for Persons

Respect for persons refers to the requirement that individuals be treated as autonomous agents and that those with diminished autonomy be provided with additional protections. Respect for persons encompasses issues of informed consent and voluntariness. The informed consent process requires (1) an assessment of the prospective participant's legal capacity to provide informed consent, (2) the provision of sufficient information to allow the prospective participant to decide whether or not to enroll in the study, (3) the individual's comprehension of the information that is provided, and (4) the individual's voluntary decision to (not) participate in the study.[2,29] Issues related to these components are listed in Table 1, together with a listing of other ethical issues to be considered in HIV prevention research.

Determining Whose Consent Is Needed

A threshold question to be addressed, sometimes even prior to a determination of capacity, is the issue of whose consent is to be obtained. As indicated, the Nuremberg Code mandates that each individual participant provide informed consent prior to his or her enrollment in a research study. This requirement was modified through a provision for surrogate consent by the Helsinki Declaration, as amended. The *International Guidelines for Ethical Review of Epidemiological Studies*[7] recognizes that unlike many Western cultures, which define autonomy in terms of individual sovereignty, some cultures define the individual in the context of a family of community. Accordingly, the guidelines permit, under some circumstances, a researcher to rely on the consent of a community leader. Reliance on a community leader for consent, however, does not resolve the issue of voluntariness. For instance, an individual may feel pressured to participate in a study by the status of the community leader, or pressures may have been exerted on individuals to participate.

A strictly principlistic approach, such as that adopted by the United States, demands that informed consent be obtained from each prospective participant, with the exception of those circumstances in which consent from a surrogate is permitted. This would include, for instance, minor children and the mentally ill. In contrast to the US approach, Uganda's modified casuistic approach requires the informed consent of all individual prospective participants, with the exception of children, the mentally ill, and the behaviorally disordered, for whom surrogate consent can be obtained. Uganda further requires that prospective participants in health research be afforded sufficient opportunity to confer with persons of their choosing prior to deciding whether or not to enroll in a research study.[30] This provision for "sufficient opportunity" to consult with others recognizes and incorporates a cultural view of the individual in the context of his or her family and community.[13]

Surrogate consent permits the participation in research of persons who, either individually or as a class, would otherwise be unable to participate due to lack of capacity to provide informed consent. (Lack of capacity is discussed in detail below.) Surrogate consent addresses the issues of beneficence and nonmaleficence, by providing protection to those unable to consent themselves, and of justice, by distributing the benefits and burdens to classes of persons who would not otherwise receive them. Reliance on surrogate consent, though, raises additional ethical issues. The investigator cannot be certain whether the surrogate has a conflict of interest that will affect his or her judgment regarding participation. Consider the situation facing an HIV-infected child participant in a clinical trial:

Table 1. Ethical Issues To Be Considered in Conducting HIV Prevention Research

- Who may participate in the study? What are the implications of excluding specific individuals or classes of individuals from the study?
- Is informed consent needed? If so, from whom?
- What process should be utilized for informed consent?
  1. What information must be provided?
  2. How should the information be provided to prospective participants?
  3. How should capacity be assessed? If a particular participant is found to lack capacity, should he or she be excluded from the study or should there be alternative mechanisms for consent established?
- What is the risk-benefit ratio? From whose perspective?
- What measures have been taken to protect participants' privacy and the confidentiality of the data?
- If individuals are to be tested for HIV in the context of the study:
  1. Are the results of those tests to be linked or unlinked?
  2. Who will be given these results and who will have access to these results?
  3. What procedures have been established for pre- and posttest counseling and referral of participants?
- How is voluntariness to be evaluated?
- Are participants to receive a stipend or incentive? What is the effect of that payment?
- Are there circumstances that preclude the possibility of voluntary informed consent?
- Are there conflicts of interest in the recruitment of participants?
- What provisions have been made to address harm arising to the participants during the course of the study?
- If this is an experimental study:
  1. What is the experimental condition? The comparison condition?
  2. Are the experimental and comparison conditions in a state of equipoise in that we do not know which is "better"?
  3. In formulating the comparison condition, what standard of care is to be used? How is that standard determined? If the comparison condition is placebo or the standard of care at the location of the study, what are the implications of using this?
  4. What mechanisms are in place that will identify any harm arising to participants during the course of the study in conjunction with their participation in the study? What procedures are in place to reduce such harm once it is identified?
  5. If the intervention is found to be effective, what obligation exists to the study participants and the larger community to continue to make that intervention available following the conclusion of the study?
- How will you communicate study results and to whom? How will you acknowledge uncertainty?

> First, children recruited for phase I trials will be in the later stages of their illness, since they are usually not eligible until phase II or III drugs have proven ineffective or unacceptably toxic in their treatment. As a result, they will have incurred a substantial burden of prior suffering and may be significantly debilitated. Second, many subjects in phase I trials do not receive potentially therapeutic doses of the drugs being studied, because the increments in dosing for consecutive groups of subjects usually begin with a very conservative low dose. Third, exposure to unexpected toxicities and additional monitoring procedures may compound the suffering.... Further, many drugs that enter phase I testing do not yield evidence of potential efficacy.[31]

The parent–surrogate may consent to the child's participation in the belief that it will potentially help the child or others suffering from HIV. Alternatively, the parent may consent because of a monetary incentive or because participation will necessitate long periods of the child's absence from the home and provide the parent with an expense-free respite from caregiving responsibilities.

Assessing Capacity

In general, a person is believed to have the capacity to give informed consent if he or she can understand the nature of the research, the nature of his or her participation in the research, the risks and benefits that may result from participation, and alternatives to participation.[32,33] In some instances, the prospective participant is presumed to be incapable of giving informed consent, for instance, where the prospective participant is a minor child or is mentally ill. In such circumstances, the participant must be provided with additional protections. US regulations specify that the following classes of persons are to be considered as requiring special protection: children, pregnant women, prisoners, and the mentally disabled. It should be noted here that compliance with US regulations constitutes a *legal* obligation. *Ethical* analysis may demand that additional classes of persons be provided with special protections due to diminished autonomy.

In most circumstances, the law will not provide rigid rules by which to determine capacity. A researcher can assess whether a particular individual has the mental capacity to consent by conducting a short mental status examination. This will provide information relating to the prospective participant's orientation to time and place, his or her ability for immediate recall, his or her short- and long-term memory, and the ability to perform simple calculations.[33] This strategy may be particularly helpful in situations where the researcher has reason to believe that the prospective participant is mentally ill or is under the influence of a controlled substance. The examination will not reflect, though, the individual's capacity if the questions are culture-based or in a language that the participant does not understand.

Providing Adequate Information

The informed consent process must provide prospective participants with information about the study, the fact that it is a study, the methods to be used during the study, the potential benefits to the participant and others that may result from the research, and any foreseeable risks or discomforts associated with the research.[34,35] Participants also must be informed of any existing alternatives to participation, of the extent to which confidentiality will be maintained, and of the extent of care that would be available to the participant in the event of a study-related injury. The individual must be told that his or her participation is voluntary and that he or she may withdraw from the study at any time without the loss of any benefit to which he or she is otherwise entitled.[36] Clearly, the information must be provided to participants in a language and format and at a level that they can understand.

Assessing Voluntariness

Issues relating to the voluntariness of consent arise most frequently in situations where the individual's consent to participate in the proposed research could result from coercion or duress. Some situations may be inherently coercive, such as those involving prisoners or the terminally ill, those involving individuals suffering from cognitive impairment, and those in which individuals are being provided with an incentive to participate in the research.

Prisoners' situations provide an excellent example of this dilemma. Health care services in a prison setting may be inadequate and an inmate's only hope of obtaining ongoing care may be in the context of a research study.[37,38] An inmate may be willing to risk the stigmatization that may result from awareness of his or her HIV status in order to obtain the desired treatment.[37,39] The complete exclusion of prisoners for all research, though, would result in the denial of both the potential medical[39,40] and nonmedical benefits associated with participation in the research.[41]

The voluntariness of consent cannot be assessed apart from the factual context in which the issue arises, and there is no clear standard by which to make this determination, regardless

Table 2. Factors to Consider in Evaluating Voluntariness

- Are there circumstances or conditions external to the study, such as absence of any alternative source of education or care, that would significantly decrease the likelihood that individuals would refuse to participate?
- Is the situation so inherently coercive that refusal is perceived as not an option?
- Is the individual soliciting consent from the participant in a position of relatively greater power or authority, or does the prospective participant depend on the recruiting individual for the receipt of a benefit, such as medical care?
- Can special protections be instituted to insulate prospective participants from potential coercion or duress?
- Are the perceived benefits of participation so great that participants may not consider the risk of participation?
- If participants are to receive an incentive:
  1. Does the incentive represent compensation for participants' costs, such as travel, or is it a payment?
  2. Is the payment, whether in the form of money or goods, proportional to the time and activities expected of participants?
  3. Does the incentive offered represent a windfall to participants?

of the approach used. Table 2 provides a list of factors to be considered in evaluating the potential for duress or coercion and the voluntariness of consent.

Various strategies may be used to reduce the likelihood of coercion or duress. The United States has implemented regulations that prohibit consideration of prisoners' participation in research in making parole decisions.[42] If the study is recruiting participants through health care settings, it may be advisable to have someone other than the patient's regular care provider discuss the possibility of study participation, in order to reduce any pressure that the patient may feel.

Beneficence and Nonmaleficence

Beneficence refers to respect for individuals' decisions and to the protection of research participants from harm. This principle requires that researchers secure the well-being of the participants and that there is a favorable balance between the risks and the benefits of the proposed research.[29] It is important to note that although the risks and benefits to the participant can be physical, they also can be economic, social, or legal and can relate to any number of substantive concerns.[43]

Nonmaleficence refers to the obligation to refrain from inflicting harm on another.[20] This obligation not to do harm is distinct from the obligation to help others.

Special Protections

Special protections are often instituted in situations where individuals are particularly vulnerable, such as those with limited capacity, in order to prevent harm to them in the context of the research. Exactly which classes of persons should be entitled to special protection must be determined on the basis of the factual situation. The United States has defined children, the mentally ill, and prisoners as vulnerable classes by regulation. This does not, however, preclude consideration of other classes of individuals as vulnerable.

In contrast to the US approach, Uganda utilized a casuistic approach in determining that the following classes of persons are deserving of special protections: children, pregnant women, the mentally ill and behaviorally disordered, refugees, prisoners, and soldiers. Street children and orphans are classified as a special category of children, meriting an increased level of protection. The impetus for these categories came from an examination of Uganda's current situation. As of the end of 1997, Uganda had estimated that 930,000 of its adults and children currently alive were infected with HIV, including approximately 9% of its adult population. A total of 1,700,000 children had been orphaned through the deaths of their parents due to HIV; 1,800,000 adults and children had already died from HIV; and by June 1998, Uganda had reported a total of 1,900,000 cases of AIDS among its women and children.[44] Women are especially vulnerable socially due to the traditional authority of the husband and father over his wife and children,[45] and are vulnerable to HIV transmission due to cultural practices such as polygamy, wife inheritance,[46] and male infidelity.[47] Thousands of refugees have flowed into Uganda from Rwanda and what was Zaire, many of whom are malnourished and traumatized.[48] Uganda has suffered through long years of instability, tyranny, and torture under the successive regimes of Idi Amin and Milton Obote,[49] prompting the inclusion of soldiers and prisoners as vulnerable classes.

Special protections can take a variety of forms. The United States provides for varying consent requirements of a child's parents or guardians commensurate with the level of risk involved.[42] Uganda prohibits almost all research involving street children and orphans unless the research will benefit them as a class and the research question cannot be answered without their participation.[30]

It is important to recognize that in attempting to maximize respect for persons, beneficence, and nonmaleficence, justice may be minimized. As an example, a prohibition against the involvement of street children in research recognizes their lack of capacity and minimizes the risk of harm. However, it also precludes them from sharing the benefits and burdens of research.

Confidentiality Concerns

The assessment of risks and benefits often may involve issues related to the confidentiality of the information provided by the participants to the researcher. Respect for persons and autonomy requires that the confidentiality of the information provided be respected and safeguarded. However, there may be legal and ethical limitations on the extent to which that confidentiality may be safeguarded. Depending on the law of the state in which the study is being conducted, the researcher may be required to report the research participant's behavior pursuant to abuse and neglect laws, public health reporting requirements, and partner notification laws and duty to warn provisions.[50]

Partner notification refers to the notification of an HIV-infected individual's current sexual or needle-sharing partner that he or she may have been exposed to HIV. It must be distinguished from contact tracing, which is a form of medical investigation that involves contacting all known sexual or needle-sharing partners within a defined period of time to advise them of possible exposure to HIV and to ascertain their possible sexual and needle-sharing partners who may have been exposed.[51]

Apart from state statutory provisions mandating or permitting the notification of specific classes of individuals of possible exposure to HIV a "duty to warn" may exist as the result of a line of court cases that began in 1976 with *Tarasoff v. Regents of the University of California*.[52] The Tarasoff family sued the University of California and a psychologist at the Berkeley campus of the university for the death of their daughter Tatiana. Tatiana had refused the advances of another graduate student at Berkeley. The student sought counseling from a psychologist at the school's counseling service. He advised the psychologist that he intended to kill Tatiana. The psychologist and several colleagues sought the involuntary hospitalization of the student for evaluation purposes. The student was released after a brief observation period, during which it was concluded that he was rational. The student subsequently shot Tatiana.

The psychologist claimed that he could not have advised the family or Tatiana directly of the threat, because to do so would be a breach of the traditionally protected relationship between therapist and patient. The majority of the court, however, rejected this contention and held that when a patient "presents a serious danger ... to another [person], [the therapist] incurs an obligation to use reasonable care to protect the intended victim against such danger."[52(p.431)] That obligation could be satisfied by warning the intended victim, by notifying authorities, or by taking "whatever other steps are reasonably necessary under the circumstances."[52(p.431)] The court specifically noted that the therapist–patient privilege was not absolute.

Later cases have followed the *Tarasoff* court's reasoning. A New Jersey court ruled in *McIntosh v. Milano*[53] that the doctor–patient privilege protecting confidentiality is not absolute, but is limited by the public interest or the private interest of the patient. In reaching this conclusion, the court relied on the 1953 case of *Earle v. Kuklo,*[54] in which the court had stated that "a physician has the duty to warn third persons against possible exposure to contagious or infectious disease (p. 475). A Michigan appeals court held in *Davis v. Lhim*[55] that a therapist has an obligation to use reasonable care whenever there was a person who was foreseeably endangered by his or her patient. The danger would be deemed to be foreseeable if the therapist knew or should have known, pursuant to his professional standard of care, of the potential harm. Courts are divided, though, on the issue of whether the patient must make threats about a specific, intended victim to trigger the duty to warn. The court in *Thompson v. County of Alameda*[56] found no duty to warn where there was no identifiable victim. Another court, however, found that such a duty existed even absent specific threats concerning specific individuals, where the patient's previous history indicated that he would be likely to direct violence against a person.[57]

Analogous conduct may occur in the HIV setting. A research participant may discover that he or she is HIV-infected. Angry, and refusing to accept the diagnosis and recommended changes in behavior, the individual decides to continue engaging in unprotected sex with his or her current sexual partner or to continue sharing needles for injecting drugs. This type of situation is most similar to the *Tarasoff* situation: there exists a specific person who is at risk of exposure. Less clear is the situation where an individual resolves to "take as many people" with him or her by engaging in unprotected sexual relations with multiple, anonymous partners. Who, in this situation, can realistically be warned?

Legally, there is no consensus on the applicability of the *Tarasoff* doctrine to HIV-related situations. *Tarasoff* generally has been applied in situations involving violence rather than communicable disease. HIV is less likely to be contracted through intercourse than death is likely to occur as the result of a fatal bullet. Even if an individual is exposed to HIV, it is unclear whether an individual might be able to clear the virus from his or her system. Additionally, those with HIV infection may live for substantial periods of time, unlike individuals killed with a single shot.[58]

There are many questions involving both legal and ethical issues that remain unresolved.[59–60] First and foremost is the issue of whether confidentiality should ever be breached, regardless of the circumstances. Francis and Chin[61] support the maintenance of confidentiality:

> Maintenance of confidentiality is central to and of paramount importance for the control of AIDS. Information regarding infection with a deadly virus, sexual activity, sexual contacts and the illegal use of IV drugs and diagnostic information regarding AIDS-related disease are sensitive issues that, if released by the patient or someone involved in health care, could adversely affect a patient's personal and professional life. (p. 1364)

The American Medical Association[62] takes a different view, balancing the patient's expectation of confidentiality against social concerns:

> The obligation to safeguard the patient's confidences is subject to certain exceptions which are ethically and legally justified because of overriding social considerations. Where a patient threatens to employ serious bodily harm to another person, and there is a reasonable probability that the patient may carry out the threat, the physician should take reasonable precautions for the protection of the intended victim, including notification of law enforcement authorities.

To what extent can a trained researcher predict the behavior of a research participant? There are no generally accepted standards for the evaluation of dangerousness.[63,64] To what extent should a participant's behavior provide the foundation for a breach of confidentiality? Psychotherapists have been found to differ in their assessments of the extent to which the dangerousness of an HIV-infected individual and the identifiability of a victim should mandate a breach of confidentiality.[65] Clinicians may function at various levels within a study. Are clinicians responsible only for the development of assessment instruments to be held to the same standard as the clinician–principal investigator of the study? From an ethical perspective, how does the researcher balance the harm that may befall the research participant as a result of disclosure against the benefit to others of that disclosure? It can be argued that the same obligation does not run to past sexual and needle-sharing partners as it does to current partners, who are more clearly at risk of exposure.[66]

Balancing the Risks and Benefits

The principles of beneficence and nonmaleficence require that there be a favorable balance of the benefits of participation against the risks of participation. This appears significantly simpler than it actually is. A researcher conducting an HIV prevention intervention trial may view a participant's time away from work to participate in the initial interview and follow-up sessions as a minor inconvenience when balanced against the benefits to be gained by not contracting HIV. The prospective participant, however, may fear the loss of employment due to these absences and/or the inadvertent disclosure of participation in an HIV-related research study, potentially resulting in his or her stigmatization. It is critical that the assessment of risks and benefits be conducted from multiple perspectives.

Significant controversy has been raised by the use of placebo controls in the conduct of clinical trials designed to assess simplified regimens for the prevention of maternal–child HIV transmission.[9,67–69] The controversy relates specifically to the operationalization of beneficence and nonmaleficence and stems, in part, from varied interpretations of the Helsinki Declaration's provision requiring that "[i]n any medical study, every patient—including those of a control, if any—should be assured of the best proven diagnostic and therapeutic method."[6] The "best therapeutic treatment" may include an inert placebo if no proven diagnostic or therapeutic method exists.[6] Proponents of placebo-controlled trials have argued that they are necessary to assess the safety and value of the proposed prevention intervention in the specific setting in which it is to be used.[69] Opponents have countered that the control group must receive the highest available standard of care, even if it is not now and never will be available at the study site.[9] These arguments, in turn, raise questions related to the foreseeable but unintended development of drug resistance among trial participants following cessation of the trial; the abandonment of patients if ongoing care is unavailable at the study site on conclusion of the trial[9,70,71]; and exactly what constitutes the best therapeutic treatment in situations where the recommended regimen varies even between developed countries.[72,73]

Although the relevant provision of the Helsinki Declaration applies to medical studies, the question must be raised as to whether the comparison group in any trial, including a behavioral trial, must receive the "best treatment" and by what standard best is to be identified. As an example, consider a behavioral prevention intervention trial with women at high risk of HIV transmission. The usual prevention activity in the community of the trial site is the provision of HIV prevention information through the distribution of brochures. We know, however, that the use of condoms reduces the risk of HIV transmission and that various strategies have been effective in reducing HIV transmission within specific groups, such as gay men. We do not know if such strategies are effective at reducing HIV transmission among all other subgroups. One must ask (1) whether the provision of accurate information to the comparison group is sufficient, (2) whether the participants must receive, at a minimum, free condoms, and (3) whether it can be assumed, in the absence of research, that a strategy that effectively reduces HIV transmission in one subgroup will be effective in another, thereby constituting the "best treatment." There is no clear resolution to such issues.

JUSTICE

The principle of justice requires that the benefits and burdens of research be distributed equitably among individuals or communities. No single group should bear a disproportionate share of the risk or a disproportionate share of the benefits. For instance, the maximization of beneficence and nonmaleficence through the complete exclusion of children from research due to their lack of capacity would contravene the principle of justice by depriving children of participation in the benefits and burdens of research.

AIDS research in general has been criticized for its inclusion of white male homosexuals in many studies[74] and its exclusion of women, persons of color, and injection drug users.[75] Four reasons have been advanced for the exclusion of women from drug trials: (1) women may be pregnant or become pregnant,[76,77] (2) women may lack access to the health care system in general and to research in particular, (3) women who are drug users are perceived as "noncompliant" and therefore are undesirable as participants, and (4) women who have been infected more recently have not progressed to AIDS and many studies focus on AIDS rather than HIV.[11,78] Women's participation in HIV research is restricted as well due to pharmaceutical manufacturers' fears of liability for the potentially teratogenic effects of a drug.[77,79] The fear of harm to an unborn fetus and resulting liability may be misplaced, as these potentialities rest on an assumption that all women who would want to participate in HIV research in general and in clinical trials in particular are heterosexually active and fertile.[80] Ultimately, the exclusion of women, injecting drug users, and persons of color is scientifically unwise, as well. Medications tested on non-drug-using white males may not produce the desired effects in other populations[81,82] due to differences in pharmacokinetics and pharmacodynamics.[83]

Clearly, the simultaneous maximization of beneficence, autonomy, and justice in this situation is problematic. Beneficence refers to a responsibility not to do harm, including harm to unconsenting future children. That harm is difficult to measure. However, the exclusion of women of childbearing age places greater importance on the consequences to the unborn and perhaps never-to-be-born children than on women's autonomy. Others argue that if women of childbearing age are to be excluded from participation in clinical trials, justice and beneficence demand the similar exclusion of men of reproductive potential.[84]

The issue of the exclusion of women and persons of color from participation in HIV research, however, is not limited to the context of clinical trials. For instance, a researcher conducting a behavioral intervention trial may want to maximize the homogeneity of the study population in order to reduce or eliminate sources of variance, such as sex and ethnicity, that are not under his or her control and that may be difficult to control for if the sample size is small. The successful recruitment and retention of women and other groups also may require the provision of additional services, such as child care, to facilitate continuing participation. These services may substantially increase the cost of the study and investigators may simply wish to avoid these additional methodological and logistical difficulties and their associated costs.[85]

REFERENCES

1. Applebaum PS, Lidz C, Meisel A. *Informed Consent: Legal Theory and Clinical Practice*. London: Oxford University Press; 1987.
2. Grodin MA, Kaminow PV, Sassower R. Ethical issues in AIDS research. *QRB Qual Rev Bull* 1986; 12:347–352.
3. World Medical Association. The Nuremberg Code. *Law Med Health Care* 1991; 19:266.
4. Perley S, Fluss SS, Bankowski Z, Simon F. The Nuremberg Code: An international overview. In: Annas GJ, Grodin MA, eds. *The Nazi Doctors and the Nuremberg Code*. London: Oxford University Press; 1992: 149–173.
5. Christakis NA, Panner MJ. Existing international guidelines for human subjects research: Some open questions. *Law, Med Health Care* 1991; 19:214–221.
6. World Medical Association. Declaration of Helsinki. *Law, Med Health Care* 1991; 9:264–265.
7. Council for International Organizations of Medical Sciences. *International Guidelines for Ethical Review of Epidemiological Studies*. Geneva: Council for International Organizations of Medical Sciences; 1991.
8. Council for International Organizations of Medical Sciences, World Health Organization. *International Ethical Guidelines for Biomedical Research Involving Human Subjects*. Geneva: Council for International Organizations of Medical Sciences; 1993.
9. Cohen J. Ethics of AZT studies in poorer countries attacked. *Science* 1997; 276:1022.
10. Gambia Government/Medical Research Council Joint Ethical Committee. Ethical issues facing medical research in developing countries. *Lancet* 1998; 351:286–287.
11. Levine RJ. Informed consent: Some challenges to the universality of the Western model. *Law Med Health Care* 1991; 19:207–213.
12. Newton LH. Ethical imperialism and informed consent. *IRB: Rev Human Subjects Res* 1990; 12:10–11.
13. Loue S, Okello D. Kawuma M. Research bioethics in the Ugandan context: A program summary. *Ethics Law Med* 1996; 24:47–53.
14. Jonsen AR. Casuistry and clinical ethics. *Theor Med* 1986; 7:65–74.
15. Arras JD. Getting down to cases: The revival of casuistry in bioethics. *J Med Philos* 1991; 16:29–51.
16. Jonsen AR, Toulmin S. *The Abuse of Casuistry: A History of Moral Reasonings*. Berkeley: University of California Press; 1988.
17. Dworkin R. Spheres of justice: An exchange. *NY Rev Books* 1983; 30:44.
18. Habermas J. The hermeneutic claim to universality. In: Bleicher J, ed. *Contemporary Hermeneutics*. London: Routledge & Kegan Paul; 1980:181–211.
19. Nisbet R. The problem of community. In: Daly M, ed. *Communitarianism: A New Public Ethics*. Belmont, CA. Wadsworth, Inc; 1994:139–153.
20. Beauchamp TL, Childress JE. *Principles of Biomedical Ethics*, 4th ed. New York: Oxford University Press; 1994.
21. Bentham J. *An Introduction to the Principles of Morals and Legislation*. Oxford: Clarendon Press; 1970.
22. Moore GE. *Principia Ethica*. Cambridge: Cambridge University Press; 1903. Cited in Beauchamp TL, Childress JE. *Principles of Biomedical Ethics*, 4th ed. New York: Oxford University Press; 1994.
23. Griffin J. *Well-Being: Its Meaning, Measurement, and Moral Importance*. Oxford: Clarendon Press; 1986.
24. Carse AL. The "voice of care." Implications for bioethics education. *J Philos Med* 1991; 16:5–28.
25. Jaggar AM. Feminist ethics: Projects, problems, prospects. In: Card C, ed. *Feminist Ethics*. Lawrence, KS: University of Kansas Press; 1991:78–104.
26. Baier A. What do women want in a moral theory? *Nous* March 1985:53–63.
27. Held V. Noncontractual society. In: Hanen M, Nielsen K, eds. *Science, Morality, and Feminist Theory*. Calgary: University of Calgary Press; 1987:111–137.

28. Gilligan C. *In a Different Voice: Psychological Theory and Women's Development.* Cambridge, MA: Harvard University Press; 1982.

29. Mendelson JH. Protection of participants and experimental design in clinical abuse liability testing. *Br Med J* 1991; 86:1543–1548.

30. Uganda National Council on Science and Technology. *Guidelines for the Conduct of Health Research Involving Human Subjects in Uganda.* Kampala, Uganda: Uganda National Council on Science and Technology; 1998.

31. Ackerman TF. Protectionism and the new research imperative in pediatric AIDS. *IRB: Rev Hum Subjects Res* 1990; 12:1–5.

32. High DM. Research with Alzheimer's disease subjects: Informed consent and proxy decision making. *J Am Geriatrics Soc* 1992: 40:950–957.

33. Lo B. Assessing decision-making capacity. *Law Med Health Care* 1990; 18:193–201.

34. Herxheimer A. The rights of the patient in clinical research. *Lancet* 1988; 2:1128–1130.

35. Portney LG, Watkins MP. *Foundations of Clinical Research: Applications to Practice.* Norwalk, CT: Appleton & Lange; 1993.

36. Owens JF. Informed consent in the clinical research setting: Experimentation on human subjects. *Med Trial Techniques* 1987; 33:335–350.

37. Dubler NN, Sidel VW. On research on HIV infection and AIDS in correctional institutions. *Milbank Q* 1989; 67:171–207.

38. Siegel HA, Carlson RG, Falck R, et al. Conducting HIV outreach and research among incarcerated drug abusers: A case study of ethical concerns and dilemmas. *J Subst Abuse Treat* 1993; 10:71–75.

39. Hammett TM, Dubler NN. Clinical and epidemiologic research on HIV infection and AIDS among correctional inmates: Regulations, ethics, and procedures. *Eval Rev* 1990; 14:482–501.

40. Schroeder K. A recommendation to the FDA concerning drug research on prisoners. *Southern Cal Law Rev* 1983; 56:969–1000.

41. Woody KJ. Legal and ethical concepts involved in informed consent to human research. *Cal West Law Rev* 1981; 18:50–79.

42. 45 Code of Federal Regulations, sections 46.305, .404–.408; 1997.

43. Sieber J. *Planning Ethically Responsible Research: A Guide for Students and Internal Review Boards.* Beverly Hills, CA: Sage; 1992.

44. Joint United Nations Programme on HIV/AIDS. *Report on the Global HIV/AIDS Epidemic.* Geneva: World Health Organization; June 1988.

45. Barton J, Wamai G. *Equity and Vulnerability: A Situation Analysis of Women, Adolescents, and Children in Uganda.* Kampala, Uganda: Uganda National Council for Children; 1994.

46. Nzita R, Niwampa M. *Peoples and Cultures of Uganda,* 2nd ed. Kampala, Uganda: Fountain Publishers; 1995.

47. Wallman S. *Kampala Women Getting By: Well-being in the Time of AIDS.* London: James Currey; 1996.

48. Pirouet L. Refugees in and from Uganda in the post-independence period. In: Hansen HB, Twaddle M, eds. *Uganda Now: Between Decay and Development.* London: James Currey; 1988:239–253.

49. Mutibwa P, *Uganda since Independence: A Story of Unfulfilled Hopes.* Kampala, Uganda: Fountain Publishers; 1992.

50. Loue S. *Legal and Ethical Aspects of HIV-Related Research.* New York: Plenum Press; 1995.

51. Falk TC. AIDS public health law. *J Legal Med* 1988; 9:529–546.

52. *Tarasoff v Regents of the University of California,* 17 Cal. 3d 425 (1976).

53. *McIntosh v Milano,* 168 N.J. Super. 466 (1979).

54. *Earle v Kuklo,* 26 N.J. Super. 471 (App. Div. 1953).

55. *David v Lhim,* 124 Mich. App. 291 (1983), *aff'd on rem* 147 Mich. App. 8 (1985), *rev'd on grounds of government immunity in Canon v Thumundo,* 430 Mich. 326 (1988).

56. *Thompson v County of Alameda,* 27 Cal. 3d 741 (1980).

57. *Jablonski v United States,* 712 F.2d 391 (9th Cir. 1983).

58. Traver LB, Cooksey DR. Defense argument. In Girardi JA, Keese RM, Traver LB, Cooksey DR, eds. Psychotherapist responsibility in notifying individuals at risk for exposure to HIV. *J Sex Res* 1988; 25:1–27.

59. Knapp S, Van de Creek L. Application of the duty to protect to HIV-positive patients. *Profess Psychol Res Pract* 1990; 21:161–166.

60. Appelbaum PS, Rosenbaum A. *Tarasoff* and the researcher: Does the duty to protect apply in the research setting? *Am Psychol* 1989; 44:885–894.

61. Francis D, Chin J. The prevention of acquired immunodeficiency syndrome in the United States. *JAMA* 1987; 257:1357–1366.

62. American Medical Association. Current opinions of the Judicial Council, Current Opinion 5.05. In: McDonald

BA, ed. *Ethical Problems for Physicians Raised by AIDS and HIV Infection: Conflicting Legal Obligations of Confidentiality and Disclosure.* Davis: University of California; 1989:557–592.

63. Lamb DH, Clark C, Drunheler P, et al. Applying *Tarasoff* to AIDS-related psychotherapy issues. *Profess Psychol Res Pract* 1989; 20:37–43.

64. Public Health Service, United States Department of Health and Human Services. *A Public Health Challenge: State Issues, Policies, and Programs*, vol. 1. United States Department of Health and Human Services 1987: 4-1–4-31.

65. Totten G, Lamb DH, Reeder GD. *Tarasoff* and confidentiality in AIDS-related psychotherapy. *Profess Psychol Res Prac* 1990; 21:155–160.

66. Fruman LS. AIDS and the physician's duty to warn (part 2). *Med Law* 1991; 10:515–526.

67. Angell M. The ethics of clinical research in the Third World. *N Engl J Med* 1997; 337:847–849.

68. Lurie P, Wolfe SM. Unethical trials of interventions to reduce potential transmission of the human immunodeficiency virus in developing countries. *N Engl J Med* 1997; 337:853–856.

69. Varmus H, Satcher P. Ethical complexities of conducting research in developing countries. *N Engl J Med* 1997; 337:1003–1005.

70. Pellegrino ED. Nonabandonment: An old obligation revisited. *Ann Intern Med* 1995; 122:377–378.

71. Quill TE, Cassel CK. Nonabandonment: A central obligation for physicians. *Ann Intern Med* 1995; 122:368–374.

72. British HIV Association. Guidelines. *Lancet* 1997; 349:1086–1092.

73. Carpenter CC, Fischl MA, Hammer SM, et al. Antiretroviral therapy for HIV infection in 1997. Updated recommendations from the International AIDS Society-USA panel. *JAMA* 1997; 277:1962–1969.

74. Macklin R, Friedland G. AIDS research: The ethics of clinical trials. *Law Med Health Care* 1986; 14:273–280.

75. Freedman B. Suspended judgment: AIDS and the ethics of clinical trials: Learning the right lessons. *Controlled Clin Trials* 1992; 13:1–5.

76. Halbreich U, Carson SW. Drug studies in women of childbearing age: Ethical and methodological considerations. *J Clin Psychopharmacol* 1989; 9:328–333.

77. Murphy TF. Women and drug users: The changing faces of HIV clinical drug trials. *QRB Qual Rev Bull* 1991; 17:26–32.

78. Levine C. Women and HIV/AIDS research: The barriers to equity. *Eval Rev* 1990; 14:447–463.

79. Levine C. Women and HIV/AIDS research: The barriers to equity. *IRB: Rev Hum Subjects* 1991; 13:18–23.

80. Buc NL. Women in clinical trials: Concluding remarks. *Food Drug Law J* 1993; 48:223–226.

81. Merton V. The exclusion of pregnant, pregnable, and once-pregnable people (a.k.a. women) from biomedical research. *Am J Law Med* 1993; 19:369–451.

82. Murphy D. Women in clinical trials: HIV-infected women. *Food Drug Law J* 1993; 48:175–179.

83. Merkatz RB, Temple R, Subel S, et al. Women in clinical trials of new drugs: A change in Food and Drug Administration policy. *N Engl J Med* 1993; 329:292–296.

84. Moreno JD. Ethical issues relating to the inclusion of women of childbearing age in clinical trials. In: Mastroianni AC, Faden R, Federman D, eds. *Women and Health Research: Ethical and Legal Issues of Including Women in Clinical Studies*, vol. 2. Washington, DC: National Academy Press; 1994:29–34.

85. Mastroianni AC, Faden F, Federman D, eds. *Women and Health Research: Ethical and Legal Issues of Including Women in Clinical Studies*, vol. 1. Washington, DC: National Academy Press; 1994.

17

Looking Forward
Future Directions for HIV Prevention Research

RALPH J. DICLEMENTE

INTRODUCTION

Recent advances in combination antiretroviral therapy have been encouraging. The advent of highly active antiretroviral therapy (HAART), a combination therapy that includes protease inhibitors, has revolutionized treatment and enhanced the prospects for survival for people living with human immunodeficiency virus (HIV).[1] While HAART can markedly suppress HIV in plasma to undetectable levels, considerable uncertainty remains whether reductions in plasma levels correspond to decreased risk of transmission and whether treatment advantages can be sustained. Recent findings indicate that individuals undergoing treatment with HAART, with nondetectable HIV levels in plasma, may still have the virus present in seminal cells.[2] Thus, the potential to sexually transmit HIV persists despite effective suppression of viral replication.[3] From an international perspective, irrespective of the effectiveness of HAART in managing disease among people living with HIV in developed countries, the availability of HAART in less developed countries in all likelihood will be severely limited due to its prohibitive cost.

While developing a more effective therapeutic regimen represents one research focus, development of an effective vaccine to prohibit HIV infection represents a second major research agenda. A safe and effective vaccine would represent a significant advance in disease prevention. While major strides have been made in the development of a prophylactic vaccine, developing a vaccine is a complex research challenge and significant hurdles remain to be surmounted.[4,5]

While great strides have been taken in the search for more effective therapies and, to a lesser extend, in the development of a prophylactic vaccine, an overriding urgency to develop and implement HIV prevention interventions remains. Prevention programs designed to motivate individuals to adopt and maintain HIV preventive practices, particularly condom use during sexual intercourse and safer injecting drug use practices, represent the most practical strategy for controlling the HIV epidemic. While modifying individuals' HIV risk taking behaviors is admittedly a formidable challenge, recent reviews and meta-analyses[6–8] and rigorously conducted large-scale multisite trials[9,10] suggest that such changes are achievable.

The chapters in this book describe promising advances in the field of HIV prevention, with respect to theory, design, implementation, evaluation, cost-effectiveness analysis, and

RALPH J. DICLEMENTE • Department of Behavioral Sciences and Health Education, Rollins School of Public Health, Emory University, Atlanta, Georgia 30322.

Handbook of HIV Prevention, edited by Peterson and DiClemente.
Kluwer Academic/Plenum Publishers, New York, 2000.

technology transfer. Intervention approaches are discussed that address different risk behaviors (i.e., injection drug use, sexual risk behaviors) across cultures (more and less developed countries), in diverse settings (i.e., schools, communities, clinics), and with different populations (men who have sex with men, adolescents, women, injection drug users). This chapter, unlike its predecessors, attempts to highlight key areas of prevention research and discern fruitful directions for future HIV prevention research.

It is beyond the scope of this chapter to reiterate the richness of diversity or depth of information captured and articulated so skillfully in previous chapters. It is useful, however, to understand our successes and, as importantly, to identify and confront existing challenges. By so doing, we hope to bring into sharper focus those areas that hold considerable promise for HIV prevention and as such warrant vigorous exploration. Only by understanding the past, its successes and its failures, and gazing toward the future, its opportunities and its challenges, can we as prevention scientists move forward with unwavering determination to capitalize on history and create promising and more effective interventions in the future.

HIV PREVENTION—BUILDING A SCIENCE OF PREVENTION FROM AN INTERDISCIPLINARY PERSPECTIVE

The success of prevention efforts to a large extent is attributable to the heterogeneity of disciplines that are actively involved in the science of HIV prevention. Disciplinary diversity is a research strength. Because of this diversity, advances in prevention are being made by transcending disciplinary boundaries, in terms of theory, methodology, and evaluation strategies. These advances have been most readily made with true interdisciplinary approaches that involve not just individuals who are contributing to a particular project or addressing a particular research question from social and behavioral science disciplines, but from the active involvement of all relevant disciplines in an effort to integrate the disciplines into a science of HIV prevention. Continued integration and collaboration between researchers in the behavioral and social sciences, with clinicians, policy analysts, epidemiologists, and biostatisticians, represent the best opportunity to develop a coherent, effective, and interdisciplinary approach to HIV prevention research.

HIV PREVENTION NEEDS TO TARGET MULTIPLE LEVELS OF CAUSALITY

Historically, the HIV epidemic had been largely viewed as an individual-level health phenomenon. This perspective has dominated the field of HIV prevention. More recently, prevention scientists have realized that there are a host of environmental and structural influences that make a significant contribution to sustaining the HIV epidemic.[11] Researchers and practitioners alike are increasingly acknowledging the importance of social contextualism; the need to understand an individual's behavior within their social environment and intervene not only on the individual level but with broader social structural levels. It is clear, for example, that individual-level interventions, while effective at motivating behavior change, may not be sufficient to sustain behavior changes over protracted periods of time, particularly in the face of pervasive countervailing pressures that promote or reinforce risk behavior. Further, addressing behavior change at the individual-level lacks sufficient breadth to reach large segments of the at-risk population. Community-level interventions are needed which create an atmosphere supportive of prevention norms.[12–14]

Interventions targeted at the community level are designed to promote HIV preventive behavior change by providing individuals with information and skills to change behavior through naturally occurring channels of influence in the community and simultaneously to provide a supportive environment that encourages HIV preventive behavior. Changing community norms also reinforces and maintains the practice of health-promoting behaviors. This provides one avenue for ensuring a social context in which individuals will be reminded that the healthier alternative (safer behavior) is preferred according to community standards and norms.

Community-level interventions may have four interrelated outcomes. First, they may promote the adoption of HIV preventive behaviors among persons engaged in risky behaviors. Second, they may help sustain newly acquired HIV preventive behaviors and hopefully solidify these changes. Third, community-level interventions also may serve to amplify individual-level program effects over extended time periods, reducing the potential for relapse to high-risk behaviors. Finally, community-level interventions may foster an atmosphere that discourages the initial adoption of high-risk behaviors.

While community-level intervention programs represent one area for increased research, it is crucial that broader structural changes take place to ensure that persons are enabled to make the desired changes in behavior. These can include changes in laws, public health policy, and the context and circumstances in which sex and injecting drug use occur. Therefore, future HIV prevention programs will need to examine in greater detail the effects of social, cultural, institutional, political, and economic forces as they promote or reinforce risky behavior and impeded the adoption and maintenance of HIV preventive behavior. By understanding these broader, pervasive influences, it may be possible to develop community-level interventions, initiate policy changes, design institutionally based programs, and promote the development of broader, macro-level societal changes that access many more persons and promotes a social environment conducive to adopting and sustaining health-promoting behaviors while supporting the development and implementation of HIV prevention activities.

LINKING HIV PREVENTION WITH SEXUALLY TRANSMITTED DISEASE DETECTION AND TREATMENT

Sexually transmitted diseases (STDs), excluding HIV, pose a serious health threat to the United States. While the STD epidemic has been masked by the HIV epidemic, the cost of STDs in terms of morbidity, mortality, and medical care expenditures is substantial.[15] Moreover, there is a significant intersection between the STD and HIV epidemics.

Converging lines of research indicate that STDs, both inflammatory and ulcerative, may increase HIV infectivity and susceptibility.[16] An effect on HIV infectivity is supported by the presence of HIV in genital ulcers,[17] by the increased rate of detection of HIV in cervical specimens among women with cervical inflammation,[18] and by the increased prevalence of HIV in specimens from men with gonococcal urethritis.[19] With respect to enhanced susceptibility to HIV, there is empirical evidence from discordant couple studies suggesting that HIV-seronegative partners who developed genital infections were more likely to become infected with HIV than were those HIV-seronegative partners who did not have genital infections.[20,21]

Several studies provide evidence that early detection and treatment of STDs can have an impact on sexual transmission of HIV. Moss and colleagues[19] observed significant reductions in the rate of detection of HIV in urethral specimens following curative treatment. Marked reductions in HIV also have been observed in semen following treatment for STDs.[22,23]

Although appropriate treatment of these conditions resulted in significant decreases of genital HIV levels, concomitant reductions in serum HIV levels were not observed.

The integral role of STD detection and treatment for HIV prevention cannot be overestimated. From a clinical perspective, there is ample evidence that individuals seeking treatment for STDs represent a high-risk population for acquisition of HIV.[24] Given their elevated risk, sexual risk-reduction interventions need to be implemented in clinical settings where individuals are screened and treated for STDs. Recent studies provide evidence that intensive counseling at STD clinics can significantly reduce subsequent STD infections.[10,25,26]

One study, Project RESPECT, was a multicenter randomized controlled trial conducted in five public STD clinics designed to evaluate the efficacy of counseling to prevent HIV/STD by comparing the effects of two interactive counseling interventions with didactic prevention messages typical of current practice.[10] In this trial, at 3- and 6-month follow-up, self-reported consistent condom use was significantly higher in both the enhanced counseling (4 interactive theory-based sessions) and the brief counseling (2 interactive risk-reduction sessions) interventions compared with participants receiving didactic prevention messages (comparison condition). Through the 6-month interval, significantly fewer STDs were detected among participants in the counseling interventions; 30% fewer participants had new STDs in both the enhanced counseling and brief counseling interventions compared with those in the comparison condition. Through the end of the 12-month study, significantly fewer STDs were detected among participants in the counseling interventions; 20% fewer participants in each counseling intervention had new STDs relative to those in the comparison condition. Likewise, Shain and colleagues[25] observed significant reductions in STD rates at 6- and 12-month follow-up among Latino and African-American women randomized to receive three 4-hour small-group sessions designed to promote the adoption of preventive behaviors versus women randomized to a comparison condition. Similarly, Branson and colleagues[26] observed comparable decrease in STD/HIV-associated risk behaviors (i.e., poor condom use and multiple sex partners) and reductions in STD incidence for clients randomized to either two 20-minute counseling sessions or four 1-hour group sessions. The findings suggest that relatively brief interventions can be effective at modifying high-risk behaviors and, more importantly, reducing STDs.

Sexual risk reduction interventions need not be restricted to public STD clinics. Much of STD treatment is provided by nonpublic facilities; thus, it is imperative that we implement and evaluate interventions in managed care organizations and other private practice environments as well as other nontraditional settings (i.e., detention facilities, prisons, jails, and drug treatment facilities). STD screening also is facilitated by the advent of new and less invasive detection assays using urine as a specimen. While one advantage of these newer assays is their increase in sensitivity and specificity, the primary advantage lies in their capacity to be used in nonclinical settings.

The concept of early detection and treatment of STDs need not be limited to clinical environments. There is evidence from a community trial that aggressive case detection and treatment of STDs can markedly reduce HIV incidence.[27] In the Mwanza trial, the number of new HIV infections was reduced by 40%. Notwithstanding potential methodological biases, the concept of STD control for HIV prevention may be an effective strategy that can be implemented at the community level as well as the clinic level. However, while improving STD case management is an important additional HIV prevention strategy, its potential benefit will depend in large part on the prevalence of STDs in the community and the effectiveness of the STD program to identify and treat infected individuals.[28] In addition, such a communitywide intervention also may be dependent on the level of maturity of the HIV epidemic in the community. Overall, the accumulating empirical evidence suggests that a focus on STD prevention, detection, and management may be a cost-effective approach that has a significant collateral effect for HIV prevention.[29]

PREVENTION INTERVENTIONS FOR PEOPLE LIVING WITH HIV REMAINS AN UNDERSTUDIED AREA

In more developed countries, advances in HIV treatment have resulted in significant decreases in HIV-related mortality. These treatment advances have had and are likely to have little impact in lesser developed countries, given that the cost of HAART represents a significant obstacle to widespread use. However, while the therapeutic landscape of HIV treatment has rapidly evolved, a lack of emphasis on prevention strategies for persons living with HIV and a lack of prevention research among this population remains.

It should be axiomatic that prevention does not stop with HIV infection. On the contrary, prevention efforts need to be intensified for those living with HIV. Indeed, there are several cogent and compelling clinical and public health reasons to reduce high-risk sexual behavior in persons living with HIV. First, there is accumulating evidence to suggest that acquisition of an STD may facilitate HIV disease progression. Second, it may be possible to acquire different strains of HIV (reinfection). Third, with the advent of HAART there is an emergence of drug-resistant viral strains. Thus, exposure to drug-resistant strains may seriously compromise the efficacy of HAART therapy. Finally, acquisition of an STD also may facilitate transmission of HIV to seronegative sexual partners.

While there is ample rationale for designing and implementing prevention interventions tailored for persons living with HIV, few studies have been evaluated with this population. This area of prevention research, rapidly emerging as critically important for the control of the HIV epidemic, remains understudied.

IDENTIFYING STRATEGIES TO IMPROVE THE SUSTAINABILITY OF HIV PREVENTION PROGRAM EFFECTS

Another key area of investigation is in the development of strategies to sustain intervention treatment or program effects over extended time periods. There is ample evidence that both individual-level as well as community-level interventions can modify risk behaviors. However, there also are data suggesting that intervention–treatment effects decay over time. In individual-level prevention interventions, one strategy that is frequently used to minimize decay (or attenuation of treatment effects) is to use booster sessions subsequent to delivering the primary "dose" of the intervention. While this has shown efficacy in reconstituting treatment effects in long-term follow-up, it is clearly labor- and time-intensive, and thus costly. Alternative approaches are needed. One strategy that holds promise is the use of social marketing or media interventions to motivate adoption of HIV preventive behaviors, reinforce prevention messages, and sustain behavior change.

There is evidence that mass media may help to create an environment conducive to HIV prevention. In particular, mass media can help increase awareness of the HIV epidemic and its impact and encourage public funding for prevention, treatment, and social services. In a number of European countries, as well as in Canada, New Zealand, and Australia, the media has been instrumental in creating a social climate that makes a wide spectrum of prevention strategies more acceptable. Additionally, messages about HIV disseminated through the mass media may facilitate more open discussion of drug use and sexuality in circumstances where heretofore this was not possible. The widespread promotion of condoms, for example, which is commonplace now in most countries of Western Europe, may reflect to some extent the attention given to the HIV epidemic by mass media.

Evidence for the efficacy of media interventions can be gleaned from the campaigns undertaken in Switzerland. Evaluation of media-based interventions in Switzerland have observed marked reductions in risk behaviors. For example, between 1987 and 1991, an aggressive marketing campaign aimed at 21- to 30-year-olds observed an increase in condom use with casual sex partners from 8% to 50%. Among a younger subgroup, 17- to 20-year-olds, effects were even more marked; condom use increased from 19% to 73%. Equally important from a health policy perspective, the Swiss study found that rates of sexual activity remained unchanged over the time period during implementation of the media campaign. More recently, evidence from an evaluation of HIV prevention messages diffused through a radio soap opera in Tanzania support the efficacy of media for promoting behavior change. Evaluation of HIV-associated risk behaviors among people residing in the broadcast area and those in the control area indicate that condom use markedly increased in the intervention areas. While media-based interventions may be effective at promoting the adoption of HIV preventive behaviors, they need not be limited to public service announcement-type interventions; but they also may be innovative and entertaining.

Media interventions are not a panacea. It is clear that media-based interventions remain an understudied intervention modality in the United States. Whether such media campaigns would enjoy support and success in the United States is arguable. However, media programs, even those that may be less candid or innovative, still may serve to create a social climate conducive to open discussion about sex, STDs, and HIV. Media messages also may reinforce prevention messages for individuals exposed to other, more intensive interventions. In this way, media campaigns may directly impact individuals' behavior and may indirectly influence behavior by affecting social norms to help sustain newly adopted HIV preventive behaviors or reinforce maintenance of low-risk behaviors in the face of countervailing social pressures.

IN SEARCH OF NEW AND PROMISING THEORETICAL ORIENTATIONS

As in any science, theories are developed to explain phenomena under study. In HIV prevention, theories of human behavior are useful in explaining why people do or do not engage in certain behaviors that lead to HIV infection. Many theories have been used to guide exploratory research designed to identify the antecedents and determinants of HIV risk behaviors. Likewise, theory has played an integral role in guiding the development of programs designed to eliminate or reduce risk behaviors associated with HIV infection.

The range of theoretical approaches in HIV prevention is a reflection of the field itself: eclectic and diverse. Theoretical approaches from a broad spectrum of disciplines have been used. The scales of evidence suggest that theory-based interventions are effective at promoting the adoption of HIV preventive behaviors. However effective our current array of theories, it would be premature to foreclose on the utility of other as of yet untested theories. Only by constantly reevaluating the explanatory and predictive capacity of theories does the field of HIV prevention mature.

Part of the maturation process involves change. As theories become less useful, that is, they explain an insufficient amount of variance in particular risk behaviors, or they are found wanting as a foundation for guiding the design and implementation of behavior change interventions, they are modified or even discarded in favor of potentially more useful theories. This process of development, elimination, and replacement is gradual. New theories are synthesized and embraced. They, too, are subject to empirical validation, and if found lacking are similarly discarded. This evolutionary process builds on the past as a way of contextualizing the present and predicting the future.

The current theoretical armamentarium has been quite useful, particularly the social cognitive theories, in furthering our understanding of the interplay of factors that affect both risk and preventive behavior as well as informing development and implementation of prevention interventions. Despite the utility of current models, much of the variance of behavior change remains unaccounted for in intervention studies. Thus, other theoretical models may prove useful and should be empirically tested. Diversity in terms of theory selection needs to be embraced and indeed encouraged. The field needs to be open and receptive to new models from other disciplines. Likewise, as the focus of intervention research shifts from individual-level to broader community-level interventions, a different array of theories may be sought to help guide these interventions. As in any science, we need to be receptive to innovation and we need to maintain rigorous evaluation standards to cull those theories that are useful from those that are not.

THE NEED TO IMPROVE HIV PREVENTION TECHNOLOGY TRANSFER

No HIV prevention intervention is perfect. Not every individual exposed to an intervention will adopt HIV preventive behaviors. Such a goal is unrealistic and, most important, unnecessary to significantly impact the course of the HIV epidemic. Such an approach in fact may be counterproductive, creating inertia among consumers of prevention research while they search for the "magic bullet" intervention.[30]

This does not mean that we lower the standard for determining "effective" HIV prevention interventions. Quite the contrary. A failure to adopt and maintain rigorous standards for identifying effective HIV prevention interventions is bought at the cost of wasting scarce resources on ineffective programs. It does mean, however, that while the continued efforts of prevention scientists need to be directed at developing more effective HIV prevention interventions, existing interventions that have demonstrated programmatic efficacy need to be widely disseminated.

Ultimately, preventing HIV infections not only depends on the development and evaluation of innovative behavior change approaches but on how effectively these interventions can be translated and integrated into self-sustaining components of clinic practice, school curricula, or community programs, particularly in those countries and populations most adversely impacted by the HIV epidemic.[31] Thus, future research efforts should be directed at identifying mechanisms for the timely translation of effective HIV interventions into sustainable community-, clinic-, or school-based programs.

While the research "output" in terms of HIV prevention technology has been remarkable, particularly in the past few years, the "uptake" and integration of the of this technology into ongoing programmatic activities have been far less effective. Understanding the barriers that impede the rapid adoption of new HIV prevention technology by organizations is critical for developing effective strategies designed to facilitate the translation of prevention technology to end users in community, clinic, and school settings. Further study is needed in advancing our understanding of how organizations, including the individual providers within those organizations, are influenced to adopt innovations in HIV prevention.

The development of sustainable systems and processes for the efficient transfer of HIV prevention technology is contingent on many factors. Foremost is the need for an infrastructure that is responsible for collecting and collating new HIV prevention technology as well as organizing, managing, and coordinating its active transfer to end users (i.e., policy analysts, elected officials, health department officials, clinical and social service providers, and prevention program managers in community-based organizations). As for any science of technology transfer, investing in the development of an infrastructure to design and continually monitor systems and processes needed to promote rapid and widespread use of HIV prevention technologies is critical. Resources will need to be identified, mobilized, and committed to the ongoing maintenance and support of infrastructure that promotes the rapid dissemination of HIV prevention technology.

There is a clear distinction between the passive transfer of HIV prevention technology versus the actions required to encourage the uptake and implementation of technology.[32] To be effective, technology transfer must not be a passive activity. Rather, it is an active and purposive application of skills, systems, and resources dedicated to supporting both the transfer and the uptake of new prevention technologies. Thus, gaps and inadequacies in the infrastructure responsible for supporting the transfer and uptake of new HIV prevention technologies will clearly limit how efficiently systems and processes can be designed, implemented, maintained, and evaluated. Without a competent and fully operational infrastructure, the primary goal of which is to guide and coordinate HIV prevention technology transfer, it is doubtful whether we can maximize our investment in prevention research and implement newly developed, innovative and effective prevention strategies and activities on a scale broad enough to impact the HIV epidemic.

With judicious planning, however, we can create an infrastructure that provides oversight, guidance, and coordination, enabling the rapid dissemination of HIV prevention technology and supporting the uptake of these technologies by consumers through appropriate training, the provision of relevant materials, and an ongoing program of technical assistance. Only by assuring that HIV prevention research is translated into usable information and materials and reaches consumers who can use this information and materials in prevention programs will prevention research realize its potential and its promise in terms of impacting the HIV epidemic.

NEED FOR PUBLIC AND HEALTH POLICY SUPPORTIVE OF HIV PREVENTION RESEARCH AND PRACTICE

The need for coherent and rational public and health policy is critical for furthering the HIV prevention agenda. One significant obstacle in disseminating HIV prevention research technology has been the reluctance to use scientifically generated evidence as a basis for health and public policy decision making, primarily attributable to perceived adverse political consequences.[33,34] Given the weight of scientific evidence demonstrating the efficacy of safer sex and needle exchange interventions and the absence of data demonstrating adverse consequences associated with these programs, it is difficult to understand the logic behind current public and health policy that constrains these interventions and limits their ability to be broadly disseminated, widely adopted, and effectively utilized.

To the detriment of HIV prevention efforts much of the public and health policy debate has been ideologically motivated rather than empirically driven, often substituting well-intentioned though misguided motives for scientific evidence. However, no matter how politically viable, widespread, or popular a program maybe, efficacy in preventing HIV-associated risk behaviors and their consequences (STDs, HIV) must remain the primary and sole criterion by which programs are judged. Priorities need to be directed away from programs that are based on persuasive philosophy, anecdotal evidence, or, as is often the case, political convenience and toward those that are based on sound empirical research and demonstrated programmatic efficacy. Policies that constrain the range of HIV prevention options severely reduce the flexibility needed to design and implement programs and negatively impact our ability to disseminate effective programs to consumers, inhibit adoption of these programs, and if adopted reduce their capacity to be effectively used.

THE NEED FOR BIOLOGICAL OUTCOMES IN HIV PREVENTION RESEARCH

Historically, HIV prevention interventions have relied almost exclusively on individuals' self-reported behavior change to assess program efficacy. Typically, individuals reported their frequency of condom use, number of different sexual partners, or frequency of drug use when engaging in sexual behavior. In the most rigorous research designs—randomized controlled trials—baseline frequency of risk measures are contrasted with postintervention measures of similar risk behaviors relative to a placebo–attention comparison group or control group. Self-reported data have been criticized as subject to potential reporting biases, inaccurate recall, and social desirability bias.[35,36] Recently, the use of prevalent sexually transmitted diseases has been advocated as a complementary measure for evaluating program efficacy.

In the past, the primary drawback of using biological markers was the logistics of data collection. Data collection was typically feasible only in a clinic environment, such as an STD clinic or other clinical venue, and often required trained clinicians using invasive procedures. Recently, however, major advances have been made in STD diagnostic procedures, in particular, the advent of DNA amplification assays that have high sensitivity and specificity. With the availability of these DNA amplification techniques that can detect bacterial STDs in urine specimen, in particular, prevalent STDs, such as chlamydia and gonorrhea, it is now possible to detect STDs in a noninvasive manner in a broad range of nonclinical settings.[37–43] The development of this diagnostic technology paves the way for greater utilization of STDs as a clinical endpoint in evaluating HIV prevention interventions.

The use of biological endpoints, while representing an objective and quantifiable marker of high-risk sexual behavior, is not without controversy, nor is it a panacea for avoiding bias associated with self-report. It is important to recognize that reliance on incident STDs as a measure of program efficacy may not be an appropriate outcome for every study. It is unlikely, for instance, that the incidence of STDs will be changed in a short- term study conducted in a population with little sexual activity or in a community with a low prevalence of STDs. Conversely, populations with a high degree of sexual activity and a high prevalence of STDs are ideal for studying the effects of behavioral interventions on STD incidence. Moreover, studies incorporating biological markers as the primary outcome measure will need to be conducted with samples that are large enough and follow-ups that are long enough to provide sufficient statistical power to detect differences in STD incidence.

A few recent studies have used biological endpoints as one component of program evaluation. These studies have demonstrated not only a capacity to reduce self-reported risk behaviors but more importantly to decrease the incidence of subsequent STDs.[10,25,26] These studies were conducted with STD clinic clients, a population that is at high risk of subsequent STD acquisition. Future HIV prevention intervention studies, when applicable and feasible, will need to seriously consider the utility of including biological markers as an objective outcome measure of program efficacy.[44]

THE NEED TO MEASURE COST-EFFECTIVENESS IN HIV PREVENTION RESEARCH

The increasing emphasis on cost containment, the emergence of the managed care environment, and the disproportionate increase in the cost of health care versus other expenditures over the past decade have prompted examining cost-effectiveness as one criterion for evaluating health promotion programs.

In our current fiscal environment, it becomes imperative that we not only evaluate program efficacy in terms of impact (e.g., changes in behavior, attitudes, norms, knowledge) and outcomes (e.g., changes in morbidity, mortality, quality of life) but also assess cost-effectiveness. Such information is vitally important to program planners, policy makers, and other persons involved in the design and implementation of health promotion and disease prevention programs who are responsible for the judicious allocation of limited financial resources so as to maximize the number of adverse outcomes (e.g., STD or HIV infection) averted through participation or exposure to an intervention program.

Arguably, one might question whether HIV prevention programs should be held accountable to the standard that a program's economic benefits to society outweigh its financial costs. This is certainly a debatable issue. However, whether or not one accepts the standard, the application of economic evaluation techniques is as appropriate to HIV prevention interventions as it is to other health programs.[45]

Unable to sidestep the issue of cost effectiveness, HIV prevention scientists and program planners need to become familiar with the theory and methods used to conduct cost-effectiveness studies.[46–48] This methodology represents an entirely different perspective for many in the field of HIV prevention research. Most often, HIV prevention scientists have had their philosophical, theoretical, and methodological roots in the social and behavioral sciences. While an interdisciplinary perspective is the hallmark HIV prevention, one area that is underdeveloped is the science of economic evaluation.

In our current resource-constrained environment and for the foreseeable future, HIV prevention scientists need to become familiar with cost-effectiveness methods and analysis and plan their programs with these measures incorporated in the study design. As HIV prevention advances and more interventions are shown to be effective in reducing risk behaviors and their adverse sequelae, it will become increasingly important to establish the cost-effectiveness of these interventions.

THE NEED FOR STRUCTURED REPORTING OF HIV PREVENTION INTERVENTIONS

Some journals in the field of medicine, including the *Journal of the American Medical Association* and the *British Medical Journal*, have adopted structured reporting requirements to enhance study comparability and quality. Working groups have been convened to study and recommend reporting guidelines for biomedical clinical trial research.[49,50] One goal would be to provide similar reporting guidelines for HIV prevention intervention trials.

The increasingly rapid growth in HIV prevention intervention research has led to new challenges; namely, how to calibrate an intervention's efficacy vis-à-vis other interventions. Variability in the reporting of HIV prevention intervention trials severely limits comparability of findings between trials. Moreover, the lack of structured reporting guidelines reduces the level of certainty with which HIV prevention interventions could be carefully assessed, weighed against other interventions and replicated.

Structured reporting is meant to provide investigators and consumers of HIV prevention research with a list of essential elements necessary to adequately describe and if need be replicate the study. The purpose is to assist investigators in preparing reports that will facilitate understanding of the study; its rationale, methodology, and statistical analyses, thus increasing the utility of the findings for consumers (e.g., researchers, policy analysts, and public health practitioners). A principal advantage of structured reporting is that consumers will have uniform, comparable information to review and evaluate, regardless of variability in investigator's writing styles or reviewer's and journal's policies, that is much needed in making a determination about the validity of the findings and can influence decision making about implementation of a particular HIV intervention.

The reporting guidelines specified by O'Leary et al.[44] address a number of theoretical, design, and analytic elements essential to the implementation, conduct, and evaluation of HIV prevention interventions. The intent of the proposed reporting format is not to discourage investigators from including additional elements in published reports, nor is it meant to discourage investigators in the design and implementation of innovative interventions. Structured reporting does not preclude innovation; it only requires that investigators provide a clear, accurate, and consistent structure for describing the study design, its implementation, specification of the intervention, and data analysis. With the development and evaluation of increasing numbers of HIV prevention interventions, structured reporting guidelines will provide a framework that may enhance interpretation of research findings by researchers, practitioners, and policy analysts.

INTERACTIONS BETWEEN SPHERES OF INFLUENCE: LESSONS FOR THE FUTURE

Several converging spheres will likely result in increased attention to HIV prevention research, but some important caveats must be noted if there is truly to be an increase in attention to this area of research. First, HIV prevention is an emerging science of diverse disciplines. Much will be gained by embracing the breadth of perspectives from these different disciplines. However, it is incumbent on both HIV researchers and practitioners to work toward convergence of theories and methodologies if the goal of achieving a defined science of HIV prevention is to be realized. Second, not only will the goal of converging the science of HIV prevention be advanced by using rigorous, empirically based methodologies, but such methodological rigor will soon be required as managed care organizations and governmental agencies increasingly demand demonstrable cost-effectiveness of HIV prevention programs. Third, these increasing requirements to provide documented cost-effectiveness data to support intervention programs will require that HIV prevention program planners and interventionists have adequate research training. This will require the training of scientist/practitioners who are capable of both implementing and evaluating HIV prevention programs. In fact, academic researchers who also are trained as scientist–practitioners may be best able to appreciate the barriers of service program implementation and best able to advance the field while developing empirically validated programs capable of more broadscale dissemination than at present.

LOOKING FORWARD: SUMMARY OF FUTURE DIRECTIONS FOR HIV PREVENTION

This handbook has attempted to outline the promising developments in theory and design, evaluation, and implementation methods used in HIV prevention that address different risk behaviors in varying settings and with different populations. Clearly, the field of HIV prevention is rapidly growing in depth and breadth as new theoretical models and innovative intervention strategies are identified and as societal, health care, and regulatory influences have increased the focus on prevention. Despite great diversity in disciplines involved in HIV prevention research and practice, some convergence of the science of HIV prevention is occurring as advances are being made in theories and methods. Certainly, the variety of spheres of influence that are converging suggest that in the foreseeable future the field of HIV prevention and practice will continue to rapidly expand.

Future HIV prevention intervention programs must build on their historical roots. Programs must be developed and evaluated on an ongoing basis to monitor programmatic efficacy; not only by measuring statistically significant self-reported changes in risk behaviors, but other more meaningful changes as well, such as changes in the incidence of disease. Whenever possible, however, additional outcome measures that avoid individuals' self-report of behavior change need to be included in the evaluation of interventions. In some cases, HIV incidence rates, over time, can serve as one index of program efficacy. In some countries and among some populations in the United States the incidence of HIV infection may not be a suitable outcome measure. In these instances, surrogate biological markers (for example, STDs and secondary indicators of preventive behaviors, such as possession of condoms, bleach, or clean injection needles) could be employed in behavior change interventions. Programs also must be modified according to evaluation feedback, further refining the intervention and strengthening its potential to effectively promote behavior change. Equally important as program development, there is a need for effective program technology transfer. Programs that are evaluated and identified as effective should be widely disseminated through diverse channels and adequate training and program materials should be provided to encourage the adoption and appropriate use of these intervention programs. Finally, for HIV prevention interventions to progress more rapidly, the development of a comprehensive and coordinated infrastructure to conceptualize, stimulate, and support intervention research necessary to control the HIV epidemic is still of critical importance.

Given the human costs, not to mention lost productivity and medical costs associated with HIV, behavioral interventions that demonstrate programmatic efficacy will be an important component in any public health strategy to prevent HIV. Further, given the monetary expenditure involved in developing and evaluating HIV prevention interventions, it is critical that these studies be adequately designed, conducted, analyzed, and reported. While HIV prevention programs, adequately funded and innovative in design, offer the potential to effectively reduce risk behaviors and their adverse sequelae, these changes will not be radical or swift. Behavior change, on a scale large enough to impact the HIV epidemic, will not be realized as a result of a single, static intervention program administered at one time point, but rather program effectiveness is enhanced when applied and evaluated continuously over an extended time period. Further, to increase the comprehension and perhaps effectiveness of HIV prevention programs, they must be developed to address the many levels of causation and tailored to be relevant and sensitive to the intended population. Finally, without structured reporting of HIV prevention interventions, we run the risk of not identifying potentially effective intervention programs and adopting others that may not be effective. Clearly, if we are to successfully confront the challenge of HIV, then innovative program design, rigorous evaluation, rapid dissemination of effective prevention intervention programs, and community adoption and integration of preventive interventions into ongoing, sustainable programs must remain a public health priority.

As we look forward to the promise of HIV prevention, we should recognize that future generations will look back and reflect on our efforts. Let the future historians remark on our inspiration, our willingness to commit both fiscal and human resources, and our unwavering dedication to the control and eradication of HIV.

ACKNOWLEDGMENT.   Preparation of this chapter was supported by grants MH54412 and MH55726 from the Center of Mental Health Research on AIDS, National Institute of Mental Health, National Institutes of Health.

REFERENCES

1. Palella FJ Jr, Delaney KM, Moorman AC, et al. Declining morbidity and mortality among patients with advanced human immunodeficiency virus infection. *N Engl J Med* 1998; 338:853–860.
2. Zhang H, Dornadula G, Beumont M, et al. Human immunodeficiency virus type 1 in the semen of men receiving highly active antiretroviral therapy. *N Engl J Med* 1989; 339:1803–1809.
3. Haase AT, Schacker TW. Potential for the transmission of HIV-1 despite highly active antiretroviral therapy. *N Engl J Med* 1998; 339:1846–1847.
4. Nathanson N. Harnessing research to control AIDS. *Nature Med* 1998; 1:880–881.
5. Baltimore D, Heilamn C. HIV vaccines: Prospects and challenges. *Sci Am* 1998; 279:98–103.
6. Interventions to prevent HIV Risk Behaviors. *NIH Concensus Statement* 1997 Feb 11–13; 15(2):1–41.
7. Coates TJ, Collins C. Preventing HIV infection. *Sci Am* 1998; 279:96–97.
8. Kalichman SC, Carey MP, Johnson BT. Prevention of sexually transmitted HIV infection: A meta-analytic review of the behavioral outcome literature. *Ann Behav Med* 1996; 18:6–15.
9. NIMH Multisite HIV Prevention Trial Group. The NIMH Multisite HIV prevention trial: Reducing HIV sexual risk behavior. *Science* 1998; 280:1889–1894.
10. Kamb ML, Fishbein M, Douglas JM, et al. EFficacy of risk-reduction counseling to prevent human immunodeficiency virus and sexually transmitted diseases: A randomized controlled trial. *JAMA* 1998; 280:1161–1167.
11. Sweat MD, Denison JA. Reducing HIV incidence in developing countries with structural and environmental interventions. *AIDS* 1995; 9:S251–S257.
12. Coates TJ. Strategies for modifying sexual behavior for primary and secondary prevention of HIV disease. *J Consult Clin Psychol* 1990; 58:57–69.
13. Kelly J, Murphy DA, Sikkemas KJ, Kalichman SC. Psychological interventions are urgently needed to prevent HIV infection: New priorities for behavioral research in the second decade of AIDS. *Am Psychol* 1993; 48:1023–1034.
14. Kelly JA, Murphy DA. Psychological interventions with AIDS and HIV: Prevention and treatment. *J Consult Clin Psychol* 1992; 60:476–485.
15. Eng TR, Butler WT, eds. *The Hidden Epidemic. Confronting Sexually Transmitted Diseases.* Washington, DC: National Academy Press; 1997.
16. Cohen MS. Sexually transmitted diseases enhance HIV transmission: No longer a hypothesis. *Lancet* 1998; suppl 3:5–7.
17. Kreiss JK, Willerford DM, Hensel M, et al. Association between cervical inflammation and cervical shedding of human immunodeficiency virus DNA. *J Infect Dis* 1994; 170:1597–1601.
18. Ghys PD, Frasen K, Diallo MO, et al. The associations between cervicovaginal HIV shedding, sexually transmitted diseases and immunosuppression in female sex workers in Abidjan, Cote d'Ivoire. *AIDS* 1997; 11:85–93.
19. Moss GB, Overbaugh J, Welch M, et al. Human immunodeficiency virus DNA in urethral secretions in men: Association with gonococcal urethritis and CD4 depletion. *J Infect Dis* 1995; 172:1469–1474.
20. De Vincenzi I. A longitudinal study of human immunodeficiency virus transmission by heterosexual partners. *N Engl J Med* 1994; 331:341–346.
21. Deschamps MM, Pape JW, Hafner A, Johnson W. Heterosexual transmission of HIV in Haiti. *Ann Intern Med* 1996; 125:324–330.

22. Cohen MS, Hoffman IF, Royce RA, et al. Reduction of concentration of HIV-1 in semen after treatment of urethritis: Implications for prevention of sexual transmission of HIV-1. *Lancet* 1997; 349:1868–1873.

23. Atkins MC, Carlin EM, Emery VC, et al. Fluctuations of HIV load in semen of HIV positive patients with newly acquired sexually transmitted diseases. *Br Med J* 1996; 313:341–342.

24. Wasserheit JN. Epidemiological synergy: Interrelationships between human immunodeficiency virus infection and other sexually transmitted diseases. *Sex Transm Dis* 1992; 19:61–77.

25. Shain RN, Piper JN, Newton ER, et al. A randomized controlled trial of a behavioral intervention to prevent sexually transmitted disease among minority women. *N Engl J Med* 1999; 340:93–100.

26. Branson BM, Peterman TA, Cannon RO, et al. Group counseling to prevent sexually transmitted diseases and HIV: A randomized controlled trial. *Sex Transm Dis* 1998; 25:553–560.

27. Grosskurth H, Mosha F, Todd J, et al. Impact of improved treatment of sexually transmitted disease on HIV infection in rural Tanzania: Randomised controlled trial. *Lancet* 1995; 346:530–536.

28. Laga M. STD control for HIV prevention—It works. *Lancet* 1995; 346:518–519.

29. Gilson L, Mkanje R, Grosskurth H, et al. Cost-effectiveness of improved treatment services for sexually transmitted diseases in preventing HIV-1 infection in Mwanza Region, Tanzania. *Lancet* 1997; 350:1805–1809.

30. Cates W, Hinman AR. AIDS and absolutism: The demand for perfection in prevention. *N Engl J Med* 1992; 327: 492–494.

31. Peterson J, DiClemente RJ. Lessons learned from behavioral interventions: Caveats, gaps and implications. In: DiClemente RJ, Peterson J, eds. *Preventing AIDS: Theories and Methods of Behavioral Interventions*. New York: Plenum Press, 1994:319–322.

32. Valdiserri RO. Technology transfer: Achieving the promise of HIV prevention. In: Peterson JP, DiClemente RJ, eds. *Handbook of HIV Prevention*. Plenum Press; in press.

33. DiClemente RJ. Preventing sexually transmitted infections among adolescents: A clash of ideology and science. *JAMA* 1998; 279:1574–1575.

34. Hein K. Aligning science with politics and policy in HIV prevention. *Science* 1998; 280:1905–1906.

35. Zenilman JM, Weisman CS, Rampalo AM, et al. Condom use to prevent incident STD: The validity of self-reported condom use. *Sex Transm Dis* 1995; 22:15–21.

36. Ellish NJ, Weisman CS, Celentano D, Zenilman JM. Reliability of partner reports of sexual history in a heterosexual population at a sexually transmitted disease clinic. *Sex Transm Dis* 1996; 23:446–452.

37. Quinn TC. Association of sexually transmitted diseases and infection with the human immunodeficiency virus: Biological cofactors and markers of behavioral interventions. *Int J STD AIDS* 1996; 7(suppl 2):17–24.

38. Orr D. Urine-based diagnosis of sexually transmitted infections: A shift in paradigms. *J Adolesc Health* 1997; 20:3–5.

39. Smith KR, Ching S, Lee H, et al. Evaluation of ligase chain reaction for use with urine for identification of *Neisseria gonorrhoeae* in females attending a sexually transmitted disease clinic. *J Clin Microbiol* 1995; 33: 455–457.

40. Oh MK, Smith KR, O'Cain M, et al. Urine-based screening of adolescents in detention to guide treatment for gonococcal and chlamydial infections. *Arch Pediatr Adolesc Med* 1998; 152:52–56.

41. Lee HH, Chernesky MA, Schachter J, et al. Diagnosis of *chlamydia trachomatis* genitourinary infection in women by ligase chain reaction assay of urine. *Lancet* 1995; 345:213–216.

42. Chernesky MA, Lee HH, Schachter J, et al. Diagnosis of *Chlamydia trachomatis* urethral infection in symptomatic and asymptomatic men by testing first-void urine in a ligase chain reaction assay. *J. Infect Dis* 1994; 170:1308–1311.

43. Xu K, Glanton V, Johnson SR, et al. Detection of *Neisseria gonorrhoeae* infection by ligase chain reaction testing of urine among adolescent women with and without *Chlamydia trachomatis* infection. *Sex Transm Dis* 1998; 25: 533–538.

44. O'Leary A, DiClemente RJ, Aral S. Reflections on the design and reporting of STD/HIV behavioral intervention research. *AIDS Educ Prev* 1997; 9(suppl. A):1–14.

45. Kahn JG, Haynes Sanstad KC. The role of cost-effectiveness analysis in assessing HIV-prevention interventions. *AIDS Public Policy J* 1997; 12:21–30.

46. Holtgrave DR. Cost analysis and HIV prevention interventions. *Am Psychol* 1994; 49:1088–1089.

47. Holtgrave DR, ed. *Handbook of Economic Evaluation of HIV Prevention Programs*. New York: Plenum Press; 1998.

48. Holtgrave DR, Kelly JA. Preventing HIV/AIDS among high-risk urban women: The cost-effectiveness of a behavioral group intervention. *Am J Public Health* 1996; 86:1442–1445.

49. The Standards of Reporting Clinical Trials Group. A proposal for structured reporting of randomized clinical trials. *JAMA* 1994; 272:1926–1931.

50. Begg C, Cho M, Eastwood S, et al. Improving the quality of reporting of randomized controlled trials: The CONSORT Statement. *JAMA* 1996; 278:637–639.

Index